Philosophical Perspectives on Bioethics
Edited by L. Wayne Sumner and Joseph Boyle

How should we attempt to resolve concrete bioethical problems? How are we to understand the role of bioethics in the health care system, government, and academe? This collection of original essays raises these and other questions about the nature of bioethics as a discipline. The contributors to the volume discuss various approaches to bioethical thinking and the political and institutional context of bioethics, addressing underlying concerns about the purposes of its practice. Included are extended analyses of such important issues as the conduct of clinical trials, euthanasia, justice in health care, the care of children, cosmetic surgery, and reproductive technologies.

(Toronto Studies in Philosophy)

L. WAYNE SUMNER is Professor of Philosophy and Law and a member of the Joint Centre for Bioethics at the University of Toronto.

JOSEPH BOYLE is Professor of Philosohy, Principal of St Michael's College, and a member of the Joint Centre for Bioethics at the University of Toronto.

Philosophical Perspectives on Bioethics

Edited by

L.W. SUMNER *and* JOSEPH BOYLE

UNIVERSITY OF TORONTO PRESS
Toronto Buffalo London

© University of Toronto Press 1996
'Methods of Bioethics: Some Defective Proposals' © R.M. Hare 1996

Toronto Buffalo London
Printed in Canada

ISBN 0-8020-0771-6 (cloth)
ISBN 0-8020-7139-2 (paper)

Printed on acid-free paper

Toronto Studies in Philosophy
Editors: James R. Brown and Calvin Normore

Canadian Cataloguing in Publication Data

Main entry under title:
Philosophical perspectives on bioethics

(Toronto studies in philosophy)
Essays presented at sessions of a 1993–94 seminar
series sponsored by the Joint Centre for Bioethics
and the Dept. of Philosophy at the University of Toronto.
ISBN 0-8020-0771-6 (bound)   ISBN 0-8020-7139-2 (pbk.)

1. Bioethics.   I. Sumner, L.W. (Leonard Wayne),
1941– . II. Boyle, Joseph M., 1942– . III. Title.

BJ58.P55 1996   174'.9574   C96-930904-X

University of Toronto Press acknowledges the financial assistance to its publishing
program of the Canada Council and the Ontario Arts Council.

Contents

vi   Contents

Acknowledgments

All the essays in this volume were presented at sessions of a 1993–4 seminar series on the theme 'Philosophical Perspectives on Bioethics,' jointly sponsored by the Centre for Bioethics and the Department of Philosophy at the University of Toronto. The editors are grateful to the centre and the department for their funding and logistical support of that series and for their financial contributions to the present volume.

All the essays were written for presentation in the seminar series and had not been previously published, with the exception of Will Kymlicka's 'Moral Philosophy and Public Policy: The Case of New Reproductive Technologies,' which first appeared in *Bioethics* 7 (1993). A slightly revised version is reprinted here, by permission of Blackwell Publishers Ltd.

Two other essays have subsequently appeared elsewhere. R.M. Hare's 'Methods of Bioethics: Some Defective Proposals' was first published in *Monash Bioethics Review* 13 (1994); the version appearing here is slightly revised. Dan W. Brock's 'Public Moral Discourse' is reprinted with permission from *Society's Choices: Social and Ethical Decision Making in Biomedicine*, ed. Ruth Ellen Bulger et al., copyright 1995 by the National Academy of Sciences; courtesy of the National Academy Press, Washington, DC.

Finally, Norman Daniels's 'Wide Reflective Equilibrium in Practice' is appearing simultaneously in *Justice and Justification: Reflective Equilibrium in Theory and Practice* (New York: Cambridge University Press, 1996).

L.W.S.
J.B.

PHILOSOPHICAL PERSPECTIVES ON BIOETHICS

Introduction

L.W. SUMNER and JOSEPH BOYLE

The literature in bioethics has grown to such proportions, and become so specialized, that the addition to it of a collection of philosophical essays calls for an explanation. The primary purpose of this volume is not to advance public discussion of one or another substantive bioethical issue or some cluster of such issues. Rather, its aim is to raise questions about the nature of bioethics itself as a normative discipline. These questions fall into two broad categories.

First, there are questions about the proper methods for bioethical thinking, such as the following: How should we go about trying to resolve concrete bioethical problems? To what extent (if any) are general ethical principles (such as the Golden Rule or the principle of utility) or normative theories (such as consequentialism or natural law) either necessary or useful for resolving such problems? If we are not to refer to principles, or use abstract philosophical reasoning, what alternative models of moral thinking are available to help us? Should our thinking begin instead with particular cases and then work towards identifying relevant similarities among such cases? If so, how are we to identify and appreciate the moral complexities of particular health care dilemmas and policies? Can we develop a methodology that finds a place for both general principles or theories and contextual particularities?

Second, there are questions about the political and institutional context of bioethical thinking that reveal underlying concerns about the purposes of the practice of bioethics. For example: How are we to understand appropriate roles for bioethicists within the health care system, government, and academe? How are we to deal with the limitations and biases that arise from the social positions within which bioethicists inevitably work? To what extent should bioethicists take the social reality of modern health care as the given framework for their work? To what extent should they instead commit themselves to the political activities needed to alter this framework?

More than half of the contributions to this volume are explicitly concerned with questions in the first of these categories, and all the contributions take a stand on some key methodological issues. For instance, all the papers speak to some aspect or other of what we may call the generalist/particularist issue. This deserves some preliminary comment. Generalists about bioethics support an essential justificatory or deliberative role for ethical principles or theories. At their most ambitious, they argue that we need to subscribe to the best normative theory in order to do bioethics successfully. Moral justification or deliberation then operates in a 'top-down' manner – that is, from general principles to particular cases. One problem with this approach is that generalists have not managed to agree on which normative theory is the best, some defending consequentialism while others affiliate with one or another version of deontology or virtue theory. Another problem is that the rarefied abstractions of any such theory seem to do little real work in resolving the concrete problems of particular patients and institutions.

Particularists have reacted to these problems by advocating a rival 'bottom-up' approach. On this way of thinking we begin by working with, and attempting to resolve, particular cases in all of their contextual detail. Once we have managed to settle some of these cases, then we can apply these results to other, similar, cases, gradually widening our network until larger patterns begin to form. Some of these patterns we might then codify as rules or guidelines, or even principles, but any such generalizations would follow, not precede, the resolution of particular problems. This approach, too, has its fairly obvious problems: In working initially with particular cases, what resources can we call on if we are denied access to any ethical principles? How can we be confident that our 'resolutions' of these cases are anything more than a reflection of our initial biases? How are we to tell when cases are relevantly similar if we have no general criteria of relevance, of the sort that ethical principles would provide?

Daniel Callahan's paper usefully opens the discussion by explicitly addressing and connecting questions about the methods of moral thinking and the purposes of bioethics. He begins with a plea for an ethical theory capable both of being applied to practical problems and of being embodied in the life of the theorist. He then goes on to express scepticism about whether the kinds of theories typically devised by moral philosophers will ever be able to satisfy both of these requirements, largely because of the institutional isolation of professional philosophy from the real world in which ethical problems are embedded.

R.M. Hare then argues for the necessity of precisely the kind of ethical theory that philosophers typically devise. He begins with a critique of some recent tendencies in bioethics – situation ethics, virtue theory, the ethics of care and the appeal to rights – arguing that both the strengths and the weaknesses of these approaches can be accounted for by the kind of two-level normative theory he has developed over the past thirty years. In Hare's view, abstract theorizing takes place at the critical level of moral reasoning, while our everyday moral thinking, informed by the results of such theorizing, is done at the intuitive level. This thinking does not take the form of mechanically applying very general principles to particular cases; instead, it works with many of the techniques and resources that particularists have emphasized.

The particularist side of the debate is represented here by Albert Jonsen and Earl Winkler. Jonsen is well known for his advocacy of a casuistical, or case-centered, approach to moral thinking. In his contribution to this volume, however, Jonsen addresses a problem for casuistry: how are we to determine when the circumstances of a case are morally relevant? In his tentative answer to this question he finds a role for maxims – that is, relatively low-level rules or guidelines. He also suggests that these maxims can be connected in important ways to high-level principles, though he stops short of mapping these connections.

Winkler takes up much the same question in exploring how particularism (or what he calls contextualism) deals with hard cases. Like Jonsen, he finds a justificatory role for ethical principles, though the appropriate principles can emerge only after the contextual features of particular cases have been fully appreciated. Winkler then tries to fill in the missing part of the particularist picture: how to connect high-level principles with concrete moral judgments.

The most influential form of generalism in bioethics has undoubtedly been the principlism expounded by Tom Beauchamp. The four 'Georgetown principles' – autonomy, beneficence, non-maleficence, and justice – have acquired a virtually constitutional status in the bioethical realm. In his essay Beauchamp takes the opportunity to reply to particularist critics of principlism, utilizing a distinction between 'robust' and 'prima facie' principles. Agreeing with the particularists' rejection of the former, Beauchamp argues that principles of the latter, weaker sort are unavoidable within the particularists' own case-centred methodology.

Norman Daniels explores similar issues concerning the relationship between principles and considered moral judgments. He relies explicitly on the method of wide reflective equilibrium elaborated in his previous works. This approach rejects foundationalist moral epistemology in favour of a coherentist or holistic model. Using this method, Daniels finds significant areas of convergence between generalists and particularists, and he seeks to accommodate the strengths of both the top-down and bottom-up approaches to bioethical problems by suggesting the need for a division of ethical labour.

Laura Shanner's contribution to the discussion of the methodology of bioethics is a proposal for an alternative, narrative method that yields a phenomenological understanding of a moral problem in its fuller human and social contexts. She exemplifies her proposal within an extended exploration of a key area of women's health, the treatment of infertility. Her conclusion is that many of the methodological debates in bioethics could be avoided were we to take seriously the stories that subjects tell about their lives.

The six remaining papers in the volume focus primarily on questions about the purposes and social context of the practice of bioethics. Four of them present distinctively feminist perspectives on the present state of bioethics. While feminists have generally aligned themselves with particularists on matters of methodology, deploring the abstractness and acontextuality of traditional ethical theories, the authors here represented go far beyond endorsing one side or the other in the standard methodological debate. Instead, each argues in her own way for a reconceptualization, and politicization, of the entire discipline.

Laura Purdy contends that bioethics – indeed ethics in general – must accept some basic claims of justice that have been articulated by feminists. She accepts the observation that these claims are political in nature but responds that this will be equally true of any deep assumptions about justice embedded in an approach to bioethics. If one must choose among competing political views, she argues, then the views of feminists are simply more compelling than those of their opponents.

Christine Overall carries the politicization of bioethics a step further by examining its institutional culture. As long as bioethics continues to be parasitic on the health care system, she argues, then it will also continue to replicate the worst political features of that system. As an alternative to bioethics, she proposes the development of a biopolitics that would carry out a political critique of standard bioethical assumptions, especially those assumptions that entrench differences of power.

Susan Sherwin criticizes the distinction between theory and practice in bioethics and argues that each must inform the other. That relationship is to be understood within a methodology of reflective equilibrium, but the equilibrium must be specifically feminist. It must be sensitive to political context, especially relations of oppression, domination, and privilege. Therefore it is a method capable of including the voices of the powerless and the disadvantaged.

Kathryn Pauly Morgan's contribution illustrates many of these biopolitical themes by focusing on an area central to women's health care: cosmetic surgery. In her analysis of this practice, she addresses the poverty of rights-based approaches that ignore the context in which women make 'free' decisions about 'elective' techniques and affirms the need for attention to the socio-political factors that constrain women's autonomy.

The final two papers focus on one fairly specific question: How should bodies mandated to propose public policy on bioethical issues go about their business, and what contribution might philosophers make to their deliberations? Will Kymlicka approaches these issues from the perspective of his work for the Canadian Royal Commission on New Reproductive Technologies, whose 'guiding principles' he proposed. Kymlicka argues that it would be improper for public bodies to endorse any particular normative theory; instead, they must work within principles that command a social consensus. This approach limits the role to be played by philosophers in the formation of public policy, though it still leaves them with some useful tasks to perform.

Finally, Dan Brock looks at similar issues from the vantage point of his experience with the President's Commission in the United States. Examining the method of moral reasoning that public bioethics commissions ought to employ, Brock argues that it is not as different from the methods of moral philosophy as it may seem. What the two have in common, at their best, is the use of reflective equilibrium as a technique for finding coherence between ethical principles and considered moral judgments.

Plainly the papers collected here deal with a set of interconnected issues and themes. Still, as even our brief introductions to the contributions suggest, they also reflect the variety of viewpoints that is common within moral philosophy. Definitive answers, acceptable to all, are not to be expected. These papers address the questions at issue and engage both one another and the reader in ways that are remarkably diverse and provocatively complex. Any attempt we might make to synthesize them would therefore quickly cease to serve as helpful commentary and become editorial imposition, both on the authors and on the reader.

Consequently, we take brief note here of only two striking points of convergence among the contributions to this volume. As we have already noted, virtually all of them speak to some aspect of the generalist/particularist debate. The writers plainly dwell at different points along the continuum defined by the extreme positions. Still, their essays display a shared tendency to reject these extremes in favour of more moderate views that concede much to the other camp. Perhaps the methodological debate has now moved to a more mature and reflective stage, in which confrontation among the contending parties has begun to be superseded by accommodation and reconciliation. One comes away from a reading of these essays with the distinct impression that the hard-line generalist or particularist is nowadays a largely mythical creature (or caricature). The question then remains whether the generalist/particularist distinction is any longer a useful analytical device for identifying basic methodological differences.

This convergence on the middle ground is closely related to another theme running through most, though not all, of the papers. Although some contributors (particularly Daniels and Sherwin) are more explicit on this issue than others are, nearly all reject foundationalism in favour of a version of reflective equilibrium (the conspicuous exception here is R.M. Hare, whose method of supporting his two-level normative theory is neither foundationalist, properly speaking, nor coherentist). It is not surprising, therefore, that so many of the essays should be found to seek an accommodation between methodologies that assign a privileged epistemological place to general principles and those that do so to particular moral judgments.

Throughout this introduction we have stressed the attention given by the contributors to the methodology and purposes of bioethics. This emphasis is appropriate, since these are the main themes and rationale of the collection. However, such a focus is misleadingly narrow in two respects. First, although it is not the primary purpose of this volume to advance the discussion of particular normative issues in bioethics, many of the papers do offer extended analyses of important practical problems, including the conduct of clinical trials, euthanasia, justice in health care, the care of children, cosmetic surgery, and reproductive technologies. Nor is this attention to concrete issues surprising, given the emphasis on the unification of theory and practice that runs through the volume. Anyone interested in these issues in their own right will therefore find an additional reward in these pages.

Second, the methodological debates on which these papers focus are not limited to bioethics. While there are important respects in which bioethics differs from other areas in applied ethics – such as environmental ethics or business ethics – it is unlikely to be unique in its basic methodology. The lessons learned here should therefore be transferable to these cognate areas. More important, they should tell us a great deal about how to go about doing ethics unmodified, which, however theoretical it may become, remains ultimately a practical enterprise.

Professional Morality: Can an Examined Life Be Lived?

DANIEL CALLAHAN

To put the matter bluntly, I make my living as a specialist in ethics. Some people sell shoes, while others peddle computers and automobiles. I purvey ethics: it is my profession and trade. People pay money to hear me give lectures, visit me to solicit my views, and buy my books with the expectation that I will have something useful to say about making good moral judgments. I like this kind of life, but I have never been wholly comfortable with it. If the examined life is the only kind worth living, as one of my predecessors implied, then what ought to be the characteristics of someone who chooses to live *this* kind of life? Should the life of the professional moralist be different from the lives of others? If so, in what ways? This essay is an effort to describe how I have defined my problem and how I have attempted to respond to it. Despite the fact that there are a fair number of us who make our living these days in one branch or another of ethics, theoretical and applied, there is remarkably little written on this topic. While I am not certain exactly why that is so, perhaps this essay – and some of the delicate points it touches upon – might indirectly help answer that question.

I spend much of my life moving in and out of, and back and forth among, three different moral worlds. One of them is that of conventional ethical theory and analysis, a legacy of my training as a moral philosopher. I try to keep up with the philosophical literature and exchange shop-talk with other philosophers. Another world is that of the medical or policy practitioner, a consequence of my work in biomedical ethics. I read the medical literature, work to see what goes on in hospitals, and listen to doctors, nurses, and health administrators talk about their ethical problems. The third world is that of my personal moral life. Just who, I ask myself, is this person who tries to worry about ethical theory and medical practice, and what kind of a person should he be to do so best and also to live his own moral life among family, friends, and professional colleagues?

It is both exhilarating and depressing to move among such diverse worlds. The exhilaration comes from the diversity. Each of these worlds has its own terrain, native foliage, local landmarks, and different kinds of people (or the same people in different guises). Philosophers prize elegance of argument and care with concepts and logic relationships. Physicians look to empirical grounding for their judgments, clever clinical strategies, and good outcomes with their patients. Those who pursue personal moral analysis will ordinarily probe their intentions, their biases, their place in a given culture at a given time.

While movement back and forth among these realms is difficult, it also happens that confusion, stupefaction, or frustration in one realm can on occasion be relieved by moving to the other. The depression comes from the same diversity. The worlds seem so different in their folkways and customs, their language and traditions, that movement back and forth across the boundaries is always awkward and sometimes painful. The worlds coexist for me, and traffic is heavy among them, but it is extraordinarily hard to make of them a coherent universe. Is there some way that they could be made coherent? That is for me the way the problem of moral theory personally presents itself. I have come to think that it is the right problem to have. It reflects a variegated need: our need to think about ethics and to make rational sense of the subject; our need to take ethics out into some actual world and with it to help shape the practices and institutions of society; and our need to find out how to live our private and professional moral lives in ways that manifest seriousness and integrity.

In the best tradition of moral theory, let me move from the personal to the impersonal realm and put my problem more abstractly. Moral theory and analysis, I contend, should be able to integrate three elements. The first is that of our ideas of ethics and morality, what we think the subject matter is and how we believe it should be rationally grounded and interpreted. A good ethical theory is one that tries to make sense of our moral instincts, institutions, and traditions and to provide a plausible perspective on the making of moral judgments, the fashioning of rules and principles, and the devising of a virtuous life. It is 'theory' in the sense that the goal is some reasonably comprehensive way of understanding, and making rationally convincing, the enterprise of ethics; and it is 'ethical' in the sense that it bears on making judgments about what we count as good and bad, praiseworthy or blameworthy, in human relationships and human institutions – and I suppose I should amend that conventional description by including our relationship with the environment as well.

The second element is to determine how to make the move from thought to practice, from theory to application. It is necessary, in that respect, to remind ourselves constantly that ethical theory is meant to be a theory about the way human beings ought to live with each other and with themselves; it must turn its face outward. As citizens, or professionals, or workers of one kind or another, or just plain human beings, we have to live within the boundaries of various institutions, cultural practices, and political systems. How can we bring to them the fruits of moral theory, to reprove them when needed, to improve them when possible, to change them when to do so is imperative? How, in turn, should we try to learn from our workaday experience with them what we need to sharpen, enrich, and improve our moral theory?

The third element is that of shaping our personal moral life, not only that we might be decent persons for our own sakes and the good of those around us, but also that we might try in our own eyes to become exemplars of what it means to pursue the subject of ethics and morality. Part of this shaping must of course encompass professional integrity: taking care with one's writings, giving credit to others where it is due, maintaining standards of fairness and civility in commenting on the ideas of others. That is the easy part. The harder route is to become a person who recognizes that his or her own moral life should be constantly on trial, that to take up the vocation of ethical theorist is to embrace with special intensity the vocation of moral self-criticism and self-analysis. An important result of that effort should be to manifest to others the fact that one has taken up the role of moral theorist, and that one knows that such theory starts at home – constructing one's own moral life – not somewhere else.

I do not mean to suggest that this personal element will necessarily be expressed in the explicit content of the theory. More plausibly, it would be manifest in two ways: by informing the private life of the theorist, in such a way that he or she could explain, and show by behavior, the way the quest for good theory and analysis is part of that life; and by being manifest in the nuance and texture of the theory itself, suggesting that it is the fruit of someone who cares about morality and means it to be taken seriously in shaping a life.

I can sum up these three elements by speaking of ethical theory in terms of *thinking* (the rational devising of theory), *doing* (the application of theory in actual life), and *living* (the embodiment of the theory in the life of the theorist himself). Yet as attractive as I find this way for formulating the problem, and as imperative as I believe it is to integrate coherently the three elements, it is exceedingly hard to do so. The main reason, I have come to think, is that, on the one hand, the cultural and professional fragmentation of our society work powerfully against that integration; and, on the other hand, the recent practices of moral theorists no less work against it.

I begin with the culture of professional philosophy. As I move in and out of that culture, some of its features are strikingly evident. The most evident is that it is a relatively closed world. The debates in the field usually circle about a small number of dominant figures, analyze a relatively narrow range of theoretical topics (which come and go over the years of course), proceed by what appear to be set procedural rules, and are written in the private language of professional moral theory. As a rule, the references and sources used are those of the writings of other theorists, rarely the external world of human events, actions, and motives. One astonishing book a few years ago, ostensibly on the problem of evil, contained hardly a single reference, or even allusion, to evil motives, events, or deeds; it was an extended discussion of various philosophical theories of evil as found in the literature. Is moral philosophy about the moral life and moral judgment, or is it about what other philosophers have written about those topics? An observer who wandered in from some other field might well wonder.

At times the world of moral theory can seem a sealed world with tight boundaries, one that allows into that world only a carefully screened list of items, namely, the writings of other theorists. Another feature is that of the great indifference to the potential significance of the theory for some broader audience. The standard of prestige, of interest even, is that of the opinion of other theorists, not those outside the professional circle who might make use of, even live by, the theory. It is often painful to observe the anxiety of younger academics trying to publish articles that will capture the attention of their more powerful seniors. They try to figure out the rules of the game and then dutifully, even obsessively, play by those rules. The first rule is: impress those in your field by showing you can deploy their theories. The final feature I would mention is the extent to which elegance and detail of argument are prized. It is certainly not an inappropriate emphasis, of course; but it goes awry when it forces theorists to work with narrow, nervously manageable topics and methods, tailoring the problem to the available methodological paradigms. The result too often is not simply elegant overkill of topics (plentiful enough), but also a fragmentation of moral theory itself, which becomes a collection of numerous subspecialties, rarely in good communication with each other or in any communication with those outside the field.

Now these traits and folkways of the field might not matter, except that the theory itself often misses the mark by its inability to be taken outside the realm of theory, to that world of human beings and events that, supposedly, it is all about. Consider the needs of the practitioner. He or she would like to gain some guidance, or at least illumination, from moral theory. Physicians and medical researchers, for example, are eager for help; and they presume that ethical theory could, or should, be able to provide it. There is, to be sure, a catch in the kind of help they want: they want only the practical outcome of theory, not the details of the theory itself, much less the delicate workings of its internal process. That point is where theorists often balk. They rarely think through the problem of application, and, quite often, they feel that they have no obligation as theorists to do so. When I have pressed them on that point, they often plead a combination of professional privilege and professional ignorance. It is their privilege, as theorists, not to be responsible for creating a system of actual practices and institutions that would embody their theory. That is the work not of theorists, but of politicians, moralists, or preachers, and in any event they are ignorant about how it is to be done; it is a political and institutional problem which falls in someone else's professional domain.

The practitioners quickly come to give up hope that the moral theorist has anything helpful to say. Worse still, on occasion the practitioner comes to think of the moral theorist as a kind of trained evader, one who has an endless supply of reasons why he or she cannot be responsive to the practitioner's needs. He or she will not inform the practitioner what the theory would mean in practice for the practitioner or how it might be implemented. For his or her part, the theorist is all-too-nicely saved the difficult work of seeing whether the theory could have any force or depth out in some actual world. It can remain a delicate flower, one that, if lovely enough, can help gain its originator tenure or professional praise, but that cannot be transplanted outside the nursery. Does that restriction matter for the theorist? Not very much; for the flower was propagated not to live outside, but only to impress other like-minded horticulturists.

It is possible, I suppose, for someone to say at this point that I am demanding too much of the theorist, that he or she be able to do both the work of the theorist and that of the politician, clinician, or other professional practitioner. No, I do not think it too much to demand. Failing that effort, the theory itself is likely to be either beside the point or so cleaned up for elegant presentation that it falsifies the richness and complexity of ethics. By allowing ethical theory to become a private language – set in its ways, rigid in its semantics, hidebound in its syntax – a double danger is run: because they can talk with each other, theorists too easily can come to believe that they are still in the realm of common morality, when in fact they are in their own, wholly detached, world; and because that way of doing things mystifies or alienates those on the outside, it becomes readily possible to blame those outsiders for their lack of sophistication.

I might never have begun worrying about this kind of isolation had not I become increasingly aware of the odd relationship that ethical theory often bears to the moral life of many theorists, manifesting still another form of isolation. As someone who spends much of his time taking part in conference on ethics, I cannot help noting the sharp contrast between the way professional ethical theorists talk about ethics at the conference table and the way they talk about it away from the table in their private lives. Too often there seems to be no connection *whatsoever* between those two contexts: there is no evidence that reflection on their own life has informed their theory, or that their theory has made any difference in the way they manage their own moral decisions. I have long been uncomfortable, moreover, trying to find a good answer to those clinicians who say, with some dismay, that the moral philosophers they had come to know through our shared work in bioethics seemed neither any better morally than anyone else nor, worse still, any more concerned than anyone else personally to act in some better fashion.

There is, of course, a parallel. Just as there are physicians who seem utterly indifferent to patients, there are ethical theorists who seem utterly indifferent to morality. For both, it is the impersonal technical problems that interest them, the fine points of electrolyte balance for physicians or the nuances of rule utilitarianism for the philosopher. Both fields lend themselves to travesties of that kind precisely because the promotions, rewards, and peer approval go to those who can manage the intricacies of theory and in the way prescribed by the reigning authorities and paradigms. Sensitive physicians (including good medical researchers and theoreticians) are alert to discrepancies of that kind, and most work to counter it in themselves. They try to remind themselves that the point of medical theory is to benefit patients, to make a difference at the bedside. They are acutely embarrassed by those colleagues who become cold, distant, and impersonal in their dealing with patients, *especially* when such treatment is justified in the name of medical progress.

I see no comparable countervailing force or tradition working in moral theory. On the contrary, when I suggest to most philosophers that they ought to look closely into themselves when devising ethical theory, and that they should also work to manifest a personal seriousness about morality in their relationship with others, I am all too often greeted by incredulity or outright rejection. Is not good ethical theory a matter of well-honed rationality, where the emphasis falls solely upon the quality of one's technical analysis? What difference does the way someone lives his or her own life make if, in the professional sphere, one does good work, that is, work that measures up to the standards of the field?

It is not easy, I concede, to respond to questions of that kind. There is no obvious or direct logical connection between devising polished ethical theory and the personal moral life of theorists, just as there is no obvious logical connection between devising good scientific theory and a personal love of, or appreciation for, nature in the life of the scientist. Yet my own experience is that, just as the most sensitive scientists do more often than not seem to have a kind of love of, or sense of awe in the face of, the natural order, so the most sensitive moral theorists have a feel for the subject matter of ethics and morality that both transcends (and yet informs) their theoretical work. Those moral theorists who show only an ability to work through the logical implications of their starting point or premises can, in one sense, do good theoretical work; their technical skills can be well displayed. But the most serious moral problems, theoretical and practical, ordinarily turn on finding the right premises, or on discovering or creating that stance or perspective most likely to do full justice to the problem before one, not just on working through the details. I long ago fashioned the following proposition, which I believe is verifiable: the more an article or book on moral theory has propositions or people named '*x*' and '*y*' and a long chain of arguments deploying those descriptors, the softer the premises of the entire edifice.

The perennially hard task of moral theory is to find the right premises. Yet as the history of moral philosophy makes clear enough, there are no standard techniques, much less technical rules of thumb for finding those premises or knowing at first sight how valid and viable the various candidates may be. We can only judge them over the long term, and we do so by virtue of the kinds of fruit they bear and by their capacity to take account of wide and varying human experience, including the way earlier and competing theories seemed to have made sense of things. My own supposition is that somewhere in the mystery of creating and devising premises lies the relationship to personal morality and the theorist's private struggle with good and evil in her or his own life.

Why do I say this? I offer two reasons. The first is that, in the nature of the case, our first premises do not ordinarily admit of perfect grounding. They are 'first' in the sense that little or nothing precedes them. But that 'little or nothing' is most likely to reflect our experiential reading of the world, the force of the times and culture in which we live, and our capacity or willingness to deal with competing possibilities of analysis. Unless we are extremely careful, it is all too easy to get our premises from a combination of conventionality – whatever everyone takes for granted at the moment – and self-indulgence – whatever we find to be most comfortable with the way we are living our lives and judging the world. Only a powerful effort both to spot the pressures of conventionality (not easy for a graduate student or a young professor seeking tenure and hoping to get published in the standard professional journals) and to strike back against them if necessary will be adequate here; and a no less strong effort to understand oneself and the emotional attractions and repugnances of one's life will be necessary to find the proper psychological point of departure.

The second reason is that, if we have managed to get that far, we then encounter the problem of falling in love with our own ideas. It is not easy to be honest with ourselves about the quality and character of either our moral premises or the way an argument is developed. It takes considerable self-insight, not to mention self-discipline, to be hard on our own ideas. I do not mean being 'hard' on the logic of the argument; we do that out of self-defense. I mean 'hard' in the sense of trying to see if the shape and thrust of our approach is simply a little too comfortable about the way we would like the world to be, the triumph of hope over truth. There are many ways to deceive ourselves, or seduce ourselves, as we develop moral theories and arguments, and it is precisely because of those deleterious possibilities that the relationship of character and theory shows its force. No one can see us when we fail to pursue a line of criticism we know might undermine what we would like to be demonstrating. No one can know when we have failed to look harshly at our own biases and predilections. No one can know when we have decided to be unfair to other people or other views (or merely grossly partisan), making them look as bad as possible in order that our views will look as good as possible. Precisely because no one can see what we bring to our arguments or choose to overlook in developing them, the main burden falls upon ourselves, hidden from sight.

A question I sometimes put to myself about an ethical theorist is this: would I send one of my children to that person for moral advice on a personal problem? When I decide the answer is no and try to discover why I feel that way, one reason is sometimes that I think I know in advance what that theorist might say, and I reject that approach. There is something less than reassuring about a theorist too comfortable with her or his own theory and all too able and willing to crank out judgments consistent with it. More often than not, however, the reason has nothing directly to do with the probable content of the advice. It is more likely that, however great the professional and technical skills of the theorist, I have seen little evidence that he or she is someone who struggles to find the right premises or to be the kind of person most likely to find the right premises. On the contrary, it is too often a person who has seemed slack in dealing with the deepest and hardest questions – where we take our point of departure in ethics – and has lavished attention instead on working through, in elegant and refined ways, starting points of enormous and unexamined superficiality.

I have concentrated my attention on what I believe to be the most important conditions for the creation of good moral theory. For one reason or another – the desire to ape the sciences, peer pressure, a failure in self-examination, excessive specialization, shelter from the hurly-burly of the actual world in which we live – ethical theory has too often become the private language of a private world. Within that world, the prizes go to those who can speak most tellingly to those in that world; and that means by following the given rules of technical proficiency. But the point of ethical theory, or so I have long taken it, is to find a way to think through the living of a moral life, the devising of moral societies, and the making of moral judgments that can be grounded in some adequate theory. I fail to see how that kind of grounding can be sufficient, or ultimately satisfactory, if it does not spring from a private moral life that is itself rich and struggling, and if it cannot make sense in the actual world of human affairs, where it is most needed and will have its only real meaning.

Methods of Bioethics:
Some Defective Proposals

R.M. HARE

1

In these days of intense academic competition, which is supposed to keep us all on our toes, one has to publish or be damned; and for advancing one's career it is more important that what one publishes should be new, than that it should be true. Often it is not as new as one thinks it is; sometimes, if one looks back to the great philosophers of the past, one finds that one's bright new ideas have been anticipated by them. This has happened often enough to me.

As to being true, that is not so difficult. Most philosophical truths are fairly obvious, though people obscure them by their inability or unwillingness to express themselves clearly. The difficult thing is to grasp the *whole* truth. If you take a bunch of supposedly divergent theories on almost any philosophical question, you will find in each of them some points which are right, and some which are wrong. Those who criticize these theories often rightly attack the points that are wrong, but do not see that not everything in a theory is wrong; it also, usually, has hold of important truths. So, in putting forward their own opposing theories, these philosophers discard the good with the bad, denying truths that their victims had grasped. So they too land themselves in a mixture of truth and error.

The difficult thing, as I said, is to grasp the whole truth. This entails carefully disentangling the truths from the errors in *all* the theories one studies. It is the mark of the good philosopher to be able to do this. All philosophers can profit from the advice that I regularly give to my students: pinch your opponents' clothes. That is, find out what is right about what they are saying, and say it yourself. You will then be less exposed to their counter-attacks. You will end up, as I have ended up, as an eclectic – not the sort of eclectic that borrows

©R.M. Hare. Previously published in *Monash Bioethics Review* 13 (1994).

thoughts from all and sundry without seeking to make them consistent with one another, but the sort that sees that these thoughts are true, *and* that they can all be consistently held simultaneously. It is very difficult to be this kind of eclectic. It requires, above all, great clarity of thought and precision of expression.

I have called this essay 'Methods of Bioethics'. I could have called it, following Sidgwick, simply 'Methods of Ethics,' because the appropriate methods for bioethics are not, so far as I can see, going to differ from those appropriate for ethics or moral philosophy in general. But in attending to a branch of applied ethics like bioethics, we have brought home to us a requirement of which those who propound ethical theories seem often to be unaware: the requirement to say something that will help us answer important practical moral questions, on our answers to which lives may depend. I shall be showing later on that many of the theories that have recently won fame for their inventors are not of much use for this purpose.

In order to explain the scope of this paper I need to distinguish between different kinds of thing that have been called ethical or moral theories. I shall leave one of these kinds on one side, although it contains the more serious and useful sorts of ethical theory. I can do this, because I have written extensively about such theories in other places.[1] I mean theories about the nature and logical properties of the moral concepts, or the meanings of the moral words. This, I am convinced, has to be what we start with in any serious study of moral reasoning. But the advocates of the views I *shall* be discussing say little about ethical theory in this narrow sense. Perhaps if they did study these issues they would do more good. Ethical theories in the narrow sense, those that I shall be leaving aside, are such as naturalism, intuitionism, subjectivism, emotivism, and my own prescriptivist theory. These theories are grappling with serious problems about the logic of moral reasoning – problems which we have to solve if we are to make any progress in it. But, as I said, the theories I shall be discussing do not move in that world.

2

Enough, then, for these very general remarks. I will now give some examples, from moral philosophy, of how people can be led into error by denying truths which they only deny because the truths are tangled up, in the writings of those who have grasped them, with errors, and it is hard to disentangle the truths from the errors.

I will start with an example which I can deal with briefly, because it is a fairly familiar one and I have discussed it before, though many people seem not to have taken in what I said.[2] This is the theory commonly known as situation ethics.

Admirers of the existentialists often say the same sort of thing. The situation ethicists have hold of an important truth, that one has to judge each situation on its merits. Situations differ one from another, and the differences may be morally relevant. One cannot assume that they are not. But the situation ethicists go on from asserting this truth to asserting a dangerous falsehood. They say that in morals one cannot appeal to what they call 'general principles' or 'general rules'.

In order to see what is wrong with this one has to make a distinction of which, even now, many of our philosophical colleagues seem to be unaware. This is the distinction between universality and generality. Many people think that 'universal' and 'general' mean the same thing. Many philosophers do indeed use them as if they meant the same. Aristotle was, I think, the first offender, because he used his expression *kath' holou*, usually translated, indiscriminately, 'general' and 'universal,' without making clear that the term can have two entirely different meanings.[3]

Consider the two statements, that one ought never to tell lies, and that one ought never to tell lies to one's business partners. Both these statements are *universal*. They start with a universal quantifier ('never') and contain no individual references. They apply, the first of them to *anyone* who says anything, and the second of them to anyone who says anything to a business partner of his. But the second is less *general* than the first. It is more specific, though no less universal.

We can now see the first thing that is wrong with what the situation ethicists say. 'Considering each situation on its merits' does entail not judging it by the simple application of very *general* rules or principles. The situation ethicists have a point there. But it does not entail refusing to judge it on highly specific but still *universal* principles. Suppose one goes into the utmost detail about the specifics of a situation, carefully noticing all the features of it which might be morally relevant. Suppose, even, if that were possible, that one *describes* the situation at enormous length, leaving out nothing that could possibly be relevant to a moral decision about it. Suppose, for example, that it is a situation in a short story – or even a very long story in several volumes. And suppose that one comes to a decision as to what one of the characters ought to have done at some point in the narrative. The moral statement that one then makes is still universal, logically speaking. It can begin with a universal quantifier, and not contain individual constants or references to individuals. It can say that anyone of a certain kind, in a situation of a certain kind (the kinds being as minutely specified as you like) ought to do a certain thing.

It is true that the character is represented in the story as an individual. But in order to represent him (or her) the novelist has to describe him. And the descriptions have all to be in universal terms, because there are no other terms available for the purpose. We cannot identify the person by *pointing at him*. What we have in the novel is a description, in universal terms, of a person of a very minutely specified kind, in a situation of a very minutely specified kind. Any moral statement that we make about him (or her) has to be of the form, that a person of that kind in that kind of situation ought to act in such and such a way.

The confusion between universality and generality, which I have been exposing, leads people to think that if one makes a universal judgment about a situation, one must be making a very general judgment about it. This is not so. The judgment can be specific enough to take in any details of the situation that anybody thinks relevant. Only a victim of the confusion I have been exposing will think that a statement cannot at the same time be universal and highly specific.

There is a lot more to be said on this topic, and many more mistakes that need to be pointed out. But since I have done this in other places,[4] I can skip it now. I shall be explaining later how it is that, though we have to consider each situation on its merits, rather simple and general principles do, all the same, have a use in our moral thinking.[5] I shall not have space to explain why it is important to have regard to universal but highly specific principles, although in the actual world no two situations are ever exactly alike.[6] And I shall omit here any discussion of the familiar confusion between singular prescriptions like '*He* ought to keep *his* promise to *her*', and universal relational prescriptions like '*One* ought to keep *one's own* particular promises to the *individual* to whom *one* has made them'. The second, like '*One* ought to be faithful to *one's own* wife', is a universal prescription, even though in most countries one can have only one wife.[7]

3

I am going on now to my next example of a theory that has hold of part of the truth, but combines it with serious errors through denying other parts of the truth. This is the theory known as 'virtue ethics'. Its adherents often appeal to the authority of Aristotle, and repudiate that of Kant; but I very much doubt, after reading those great philosophers, whether the virtue ethicists have hold of the whole truth even about what they actually said.

An ethics of virtue is often contrasted with an ethics of duty, or with an ethics of principle. Let us consider first the alleged contrast between virtues and principles. The contrast is supposed to be between having good states of character (which is what virtues are) and following good or right principles. But suppose we ask some proponent of virtue ethics to tell us what one would have to do, or what states or dispositions of mind or of feeling one would have to cultivate, in order to acquire virtue. To answer this question, he will have to *describe* the states or dispositions, or the actions to which they lead. But now we have to ask, what is the difference between such a description, and a statement of the principles for living a good life. I cannot see any. It looks as if any ethics of virtue would have to borrow extensively from an ethics of principle in order even to tell us what virtue consists in.

To put it another way: suppose we have a *description* of one way of being virtuous (there are no doubt many ways). By a very simple grammatical manoeuvre, one can change the mood of this descriptive statement and put it into the imperative. It will then be a *prescription*. Or one could change it instead into an 'ought' statement; it will then be another kind of prescription. Both these prescriptions will be different kinds of *principles*. They will be principles prescribing how one should behave, and how one should be feeling, in certain kinds of situation. Behaving and feeling like that is one way of displaying virtue. Neither an ethics of virtue nor an ethics of principle has to assume, though many do assume, that there is only one way of leading a good life. Both virtues and principles could be like recipes in a cookbook; one does not have to cook them all at the same time. It is another question whether the good life *is* like that (that is, whether there are alternative possible kinds of good life); but that is a question which affects both an ethics of virtue and an ethics of principle, so I do not need to discuss it here.

It is not surprising, in the light of what I have said, that Aristotle has a lot to say about principles, and Kant a lot to say about virtues (he devoted, after all, half of his *Metaphysic of Morals* to his *Tugendlehre (Doctrine of Virtue)*).[8] These great philosophers were not so one-sided as their modern self-styled disciples. To illustrate Aristotle's belief in principles, we have only to notice that the first premises of his practical syllogisms were universal prescriptions, that is, principles – though not all of them were *moral* principles. For Aristotle the better sort of people are those who 'desire and act in accordance with a rational principle'. They are contrasted with those immature people who 'live and pursue things in accordance with feeling'.[9] And in the most famous passage of all he says, rightly, that virtue itself is 'a disposition governing our choices, lying in a mean, which is determined by a rational principle'. The word I have translated as 'rational principle' is '*logos*' – the same word he uses for describing the universal prescriptions that form the first premises of his practical syllogisms.[10] They are the verbal expressions of the dispositions or traits of character that make us act as we do. But feelings are not left out of Aristotle's account. The mean is exhibited in feelings *and* in actions.[11]

Nor does Kant leave feelings out. His view is simply that the mere feeling without corresponding action is not enough, as he makes clear in his contrast between what he calls (unfortunately to modern ears) 'pathological' and 'practical' love.[12] 'Pathological' means, of course, consisting in having *pathê*, or feelings. Kant never denies that feeling is supportive of action, nor that it is important to have the right feelings. He says that one can do the right thing, fulfilling one's duty, even if one does not have them; but of course he could agree that this is much more difficult.

If virtue is contrasted with duty, the same happens. 'Duty' is thought nowadays, though it was not in either Kant's or Aristotle's days, to be a somewhat pompous expression. But Nelson was not being pompous when he said that England expected every man to do his duty. Come to that, 'virtue' is a pretty pompous expression too, if one uses it that way. When Aristotle says that both with virtuous action and with virtuous habits of mind it is a question of 'when one ought, and under what conditions, and towards whom and for what purpose and in what manner', he was speaking of duty, or of what one ought to do or feel. One has a duty to cultivate the right feelings and to do the right actions. I can see no essential difference from Kant here. To delineate virtue is to say *what* feelings one ought to cultivate, and what actions one ought to do. This is a delineation of our duties, and requires statements of moral principles. The virtue ethicists, it appears, have, perhaps in the interests of novelty, been making a distinction without a difference. At the most they are emphasizing the importance of character for the moral life; but did Kant deny this?

4

Feelings are also stressed, to the exclusion of much else that is important, by the advocates of what we may call 'caring ethics', I include in this class such writers as Gilligan and Noddings, as well as more professional philosophers like Lawrence Blum, who has written a good book in a somewhat similar vein.[13] He has also published recently an article explicitly supporting Gilligan.[14] Though I shall not have space to discuss Blum's arguments in detail, I must say that I think his choice of antagonists was a pity. Neither Gilligan nor Kohlberg is a very clear thinker, important as their ideas are. I do not know Gilligan, but I knew Kohlberg quite well and learnt a lot from him. However, he lacked the analytical skills to give a clear account of his higher stages of development. In particular, I think he failed to make clear the crucial distinction between universality and generality that I explained earlier. As a result he gets accused by Gilligan, not unfairly, of putting in his highest stage of development people whose morality depends on very general rules, and of neglecting the special relations (especially of caring) that we ought to have with particular people. But there is nothing in the universalizability of moral judgments to prevent our being guided in our actions by very specific attachments to particular people with whom we have formed caring relations. I would not myself put in the highest moral class people who cannot manage this. I have already spoken about the confusion (that between singular prescriptions and universal relational prescriptions) involved here.

The fault of the advocates of caring, as before, is not that the virtues they emphasize are not virtues. Everyone can agree that caring, and friendship on which Blum lays so much stress, are important features of the morally good life. Helga Kuhse, in an important paper,[15] has pointed out the baffling ambiguity of the notion of caring, which its advocates have not done enough to clear up. She also points out how little guidance the notion, even if clarified, gives to our moral decisions as to what actually to do when faced with difficult choices. But the main fault of the proponents of caring ethics is that they give a completely unfair and unbalanced caricature of the views they are attacking. One would think from the way they write that no philosophers before them had said anything about caring.

Gilligan thinks that the lack of attention to caring is a symptom of male domination of philosophical thought. Peter Singer has a useful discussion of the relation between gender and approaches to philosophy in his new book.[16] It has to be admitted that nearly all famous philosophers until recently have been male; but it is simply not true that they have ignored caring and friendship. People who think they have might start by reading Anthony Price's excellent book *Love and Friendship in Plato and Aristotle*,[17] and looking at the texts he refers to. Aristotle *EN* 1168a 28 – 69b 2 is especially relevant. After that they might go on to what Hume says about sympathy. Even Kant thought that we ought to treat the ends of other people as if they were our own. He says that we shall not be treating humanity as an end in itself, 'unless every one endeavours also, so far as in him lies, to further the ends of others'.[18] If this is not caring, I do not know what is.

I shall be arguing later that it is quite easy to accommodate caring within a Kantian framework, as I have tried to do. I shall be arguing also, as I have argued elsewhere,[19] that there is no inconsistency between a carefully formulated Kantianism and a carefully formulated utilitarianism. Within such a framework the carers can have all the caring they need or desire; only they must not think (and I do not suggest that they do think) that caring is the *whole* of morality. Blum in particular is very fair about this: he thinks he is simply redressing the balance; but it needs to be asked whether he is not actually (again in the interests of novelty) tilting it too far in the opposite direction.

This is particularly clear if we consider what the carers say about impartiality. Wishing to stress the importance for the moral life of caring relationships, and recognizing the obvious fact that we cannot have such relationships with everybody, they are in danger of neglecting another important aspect of morality, namely justice and the impartial pursuit of the common good. What are we to say of the doctor who cares so much for his children that he holds back supplies of badly needed drugs in scarce supply so as to have a reserve for them? To this question too I shall return; it will prove not so difficult to answer once we have a balanced account of morality as a whole.

5

The last group of theories I shall have space to consider is that known as 'right-based' or 'rights-based' theories. There are many varieties of these, but what is common to them is the thought that we can *found* the whole of morality on an appeal to people's rights. This kind of theory too grasps one part of the truth but neglects other equally important parts. It is certainly true that rights play a significant part in morality.[20] Nobody ought to want to get rid of them. But all the same, the appeal to rights has been much abused recently, owing to the idea that one can claim a right without producing any argument to show that one has it. Such right-claims rest in the end on nothing but the claimant's intuitions (some would say 'prejudices'). We have reached the stage at which, if anybody has a mind to something, he will say he has a right to it. Without a secure way of determining who has rights to what, disputes about rights will never end. And it is certainly going to be impossible to *base* morality on rights, if they themselves are based on nothing but hot air.

Wayne Sumner has written an excellent book about this question,[21] which I recommend to anybody who wishes to understand how to argue for rights. He comes to a conclusion with which I agree almost entirely, that the most satisfactory foundation for rights is a consequentialist one. I would put it by saying that we ought to acknowledge those rights whose recognition and preservation does the best for all those affected, considered impartially. But I shall return later to the details of this suggestion.

6

I have had space to list only a few of the ethical theories that have been popular recently; and my treatment of them has been very cursory. I will now go on to show how they all fall down through ignoring important parts of the truth about morality. After that I shall show how to fill in the whole picture, and thus give the supporters of these theories what they are after, without neglecting the truths which *they* neglect.

The situation ethicists, with whom I started, say that we have to consider each situation on its merits. But they do not say how we are to judge the merits of situations. In default of some *method* for judging, everybody will be at liberty to say what they feel like saying. It is hard to see how any method for judging situations can get far without giving *reasons* for judging them one way rather than another. And any statement of the reasons is bound to bring in principles – not the very simple general principles that the situation ethicists so dislike, but universal principles all the same. If it is a reason for banning a drug from public sale that it could endanger life, then that is because of a principle that drugs which endanger life ought not to be on public sale. Of course reasons can be much more complicated than that; but they will have to state certain *features* of situations which make it right to do this or that; and these features will always have to be described in universal (though not always highly general) terms.

Even rather general principles, however, have their uses. If we had to scrutinize every situation *de novo*, we should have no time to make many decisions in the course of our lives. What sensible people do is to form for themselves some fairly general principles to deal with the general run of cases and reserve their attention for scrutinizing the difficult cases in more detail. But I shall be returning to this point.

Situation ethics does not do much good for bioethics beyond that of deterring us from oversimplification of the issues. Once we get into the really difficult problems, we find ourselves driven to give reasons for our opinions. We have, indeed, to look carefully at particular cases; but after we have done that we shall want to *learn* from these cases principles that we can apply to other cases. Cases differ from one another, no doubt; but that does not mean that we cannot learn from experience. The salient reasons for one decision may also be important for another decision. So, while avoiding oversimplification and too rigid general rules, we can still, and good medical practitioners do, form for ourselves and others general guidelines for the future. These guidelines have to be *to some degree* general, or they will apply to only one situation, and be useless for preserving the lessons of experience for later situations. I shall be coming back later to the different roles in bioethics of general principles and the careful examination of particular cases.

7

Virtue ethics, which I mentioned next, falls down for a different reason; it ignores *another* part of the truth about morality. It shares this fault with a type of ethical theory that in other respects might be thought antagonistic to it, namely that of a typical intuitionist deontologist who believes in the ultimacy of duties. Both of these kinds of theory are exposed to the question, 'How do we decide *what are* duties or virtues?'. We should most of us agree that there are duties and that there are virtues, and that both are important in morality; but it is no use the moralist saying to us just that we have to acquire virtues or perform our duties; the difficult part of morality is knowing what these are. I have written a lot in other places about intuitionism and its failings.[22] I shall be coming back later to my way of meeting this deficiency in both virtue ethics and intuitionist deontology. But it should be obvious already that neither theory is going to do much for bioethics unless it can tell us how to answer what I said is the difficult question. If we do not know what traits of character are virtues, we obviously cannot know what we have to do in order to display them.

There is also another fault in virtue ethics, which, however, may not affect all varieties of it. It does not affect Aristotle, but then that is because he is much more than a virtue ethicist. This is the fault of concentrating attention on the character of the moral agent, and diverting it from the scrutiny of what he actually does. It is possible for very virtuous people to do terrible things – and not necessarily by mistake or inadvertence.

Let me take the example of a very devout Roman Catholic missionary, a saintly man, who accepts wholeheartedly the teaching of his church about contraception. He therefore does all he can to stop the government of the African country in which he works, and in which he has some influence, from encouraging the provision of contraceptives. If successful in this, he will be contributing to the population explosion and to the keeping of women in subjection, which, we may agree, are great evils. But we may still think him a very good, though misguided, man. Devout Roman Catholics will not like this example; but they can easily find others which illustrate the same point.

The point is that very good people sometimes do things which they ought not to do, and we must preserve the possibility of saying this. If I were to confine my moral thinking to the improvement or at least preservation of my own good character, I might sometimes fail to question the morality of my *acts*. Aristotle is immune to this danger, because he explicitly says that nobody would have even a prospect of becoming virtuous by *not* doing virtuous acts.[23] A person becomes upright by doing upright acts;[24] and this can be taken in two senses; doing upright acts is *part* of the qualification for being *called* upright, and doing upright acts is a way of *making* oneself into an upright person. It is not the *whole* of the qualification, for the acts have to be done *because* one is that sort of person.[25] But for Aristotle, nevertheless, right action is a necessary condition for virtue. Like Kant, and like any balanced moralist, he appreciates the intimate link between character and action in morality. I shall be returning to the nature of this link.

8

The third on my list of ethical theories I called 'caring ethics'. If all that the proponents of such theories did was to encourage us to be more caring, in most of the senses of that ambiguous word, we could applaud them for that. But caring people, like virtuous people of all kinds, can do wrong things. I mentioned earlier the example of a doctor who cares so much for his children that he deprives other doctors' patients of drugs that are in short supply. We might condemn him even if the beneficiaries were not his children but his own patients. If there is in force a fair system for distributing the drugs, we might think that he ought not to try to cheat the system. We should say the same about a nurse who found that she was caring so much for one of her patients that she neglected the others. It is a difficult question, how to reconcile the duties or virtues of caring and justice. Many of the most difficult issues in bioethics hinge on this question, to which I shall be returning.

9

The last class of theories that I mentioned was that of rights-based theories. We have already noticed one of their faults, that they commonly give no way of deciding what rights people have. But, apart from this, it is hard to see how a rights-based theory could cover all that we want to say by way of moral judgments. Some of the aspects of morality that such theories leave out are, indeed, those emphasized by the other theories we have been discussing. For example, it is hard to see how a rights-based theory can give an adequate account of caring or of virtue. A virtuous person is much more than someone who respects other people's rights, and caring for someone is much more than not infringing his (or her) rights. So here again we have a one-sided theory which emphasizes part of the truth about morality to the exclusion of other equally important parts. An adequate theory, such as I shall be sketching shortly, will cover all these aspects of morality. It is not difficult to do this, once the structure of moral thinking is understood.

A rights-based theory is likely also to give an inadequate account of yet other moral notions besides those emphasized by caring ethics and virtue ethics. It will find it hard to give a full account even of duties. Most moral systems contain duties which are not duties *to* anybody, and which therefore generate no rights. For example, many people think that we have a duty to develop our appreciation of great art and great music and great literature; but it is extremely strained to say that this is a duty *to* anybody – for example to ourselves, or to the artists or composers or writers, most of whom are dead. Nobody, therefore, has a right to have us appreciate these things.

The matter becomes even worse when we pass from the narrow notion of duty to the wider notion of what we morally ought to do. To cite a familiar example: if when driving on a dirty night I pass someone who needs a ride and does not look like a criminal, I might think that I ought to pick him up. But I am unlikely to think that I have a duty *to him* to pick him up, or that he has a right to be picked up. Such acts of kindness are not obligations, but we may all the same commend them morally. So again, something important has been left out.

10

It is time we turned from this fault-finding to something more positive. Is there a theory that can cover *all* the aspects of morality that these different theories emphasize? I shall argue that a carefully formulated combination of Kantianism and utilitarianism, such as I have advocated in my books, can do this. In case any of you think that Kantianism is incompatible with utilitarianism, I can now refer you to a paper in which I argue that this is a mistake.[26] Kant *was* not a utilitarian: he held views which no kind of utilitarian theory could justify (for example, about punishment). But it is doubtful whether these views could be justified by his own theory either. If we look simply at his theory of the Categorical Imperative, it can be argued that this *is* compatible with a carefully formulated version of utilitarianism. What this version is, I have tried to explain elsewhere.[27]

The key to an understanding of all these problems is to see that moral thinking takes place at at least two levels. There is, first of all, the day-to-day level at which most of us do most of our moral thinking. I say 'moral thinking'; but a lot of what goes on at this level can hardly be dignified by the name of 'thinking' at all. If we have been well brought up, we often know at once what is right or wrong without doing any thinking. Philosophers call this knowledge of right and wrong that most of us have, 'moral intuition'. What intuitionists say about this intuitive level of moral thinking is mostly correct, except that they think that it is self-supporting, which it is far from being. Most of the difficult problems in moral philosophy arise because intuitions conflict: either the intuitions of one person, or the intuitions of different people. A different level of moral thinking is needed to settle these conflicts.

This higher level of moral thinking can be called the critical level. It cannot appeal to our intuitive sense of right and wrong to settle conflicts between intuitions, because that would obviously be arguing in a circle. The method of thinking to be employed in critical moral thinking is radically different from that appropriate to the intuitive level. Here we *have* to reason. *How* we have to reason remains, however, a matter for dispute. My own account of the method of moral reasoning at the critical level draws heavily on both the utilitarians and

Kant and is based on an analysis of moral language and its moral properties. It makes no appeal to moral intuitions at the critical level. However, I do not need to defend my view here, because the mere distinction between the two levels is enough to sort out our present problems, which arise mainly through neglect of the distinction.

The critical level of moral thinking is used, not only to settle conflicts between intuitions at the intuitive level, but to select the moral principles and (which comes, as we have seen, to the same thing) the virtues that we should seek to cultivate in our children and ourselves. On my own account of critical thinking, the selection is done by assessing the acceptance utility of the virtues and principles – that is, by asking what are on the whole the best for society to acknowledge and cultivate. Those who have absorbed these principles and acquired these virtues will have the corresponding intuitions about right and wrong, good and bad, and will also, unless overcome by temptations, follow the principles and display the virtues in practice. If the critical thinking has been well done, and if, therefore, the right virtues and principles have been chosen, the person who has them will be a person of good character, that is, a morally good person.

The structure that I have outlined is therefore able to give an account both of moral virtues and of moral principles. It has to be added, however, that for goodness of character or virtue it is not sufficient to do the right actions. As Aristotle saw, it is necessary that they should be done on the basis of settled dispositions, which *constitute* a person's character. The distinction between levels was anticipated by Aristotle, and indeed by Socrates and Plato. To have virtue properly so called, it is necessary to do *what* one ought to do, and to know *why* it is what one ought to do. In other words, *both* right actions and good dispositions, *and* the ability to explain why they are right and good (to give their *logos*) are necessary for virtue. The person who merely knows which actions are right and which dispositions are good, and does not understand why, lacks something, namely the intellectual virtue that Aristotle calls *phronêsis* and Plato and Socrates call *epistêmê* or understanding, as contrasted with mere right opinion. He can do only intuitive, but not critical thinking.

This two-level structure can therefore account adequately for the place of virtues *and* of principles *and* of duties in our moral thinking. But among the virtues are those on which caring ethics lays so much stress. To be a caring person is to have the disposition to feel sympathy for other people, especially when they are suffering, and to act accordingly. This is a very important virtue, but not the only one. Justice is also important, but is underemphasized by caring ethics. Sometimes justice requires us to be impartial between people for whom we care and people for whom we do not.

Here the distinction between levels is extremely important. The better of us have principles to be followed, and virtues to be exercised, at the intuitive level that require partiality to those for whom we care. A mother *should*, we think, give priority to the needs of her own children over those of other people's children. Doctors and nurses should devote themselves to their own patients more than to other people's patients. Partiality in caring is required by the intuitive principles that most of us have been taught,and probably these partial principles are sometimes innate. Here again we must avoid the confusion between singular prescriptions and universal relational ones.

However, this is all at the intuitive level. Partial principles at the intuitive level can be justified by *impartial* thinking at the critical level.[28] If we were concerned impartially for the good of all children, we should want mothers to behave partially toward their own children and have feelings which made them behave in this way. We should want this, because if mothers are like this, children will be better looked after than if mothers tried to feel the same about other people's children as about their own. The same applies to doctors and nurses. Thus, impartial critical thinking will tell us to cultivate partial virtues and principles. But it will also tell us to cultivate impartiality for certain roles and situations. These obviously include that of judges, but also those of anybody who has to distribute benefits and harms fairly, as doctors do when they have to divide scarce resources between their patients.

Lawrence Blum, whom I have mentioned already, considers the possibility that he can hive off the virtue of impartiality into these particular roles, and thus exclude it from other parts of morality.[29] This is all right at the intuitive level. But, because he seems not to understand the importance of the distinction between the levels, he misses the point that impartiality is required in all thought at the critical level, even though this impartial critical thought will bid us be partial in certain roles at the intuitive level. He does indeed consider the possibility that rule-utilitarianism (which is a kind of two-level theory) might make a distinction of levels, and thus seek to show that partial virtues should be cultivated because that is for the best for all considered impartially.[30] But his book was published before my own book *Moral Thinking*, and he probably had not come across earlier writings of mine in which I sketched a two-level theory that escapes the faults he finds in the cruder two-level theory he discusses.[31]

In that book I gave enormous emphasis to the place in moral thinking of empathy. Indeed, it is one of the crucial elements in the system of moral reasoning that I am constructing. In default of the ability to represent to ourselves fully what it is like to be the other people that our actions affect, we are not making our moral decisions with an adequate understanding of the facts of the situation in which we are acting. To enter fully into their situation, we have to think of them as if they were ourselves. And if we then universalize our prescriptions, we are led to treat their preferences as if they were our own preferences. This gets in all that the carers are asking for.

11

Coming now to rights-based theories: it is extremely easy to find a place for rights in the kind of two-level structure that I have been suggesting, but impossible to *base* the whole of morality on them. They have a place both at the intuitive level and at the critical level. I can be brief, because I have explained elsewhere what these places are.[32] At the critical level we are constrained only by the formal requirement that we eliminate all individual references from our moral principles. That is, we must not give the fact that any particular person is in a particular position in a situation as a reason for a moral judgment. This has the consequence that we have to treat all individuals on a par – to give them equal concern and respect, as some writers say. None has a greater claim on us *qua* that individual. We could, if we wished, put this in terms of rights, saying that all individuals have a *right* to equal concern and respect.

However, it has been generally recognized that from this formal requirement no substantial or contentful rights can be derived. We have to reason, in accordance with the formal requirement, counting everybody for one, as Bentham said,[33] or treating the ends of all others as our own ends, as Kant said.[34] And what *substantial* principles we then select will depend on what ends the others have. For example, since nearly everyone has the end of not being killed, we are likely to have a principle giving them a right not to be killed.

But these substantial principles will all be for use at the intuitive level. They will be defeasible or overridable. For example, if some suffering terminal patient beseeches her doctor, as happened in a recent case in Britain, to end her misery, it would be foolish to base a ban on euthanasia on the right to life of the patient.[35] The right exists because in nearly all cases people want not to be killed; in cases where a patient does want to be killed, can she not voluntarily waive the right, as we can most rights?

It will be found that by keeping substantial moral rights at the intuitive level, while preserving the formal right to equal concern and respect at the critical level, all the problems about conflicts of rights, and conflicts between rights and other duties, can be resolved. But since I have dealt with questions of rights and their place in morality at great length elsewhere,[36] I shall not go into any more details here.

12

I come back last to the theory with which I started, situation ethics. It is obvious that a distinction between levels can explain what is right and what is wrong about such a theory. Taken literally, the theory would require us to use critical thinking in all our moral decisions however straightforward. But usually we do not have time for this, nor always the necessary information about the consequences of alternative actions. We are also affected by personal bias, which, in spite of what some of the people I have discussed say, is often a source of wrong decisions.

So the sensible thing to do is to form for ourselves principles and cultivate virtues, which in the general run of straightforward cases will lead us to do the right thing without much thought, and reserve our powers of deep thought for the awkward cases. If we do not have time for this deep thought when the decision confronts us, or if we do not then have the full information needed for a right decision, we can think about it afterwards and perhaps modify our intuitive principles accordingly. When we do this critical thinking, we have to consider each situation on its merits and in detail, as the situation ethicists say we should. But it would be absurd and impracticable to do this on every occasion.

13

I will end by pointing out how important these considerations, which apply to all moral thinking, are for bioethics in particular. I have attended a lot of classes on medical ethics, such as the best medical and nursing schools make their students take. Often these classes have the form of a discussion of particular awkward cases in which doctors and others have to make agonizing decisions. The reason why they are agonizing is that principles that most of us accept conflict with one another.

For example, there are cases in which we cannot save a patient's life unless we do something to him without his consent, or even contrary to his express wishes. There is the principle requiring informed consent, and there is the principle bidding us save life if we can. Both are sound principles, but they are defeasible or overridable. The right way of handling such decisions is provided by the structure I have outlined. We have to decide what is the right decision *in this case*; and that entails examining the case on its merits and in detail. So far the situation ethicists are right. But what we decide in this case may well, and should, get incorporated into our general body of principles for use in the future. We may decide that one of the competing principles, though sound, has exceptions; and sometimes these exceptions need to be written into the rule as qualifications of it. That is what it is to learn from experience, as I said. The person who has been through such an agonizing decision ought to have learnt something, even though all situations, and all patients, are different.

In very awkward cases, we may have to use critical thinking, though our intuitive principles will probably help us decide what aspects of a case to think about first. But the cases are awkward precisely because they are not like the general run of cases, in which, if we have sound intuitive principles, they will guide us without too much thought.

Some of the cases will be awkward because different rights, whether rights of the same person or of different people, conflict. Because these rights are defeasible or overridable, we shall have to use critical thinking to determine which of them should yield in this particular case. And here again this may add to our wisdom for the future, if we incorporate the lessons of this case into our body of moral principles.

In other cases it may seem that what is required by duty conflicts with what is required by caring, or by the pursuit of some other virtue. These are all conflicts at the intuitive level; at the critical level they can be resolved by the application of the formal or logical requirements for moral thinking, in conjunction with the facts about the particular case, and especially the facts about what those affected by our decision prefer, or what their ends are. To understand these facts fully, empathy is required; otherwise we shall be making our decision in ignorance of what the outcome means for those affected. The caring ethicists do right to stress this.

It is at this higher level that the combination of Kantianism with utilitarianism that I have advocated comes into play. At the lower intuitive level we have to be guided by the sound principles that we have learnt, and by the virtues (including that of caring) that we have acquired. But when these sound principles and admirable virtues conflict in a particular case, we may need to have recourse to critical thinking to sort out the conflict, dangerous and agonizing as this may sometimes be. This thinking may even lead us to qualify one of the principles. If the students in the classes I have attended had known about the distinction between the levels of moral thinking, they would have found it easier to sort out their problems. But nobody had told them.

Notes

1   For example, R.M. Hare, 'How To Decide Moral Questions Rationally', *Critica* 18 (1987); reprinted in R.M. Hare, *Essays in Ethical Theory* (Oxford: Oxford University Press, 1989). See also 'Objective Prescriptions', in *Ethics: Royal Institute of Philoso-*

phy Lectures, 1992–93, ed. A.P. Griffiths (Cambridge: Cambridge University Press, 1993); also in *Naturalism and Normativity*, ed. E. Villanueva (Ridgeview: Atascadero, 1993).

2 R.M. Hare, *Moral Thinking: Its Levels, Method and Point* (Oxford: Oxford University Press, 1981), pp. 36, 39.

3 See R.M. Hare, 'Principles', *Proceedings of the Aristotelian Society* 73 (1972–3); reprinted in *Essays in Ethical Theory*.

4 Hare, 'Principles'; *Moral Thinking*, p. 41.

5 Hare, *Moral Thinking*, pp. 35ff., 43ff.

6 Ibid., p. 42.

7 See R.M. Hare, 'Universalizability', in *Encyclopedia of Ethics*, ed. L. Becker (New York: Garland, 1992).

8 I. Kant, *Tugendlehre (Tgl.)*, trans. M. Gregor. *The Doctrine of Virtue* (New York, 1964).

9 Aristotle, *Nicomachean Ethics (EN)*, 1095a 8–10. All references are to pages of the Bekker edition.

10 See, for example, ibid., 1147b 1ff.

11 Ibid., 1104b 13, 1106b 24, 1109b 30.

12 I. Kant, *Grundlegung zur Metaphysik der Sitten (Gr.)* (1785), BA13 = 399; *Tgl.* A118 f. = 449 f. (all references are to pages of original editions and of the Royal Prussian Academy edition).

13 L. Blum, *Friendship, Altruism and Morality* (London: Routledge, 1980).

14 L. Blum, 'Gilligan and Kohlberg: Implications for Moral Theory', *Ethics* 99 (1988).

15 H. Kuhse, 'Caring Is Not Enough: Reflections on a Nursing Ethics of Care', *Australian Journal of Advanced Nursing* 11 (1993).

16 P. Singer, *How Are We to Live?* (Melbourne: Text Publishing Co., 1993).

17 A. Price, *Love and Friendship in Plato and Aristotle* (Oxford: Oxford University Press, 1989).

18 *Gr.* BA69 = 430.

19 R.M. Hare, 'Could Kant Have Been a Utilitarian?', *Utilitas* 5 (1993); also in *Kant and Critique*, ed. R.M. Dancy (Dordrecht: Kluwer, 1993).

20 R.M. Hare, *Essays on Political Morality* (Oxford: Oxford University Press, 1989), pp. 79–120.

21 L.W. Sumner, *The Moral Foundation of Rights* (Oxford: Oxford University Press, 1987).

22 For example, Hare, *Moral Thinking*, p. 10.

23 *EN* 1105b 11.

24 Ibid., 1105b 9.

25 Ibid., 1105a 30.

26 Hare, 'Could Kant Have Been a Utilitarian?'

27 Hare, *Moral Thinking*.
28 R.M. Hare, 'Utilitarianism and the Vicarious Affects', in *The Philosophy of Nicholas Rescher*, ed. E. Sosa (Dordrecht: Reidel, 1979); reprinted in *Essays in Ethical Theory*. See also Hare, *Moral Thinking*.
29 Blum, *Friendship*, p. 46.
30 Ibid., p. 59.
31 For example, R.M. Hare, 'Ethical Theory and Utilitarianism', in *Contemporary British Philosophy 4*, ed. H.D. Lewis; reprinted in *Essays in Ethical Theory*.
32 See Hare, *Moral Thinking*.
33 Cited in Mill, *Utilitarianism* (1861), ch. 5.
34 *Gr.* BA69 = 430.
35 R.M. Hare, 'Is Medical Ethics Lost?' and letters, *Journal of Medical Ethics* 19 (1993), pp. 69–70, 237–9.
36 Hare, *Essays on Political Morality*, pp. 79–120.

Morally Appreciated Circumstances: A Theoretical Problem for Casuistry

ALBERT R. JONSEN

In recent years casuistry has reappeared in the literature of moral philosophy. It was banished at least a century ago by figures of such stature as Henry Sidgwick and G.E. Moore, who believed that the work of moral philosophy was to build a theoretically sound intellectual structure for moral reasoning. In their view, casuistry, immersed in the details of cases and foundering without solid principle and theory, was unworthy and distracting. The eminent Sidgwick once wrote, 'Although Aristotle has said that the "end of our study is not knowledge, but conduct," it is still true that the peculiar excellence of his own system is due to the pure air of scientific curiosity in which it has been developed. And it would seem that a more complete detachment of the scientific study of right conduct from its practical application is to be desired for the sake even of the latter itself.'[1] Further, everyone knew that the classical casuistry of the seventeenth-century theologians had been thoroughly discredited by the brilliant satire of Blaise Pascal's *Provincial Letters* (1656).[2] If the great systematizers and theoreticians of moral philosophy banished casuistry from their concerns, the metaethicists of postwar Anglo-American philosophy scarcely seem to have known of its existence.

In the morally heated atmosphere of the 1960s, however, when the war in southeast Asia and the civil-rights movement aroused vigorous debate about the rights and wrongs of various cases, some moral philosophers began to yearn for a way to move down from the theoretical speculation of metaethics and normative ethics to the circumstances and arguments of cases. In one particular area, the new bioethics, that interest became intense, since bioethics was about medicine and medicine is a matter of cases. It was in this atmosphere that Stephen Toulmin and I began to wonder whether the long-banished and disgraced casuists of old might have some lessons to teach us about how to get close to cases. Our book, *The Abuse of Casuistry: A History of Moral Reasoning*, reviewed the history of classical casuistry and attempted to draw some methodological lessons that might be applied to current ethical dilemmas.[3] Since it was published in 1988, it has brought the term *casuistry* back into use and stimulated debate about its usefulness and validity as a method for ethical reasoning.

This essay will focus on one feature of casuistic reasoning that may have some theoretical interest for moral philosophy and that has not been much noticed in the literature. That feature is the role of circumstances in moral judgment.

Pascal ridiculed the casuists' 'device of appealing to favorable circumstances.'[4] It was possible, he asserted, to find in any case circumstances that could be invoked to excuse the most heinous and horrible crimes. Any appeal to principles, however clear in themselves, could be countered by noting certain circumstances that soften the rigor of the principle. Pascal, of course, was right. We all are aware that the expression, 'it all depends on the circumstances,' is a common and popular maxim in moral discourse. It is rare that we accept without argument the claim that this or that principle allows of no exception under any circumstances. Even when we do, we can find only a few principles that are so impregnable.

The most widely used text in bioethics, Beauchamp and Childress's *Principles of Biomedical Ethics*, sets out various positions regarding the relationship of principles to practical decisions. They describe their approach as a 'composite theory ... in opposition to monistic or absolutistic theories' and say of it, '(it) permits each basic principle to have weight without assigning a priority weighting or ranking. Which principle overrides in a case of conflict will depend on the particular context, which always has unique features.' Again, they say that, on their approach, 'any rule may theoretically be validly overridden in a circumstance by a competing moral rule.' They then set out several requirements for justified infringements of prima facie principles, including, as their second, 'infringement of a prima facie principle must be necessary in the circumstances, in the sense that there are no morally preferable alternative actions that could be substituted.'[5]

I wish to call attention to the terms, 'particular context,' 'unique features,' 'circumstances.' These terms can slip by quickly and quietly, but in fact they are crucial players in moral reasoning. Moral philosophers hardly notice them, being much more attracted and intrigued by their showier companions, the principles and rules and theories. Despite the ubiquity of circumstances in moral thinking and discourse, moral philosophy has relatively little to say about their relationship to principle.

There are, of course, some classical references to the role of circumstances. In the Third Book of the *Nicomachean Ethics* Aristotle discusses the nature of voluntary acts. He notes that an act can be called involuntary because of 'ignorance of the particulars which constitute the circumstances and the issues involved in the action.' He spells out the principal circumstances: who the agent is, what he is doing, what thing or person is affected, the means he is using, the result intended by his action, and the manner in which he acts. He concludes that 'a voluntary action seems to be one in which the initiative lies with the agent who knows the particular circumstances in which the action is performed.'[6] This passage has spawned commentary and controversy over the centuries, and I shall not dwell on it, except to say that the role of circumstances in assessing the moral responsibility of agents has been a traditional part of moral philosophy. I tend to dwell on what has been less noticed, namely, the role of circumstances in evaluating the moral significance of action.

A tribe of scholars quite distinct from the philosophers, namely, the rhetoricians, was much more attentive to the role of circumstances in argumentation. The moral casuistry that flourished in the Renaissance was, in my view, profoundly influenced by rhetorical reasoning. Classical rhetoric took the case as the center of analysis, since the purpose of that art was to persuade citizens to choose rightly and well about civic affairs and judges to judge fairly and honestly about legal matters. It was the business of rhetoric to teach orators how 'to make the case.' For the classical rhetoricians, the case was precisely 'a collection of persons, places, times, causes, manners, events, deeds, instruments and words.'[7]

Rhetoric and casuistry combine in the work of Cicero. In his *De Officiis* he discusses at length several cases which have continued, in different forms, to be debated through the centuries: who to save in a shipwreck, whether a realtor should tell the whole truth about the house he is showing and a merchant the whole truth about the product he sells. In his *De Inventione*, however, he discusses the nature of practical argumentation. He stresses the importance of circumstances in building a case that leads to probable conclusions, the only sort of conclusion available in moral and political disputes. Later commentators summarized Cicero's list of relevant circumstances in the mnemonic, who, what, where, by what means, why, how, and when.

In a little-known corner of Immanuel Kant's work, the second part of his late work *The Metaphysics of Morals* (1797), the philosopher moves from the form of morality to the application of moral principles to the moral life. In the course of this work he poses twenty questions that he calls 'casuistical.' Among them, Kant turns bioethicist for a moment: 'Anyone who decides to be vaccinated against smallpox puts his life in danger, even though he does it to preserve his life ... is smallpox inoculation permissible?'[8] Kant does not respond to his question (he hardly ever does), but leaves it to the reader to ponder.

Let us turn to a very modern version of the same question. In March 1994 the

New York Times headlined, 'U.S. Ethics Are Questioned by Critics of Vaccine Test in Italy and Sweden.'[9] A large trial of a new vaccine against pertussis (whooping cough) is being sponsored by the U.S. National Institutes of Health. The trial is being carried out in Sweden and Italy because in both of those countries, unlike the situation in United States, most children are not vaccinated against pertussis. This provides a useful comparison or control to test the efficacy of the vaccine; children could be randomized into groups that would receive and not receive the vaccination, and the rates of subsequent disease could be compared. A leading Italian epidemiologist criticized this trial as unethical because the current pertussis vaccine, while known to have some risks, is also known to be effective, and thus all children should be vaccinated against what can be a fatal disease.

How should we analyze the ethical issue in this case? In the early 1970s the United States Congress established the National Commission for the Protection of Human Subjects of Biomedical and Behavioral Research. That commission was charged with a study of the ethical aspects of research involving human subjects. It issued a number of reports, including one on the basic ethical principles that should govern research with human subjects, known as the *Belmont Report*, and another dealing specifically with ethical issues raised by doing research with children. The *Belmont Report* stated that four basic principles should be observed in all human research: Beneficence and Non-Maleficence, Respect for Autonomy, and Justice.[10] When children are the subjects of the research, their legitimate surrogates, usually their parents, must protect them from harm and choose in their best interest; investigators cannot propose research that may raise above minimal the risks of harm to children.[11]

We must go beyond the statement of these principles, however, to an examination of the circumstances. This obligation is intimated in the principle that risks to children should not exceed the minimal. Here an important term in the principle itself begs for definition and quantification. The rules governing research with children attempt definition by analogy: minimal risks are those that children encounter in the course of their daily lives. But clearly we ask for more information relevant to this case. How serious is the disease in question? Is there treatment and how effective is it? What is the natural rate of infection? What is the incidence of adverse effects of the vaccination? Further questions about the research protocol also are relevant. How many subjects are needed for statistical validity? Is a control group necessary for validity and, if so, how large must it be? All of these questions bear on the circumstances of the case. The answers to them are integral to the ethical analysis. Circumstances are not, as the etymology of the word suggests, things that 'stand around'; they are as integral to the moral analysis as are the principles.

Note how the *New York Times* article about the vaccine trial reports the arguments. Dr Fauci of NIH says, 'a ten percent group was the smallest you can have to get statistically meaningful results.' He and other American experts say 'children in the pertussis trials who do not get the shots are not unduly at risk compared to their peers because fewer than 40 percent of the children in Italy and fewer than 10 percent in Sweden currently get whooping cough inoculations.' 'Doctors in the two countries believe the risks of the vaccine now used worldwide outweigh benefits and so do not strongly advocate its use.' American experts argue, 'if the new vaccines, which appear to have few and milder side affects, prove effective in the trials, it could lead to a resurgence of interest in having all children worldwide immunized against pertussis.' Notice how the classic circumstances of who, what, where, and by what means constantly recur. Notice as well that the quantifiable 'how many' appears.

How does the ethicist deal with circumstances? First, it is clear that the circumstances are related to the principles. The ancient Hippocratic injunction urges the physician 'to be of benefit and to do no harm.' In order to abide by that injunction, one must know what constitutes benefit and harm in a general way, but one must also know many details that measure the extent to which doing one thing or another might effect more or less of the results that are counted beneficial and harmful. Kant, in one of his casuistical questions, asks whether drinking wine can be justified and comments, 'who can determine the measure for a man who is only too ready to pass into a state where he has no clear eye for measuring.'[12] The question is not answered 'yes' or 'no,' but how much, and the how much is not a matter of principle but of judgment and prudence. Similarly, the vaccine case must balance the possibility that the unvaccinated children will contract whooping cough – which they are quite likely to do anyway – against the possibility that the vaccinated will suffer some side-effects that might be serious, against the probability that a validly proven effective vaccine will be used to inoculate many children who would otherwise not be vaccinated. This is a highly circumstantial case. The principle of beneficence is being followed, to some extent, and the principle of avoiding harm is being followed, to some extent.

The *New York Times* reporter asked an ethicist, Dr Daniel Wikler, to comment on the case. He responded, 'there is no clear answer for me because both sides have an ethical argument.' This seems to me the best one can do. The classical casuists recognized such situations, not as dilemmas, but as probable conclusions, in which sound reasons do not lead to only one judgment but support diverse conclusions. In such cases they permitted either course of action. In some situations they cautioned that the safer course must be taken, particularly when there was danger posed to life or to the certain rights of others. The ethics of research with children hew to the safer course. In this case, the question is whether the researchers are endangering the lives of the unvaccinated control group. Wikler notes, 'You as a researcher can't be responsible for the condition in which you find your subjects, but you cannot be exploitive.' It can be reasonably maintained that the researchers do not endanger children who are already endangered in the course of their daily lives.

A further question might be asked, however, and this is the question that the Italian critics are asking. Do the researchers have the obligation to protect the children who would otherwise not be vaccinated? This question directly challenges the very concept of medical research. The moral principle of medicine is to benefit and do no harm to one's patients; the moral principle of research is to derive valid generalizable science that can be useful to future patients, without at the same time doing harm. Can a researcher omit doing a good for particular individuals if, by so doing, the research is rendered more valid? Yes, say the proponents of this research, since the Italian and Swedish children would not be receiving the vaccine in the normal course of their lives and thus they are not being deprived. Here, the answer rests on a circumstance, namely, the rarity of the practice of pertussis vaccination in those countries.

The debate over this research, then, takes place at a highly circumstantial level. The broad principles may hover high in the sky above the debates and shed light on them, but the crux of the debate lies in the many minor arguments that swirl around the particulars of this problem. I say 'minor arguments' deliberately; there are in this case, as in most interesting ethical cases, many arguments that run simultaneously and are built up of certain norms and certain facts that arise only within certain concrete situations. They are 'minor' arguments, as distinguished from the large disputes that can take place at a broader level of generalization.

In this case there are minor arguments about how risky the current vaccine is, about how many unvaccinated controls are needed, about whether Swedish and Italian children are being harmed, and so on. These arguments arise because of several features of the case itself. First, it is a case of biomedical research and, within that category, a case of vaccine research. Research and vaccine research have constant, recurrent features; for example, a research intervention is determined by the design of the protocol rather than by the condition of the subject, the design cannot be one that is intended to worsen the subject's condition, the design must be capable of statistical analysis that leads to valid generalizations. Vaccine research, in particular, always requires a healthy subject and always poses the risk of making that healthy subject ill.

These constant, recurring features of the practice of research are what the ancient rhetoricians called 'topics.' They recognized that all human enterprises about which oratory was appropriate had constant, recurrent features that defined the enterprise. A speech about politics, for example, would differ from a speech about economics, or art, or religion, because each of these practices differs in its defining features, or topics. The rhetoricians used the term *topic*, that is, literally 'places,' because they recognized that these defining features were the places where the materials for argument would be found. The materials for argument were maxims and circumstances. The maxims were expressions of moral or prudential advice; the circumstances were the existential facts being addressed in the case at hand. Out of these two materials the minor arguments were constructed.

In the topics of research noted above the constants of research design not only are formed by the canons of research; they are shaped by moral maxims as well. Thus, we recognize that while research interventions are determined by the design rather than the condition of the subject, we also recognize that the intervention cannot be designed to worsen the subject's condition. This is, of course, an ethical imperative based on the principle of non-maleficence, but it is focused down, fitted to, the particular practice called research. It is, as it were, the principle of non-maleficence shaped and constrained into the practice of research.

It might have been noted that this maxim appears threatened by a constant feature of vaccine research: vaccines are tested to discover whether they will prevent infection and thus must be tested on the healthy, the not-yet-infected. Vaccines, being made from the materials of the infectious agent, may cause the very infection they are designed to prevent and may often cause some transient discomfort or illness. Thus, their investigational use appears to violate the maxim not to intend to worsen the subject's condition.

The maxim may be understood to apply, however, only if the worsening is in some sense serious, that is, very painful, leaving lasting effects, or being possibly lethal. If it is only a transitory, trivial worsening, the maxim does not apply. Thus, the slight malaise and briefly painful site of inoculation that is characteristic of vaccination are ethically tolerable. Similarly, the more serious but rare effects of testing the vaccine can be compared with the more likely possibility of having the same effects by being non-immunized in a setting or locale where the infection is rampant.

These are examples of what I called above 'minor arguments constructed from the materials of the case, the topics, the maxims and the circumstances.' I am certain that ethical evaluation of cases very often, if not always, dwells upon these minor arguments rather than on the grand arguments of principle. I am also sure that the resolution of ethical quandaries comes, not out of a vision of principles, but out of a perception of the ways in which these minor arguments work out.

How do these minor arguments 'work out'? Let me offer some rough suggestions. The circumstances of cases, the 'who, what, when, where, why, how, and how much,' are factual descriptions. They appear to be nothing but 'facts' that lie on one side of 'Hume's Hurdle,' over which philosophers must leap to get from fact to value. I have always thought this a peculiarly narrow view of moral situations. I would rather say that the circumstances function as 'morally appreciated features of a situation.' While they themselves are not derivations of moral principle, they are evaluated in relationship to principles.

By 'morally appreciated circumstances' I mean the way in which certain facts are associated with certain goals and perspectives that can themselves be subject to moral evaluation. For example, I register so many pounds on my bathroom scale. That avoirdupois can be considered overweight in relation to many perspectives: the statistical norm for my height and age in a relevant population, the cultural standards for fashionable appearance, risks associated with cardiovascular morbidity and mortality, ability to maneuvre at sports, and so on. Each of these perspectives can be morally evaluated: goals I set in relation to them can be assessed in the light of those values. The actual fact of how many pounds I weigh can be 'morally appreciated' in view of those goals and perspectives. In their light I can evaluate whether my concern about my weight arises from vanity, from responsibility for my health, from enjoyment of tennis, or from thrift about purchasing new shirts and trousers. The actual number may differ in moral relevance depending on this evaluation.

Turn from the minor matter of my avoirdupois to the more serious issue of research with children. The circumstantial observations, such as 'minor,' 'minimal over minor,' 'risks commensurate,' and so forth, that I use in the moral appreciation of my avoirdupois, are used as well in the moral appreciation of research proposals regarding children. The National Commission's *Report on Children as Research Subjects* is filled with these terms, as the commission works out a careful algorithm for evaluating the ethics of particular research protocols.

The circumstances under consideration are of quite different sorts and may seem incommensurable: the classic problem of apples and oranges. In any particular case we may be forced to evaluate a health risk, a personal preference, the protection of a person against harm, a financial cost, a scientific question. These features do not sort into the same basket. Thus, we must view the case as a whole and assess how the various circumstances affect our judgment. So, in one and the same case, we find ourselves pondering 'small risks,' 'significant costs,' 'minimal harms,' 'doubtful competence.' We must see them cumulatively, not singly. We find ourselves concluding, 'well, *all things considered*, I believe this is the right thing to do.'

We sometimes say that a particular action or choice was 'fitting.' The metaphor of 'fit' has ancient roots in western moral thought. It was a central notion in the moral doctrines of the sophists and the stoics and the key to Aristotle's concept of practical judgment (the Greek word *epikeia*, often translated as 'equity,' literally means 'fitting'). The concept has come down to recent times in the writings of authors such as D.W. Ross, F.H. Bradley, William James, and H. Richard Niebuhr. Fit implies a context, structure, or design, made up of diverse elements, into which some feature of moral discourse, either a principle or a judgment, is set. When so set, the feature is seen to be of the right measure, size, and shape, making a harmonious pattern. This old moral metaphor has been used in many ways: for the sophists, moral choice fit the situation of time and place; for the stoics, moral behavior fit the harmonious movement of the universe; for Aristotle, modifications of law suited the intent of the original legislator.

Moral judgment is a patterned whole into which principles, values, circumstances, and consequences must be fitted. The particular judgment itself must be fitted into a larger set of judgments about moral suitability of behavior and practices. Fittingness suggests how we 'morally appreciate' the circumstances of a case. Appreciation is, originally, an esthetic concept: we appreciate a painting, a landscape, a symphony, a good play, whether drama or a throw from shortstop to second to first. This sort of esthetic appreciation arises, in part, from the harmonious fitting together of various elements that may be, in themselves, heterogeneous. A moral judgment about a case is, I think, similar. Principles, values, circumstances and consequences must be seen as a whole. The judgment about them comprises all of them.

A return to the deliberations of the National Commission provides instances that illustrate this view. First, in the *Children's Report*, the maxim 'do no harm,' while never explicitly stated, is all-pervasive. Since children generally cannot give consent (a circumstance), the principle of respect for autonomy has less relevance (i.e., it does not fit) than does the principle of nonmaleficence. The principle 'do not harm' must be refined to fit, not the general context of medical care, but the particular context of medical research. It is necessary to clarify what might constitute harm and how research might do harm. The commission's deliberations bear witness to the realization that there are harms of many sorts and many degrees and that most research maneuvres do not do harm but pose risks of harm, and that these risks are of many sorts and degrees. Harms like deliberate death or maiming, such as those that took place in Nazi research, are unquestionably immoral; but how should the harm that comes from a needle stick to draw blood be judged? Is it more harmful or risky if the child is healthy and normal than if the child is a leukemia patient for whom needle sticks are routine? Is a change of daily activities for research observation a harm or risk of harm? Would it be so if the change involved placing the child for a day in the care of strangers rather than familiar caretakers? Should it be considered a harm to be randomized into a treatment regimen that turns out at the conclusion of the study to be the less effective one? These and many other variations on the theme of harm and risk are essential to any reasonable judgment that the maxim 'do no harm' is being honored or violated. It is the total picture in the instant case that allows such a judgment to be made. The moral significance of 'do no harm' is manifested only amid the greater and the less, the probables and the possibles, of quite particular circumstances.

This example illustrates how the principles and maxims that are invoked in any case of moral perplexity are 'fitted' into the contexts and patterns of circumstances. Any principle or maxim, acknowledged as morally important in itself, becomes relevant within such a factual pattern. Principles and maxims 'come into focus' against a background of circumstances. Change the background, either by addition or removal of some fact or by hightening or shading of the circumstances, and one or another maxim will appear more vividly and centrally. Seeing these patterns constitutes an essential feature of moral judgment.

Any trained moral philosopher knows the epistemological conundrums that trail such assertions. In particular, the description of moral judgment as analogous to esthetic judgment raises eyebrows. The problem of subjectivism immediately appears. One need not be a moral philosopher to recognize that if ethics is like artistic appreciation, then, 'de gustibus non est disputandum.' Also, the inevitable and somewhat unwelcome companion of ethical estheticism is ethical intuitionism, a highly problematic (though not entirely discredited) metaethical theory. I shall not confront those problems here. Instead, I shall return to the National Commission and suggest that one way of avoiding the epistemological conundrums is to put together a group of reasonably intelligent persons to argue an ethical problem, not in the abstract but in the concrete, and to demand of them a resolution, as Congress did demand from the commissioners.

At one point, the commission reflected on the hypothetical situation in which some disease seriously threatens large numbers of children; certain scientific investigations have the promise of preventing that disease but pose some risk to the very children whose lives are threatened by the disease. (The example was hypothetical, but the polio epidemics of the 1940s were a real historical analog.) Should researchers be permitted to subject children to the risk of the research in order to protect them from the disease? The commissioners struggled with the case, then they uttered the wise advice: 'rather than attempt to resolve the delemma in the abstract ... the ethical argument should be made, not over a hypothetical case, but over an actual situation, in which the real issues and likely costs of any solution can be more clearly discerned.'[12] The commission proposed that a highly visible and highly accountable body be constituted in perpetuity to deal with such situations. The situation cannot be envisioned in advance because the seriousness of the particular circumstances need concrete specification.

In January 1993 a tragic epidemic struck my own city, Seattle, Washington. Within three days 400 persons, mostly children, were struck with a devastating illness caused by Escherichia coli 051: H7, owing to undercooked, contaminated hamburger meat, provided at some fast food restaurants. Two children died and many were close to death; many who recovered will have chronic gastrointestinal and renal problems. Initially, it could not be estimated how many of the thousands of children who ate at those restaurants had ingested the pathogen and would become ill. Suppose that a pharmaceutical company had a powerful antimicrobial drug ready for testing and planned to test it in critically ill adults, who could give consent. It is known that the drug does have rare but potentially serious side-effects. Someone suggests that this drug be given prophylactically to all children who had eaten at fast-food restaurants over the previous week. Should this more than minor risk for some children who would not otherwise be infected be permitted? This is the kind of concrete problem that must be assessed in the situation in order to discern whether clear and sufficient reasons warrant a specific exception to the principle that children not be subjected to more than minor risks.

Assessment in the situation requires that a group of concerned persons must gather together all of the relevant information. Members of that group first will act as if they were epidemiologists, searching for the causes, evaluating the seriousness of the crisis, its extent, and the likelihood that it might spread, and examining the data about the investigational drug. They must then go on to act as ethicists, aware of the principles and maxims, such as protection of the innocent, respect for autonomy, avoidance of harm, the public welfare, and so forth. Each of these principles can be proposed and defined. A moment will come, however, when the group of epidemiologists and the group of ethicists must become one. The new group must answer the question: 'Can any risk of harm to an individual be permitted in order to avoid some risk of harm to the population?' The maxims about avoiding harm and about protecting the public will move into focus as answers are suggested to the questions. How much harm? How likely is it? How certain? How otherwise avoidable?'

When the group enters this debate, it merges the assessment of factual circumstances and the assertion of philosophical principles into prudent judgment. The weighing and balancing of principles does not depend on any moral equivalent of the laws of physics. It is done by practical moral judgment, discretion, prudence, or, in Aristotle's idiom, *phronesis*. Despite the recent resurgence of interest in this notion, many philosophers consider it exasperatingly vague. Indeed, it does frustrate those who are searching for the architectonic principle of morality. But vague as it is, moral judgment is moral, not merely judgment, only if it is exercised by persons who are, as Aristotle insisted, imbued with justice, friendship, and magnanimity. In more contemporary language, they are people who both hold firmly to clear principles about justice, human dignity, and welfare, and have the discretion to differentiate between the serious, the ordinary, and the trivial, in the situations of human living. We know that there are a few such persons in our world, but precious few. Thus, we hope that in the deliberations of fairly appointed committees and commissions, publicly visible and accountable, we may find something resembling the phronesis that alone can render reasonable and prudent decisions about particular moral perplexities. We are looking for principled persons who can 'appreciate circumstances.'

Notes

1 Henry Sidgwick, *The Methods of Ethics* (London: Macmillan, 1877), p. 11.
2 Blaise Pascal, *The Provincial Letters*, trans. A. Krailsheimer (London: Penguin Books, 1967).
3 Albert Jonsen and Stephan Toulmin, *The Abuse of Casuistry: A History of Moral Reasoning* (Berkeley and Los Angeles: University of California Press, 1988).
4 Pascal, *Provincial Letters*, Letter VI, p. 89.
5 Tom Beauchamp and James Childress, *Principles of Biomedical Ethics* (New York and Oxford: Oxford University Press, 1994), pp. 51, 53.
6 Aristotle, *The Nicomachean Ethics*, trans. M. Ostwald (Indianapolis: Bobbs-Merrill, 1962), Book III, 1110b16–1111a22, pp. 55–7.
7 Quintillian, *Institutiones* III, 5, 17, in Jonsen and Toulmin, *Abuse of Casuistry*, p. 132.
8 Immanuel Kant, *The Metaphysics of Morals*, trans. M.J. Gregor, Part II, The Doctrine of Virtue, I, 1, 1, vi (New York: Harper, 1964), p. 86.
9 'U.S. Ethics Are Questioned by Critics of Vaccine Test in Italy and Sweden,' *New York Times*, March 13, 1994, A 13.
10 National Commission for the Protection of Human Subjects of Biomedical and Behavioral Research, *The Belmont Report: Ethical Principles and Guidelines for the Protection of Human Subjects of Research* (Washington, DC: National Institute of Health, 1979).
11 National Commission for the Protection of Human Subjects of Biomedical and

Behavioral Research. *Research Involving Children: Report and Recommendations* (Washington, DC: U.S. Government Printing Office, 1977).

12 Kant, *Metaphysics*, I, 1, 3, viii, p. 91.

13 National Commission, *Research Involving Children*, p. 140.

Moral Philosophy and Bioethics: Contextualism versus the Paradigm Theory

EARL WINKLER

It is a familiar observation that moral philosophy in the twentieth century has been dominated by meta-ethical concerns, at least until recently. Yet there have been many notable efforts at systematic normative theory in this period, and in general faith in the possibility and power of such theory has persisted. Doubt, too, has persisted about the relevance and applicability of general ethical theory, although scepticism of this kind has tended to be both poorly articulated and perplexed about alternatives. But the current of distrust of and aversion to theory has been gathering force in the last few years. This reaction is especially noticeable within the ranks of the many philosophers, and others, who have been seriously engaged in work in practical ethics. And it has been gaining strength in relation to an increasingly well-defined rival to the 'applied ethics' model of moral reasoning that normative theory invariably invokes. I shall call this rival 'contextualism.'

I. The Rivals

My principal aim in this paper is to develop a contextualist critique of the reigning theory in bioethics, which I call the 'paradigm theory.' Using only broad strokes, I begin in this section by sketching these rivals and drawing basic conceptual and methodological contrasts between them. I also suggest that most traditional forms of normative theory face severe difficulty in accommodating the kind of domain specificity in moral reasoning common in applied ethics. In part II I develop the methodological conflict in greater detail and in relation to bioethics in particular. In part III I explore an example of the kind of philosophical reasoning that I think is most useful in bioethics and take stock of preceding results.

The Paradigm Theory

The holy grail of traditional moral philosophy is a single, comprehensive and informative theory that is based in universal principles, which, in their turn, yield particular precepts and rules that are capable of deciding concrete issues of practice. Accordingly, the ideal of moral justification is essentially deductivist, involving different levels of generalization. One justifies a particular judgment by showing that it falls under a rule, and justifies the rule by showing that it is a specification of a principle, and justifies the principle by showing that it is grounded in the most abstract levels of normative theory.

The basic philosophical conception of applied ethics has been that it is continuous with general ethical theory. Biomedical ethics, as a primary division of applied ethics, is not a special kind of ethics; it does not include any special principles or methods that are specific to the field of medicine and are not derivable from more general considerations. The practical field of medicine is governed by the same general normative principles and rules that hold good in other spheres of human life. If certain values and requirements are central to the practice of medicine, they will be explained and justified from the perspective of general moral theory. In the introduction to their seminal book, *Principles of Biomedical Ethics*, Beauchamp and Childress declare themselves as follows: 'We understand "biomedical ethics" as one type of *applied ethics* – the application of general ethical theories, principles and rules to problems of therapeutic practice, health care delivery, medical and biological research.'[1] In this same work Beauchamp and Childress go on to develop what I have called the 'paradigm theory' of bioethics. I refer to the familiar theory that comprises three main principles – those of autonomy, beneficence (including non-maleficence), and justice. It is this theory that has dominated the field of bioethics for well over a decade. General acceptance of this theoretical framework brought with it a sense of unification and definition for what was then a disparate and adolescent field struggling to identify itself. Synoptic versions of the theory became the standard fare in introductions for the most popular textbooks in bioethics; and it served repeatedly as the theoretical framework for various influential government reports in Canada, the United States, and elsewhere. The unification of theoretical vision and moral vocabulary thus sponsored by the paradigm theory gained credibility and legitimacy for the entire field of bioethics. But the ascendancy of this theoretical model has a still deeper source in the ideal of comprehensive moral understanding I sketched above.

The paradigm theory promises to bridge the logical chasm between the abstractions of normative theory – principally utilitarianism and Kantianism – and the moral complexities of the world of medical particulars. For on the one

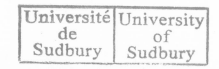

hand, its three mid-level principles are articulated and explained in relation to medical practice. This process is accomplished, first, by making connections with subsidiary principles, or rules, such as those of informed consent, truth-telling, and confidentiality; and secondly, by drawing distinctions that are crucial in applying the theory, such as those between active and passive euthanasia. The paradigm theory thus appears to provide enough substance to guide practice. On the other hand, it keeps faith with the ideal of comprehensive justification because each of its principles is linked with one or another of our central traditions in normative theory. The principle of autonomy is seen as an expression of the rights and dignity of the person that forms the foundation of Kantianism and modern deontological theory generally. The principle of beneficence, equally obviously, has its heritage in classical utilitarianism, although its specific focus is on patient welfare. And the principle of justice is most naturally connected with contractarian traditions in moral theory. The faith that is thus kept with normative theory is not, of course, perfect. The paradigm theory draws upon very different and conflicting forms of general theory. But each of these traditions is centuries old and vital today; each, therefore, is likely to have some share of the truth. So the question of the *ultimate* derivation of the paradigm theory's three principles can be left to future resolutions and reconciliations of normative theory, following perhaps upon further developments in meta-ethics.

Contextualism

The basic orientation of the paradigm theory is top down. It conceives its main principles as specifications for the field of medicine of still more basic principles taken from moral philosophy. By contrast, contextualism moves from the bottom up. Contextualism rejects the idea that universally valid ethical theory is necessary to ground moral rationality and justification. In place of this ancient quest it adopts the general idea that moral problems must be resolved within the interpretive complexities of concrete circumstances, by appeal to relevant historical and cultural traditions, with reference to critical institutional and professional norms and virtues, and by relying primarily on the method of comparative case analysis. According to this method, we navigate our way towards a practical resolution by discursive triangulation from clear and settled cases to problematic ones.

Contextualism thus begins with conventional morality and the norms and values that currently play justificatory roles in various domains of social life. These moral rules and values are presumed to be reasonable unless they can be shown to be unreasonable. Moral judgment is regarded as sufficiently justified by appeal to other moral beliefs or principles not challenged by the particular issue in question. Accordingly, relevant levels of theoretical reflection are determined by what is actually required to establish a judgment as most reasonable in the circumstances. Ultimately, contextualism tries to bring a case under a rule that can be shown to have, or properly presumed to have, instrumental validity for the social domain that contains the case.

Normative Theory and Contextual Variability

Our central traditions in normative theory share in the general idea that all moral requirements somehow derive from the most basic imperatives or principles that are binding on all of us simply as human beings or persons. Classical utilitarianism derives its basic principle from a theory of intrinsic good and evil by holding that the morality of action is completely determined by the goodness or badness of states of affairs that agents bring about or permit to occur. Utilitarianism, and consequentialism generally, is thereby committed to a particularly uncompromising form of impartiality in ethics. According to a standard utilitarian form of this commitment, equivalent human interests command equal moral consideration in every circumstance. This entrains the various, familiar efforts of utilitarians to reconcile their theoretical commitment to impartiality with commonly recognized forms of morally acceptable behaviour that violate it. There are, for example, countless situations in which we forgo opportunities to act in ways that would be of great help to others while acting instead to satisfy comparatively trivial interests of our own. We go to dinner or to a movie rather than going across town to aid the homeless. If we have a right to some of these entertainments it is hard to see how we could have a fixed obligation to attend maximally to human interests, impartially considered. Also, of course, the principle of impartiality confronts the almost universal belief that the obligation to aid and support family members is generally stronger than the requirement to help strangers and often remains so even when competing interests of strangers are in themselves more important. For my purposes, the essential point here is that classical utilitarianism has enormous difficulty with the challenge either to accommodate or to explain away commonly recognized forms of contextual variability in the force and focus of various principles and rules concerning the duty to give aid.

Besides being at odds with common morality concerning the duty to give aid, utilitarianism also faces well-known difficulties in relation to claims concerning rights, fairness, and desert. Within different domains of social life individuals are hedged around by various rules concerning rights and desert that govern action in that domain. By their very nature, such rules have a decidedly deontological force in that they are never to be violated for marginal gains in utility or, in many cases, for substantial gains. In my view, utilitarianism invariably falls victim to a familiar dilemma in attempting to deal with these common patterns of moral reasoning concerning rights and desert. In so far as classical utilitarianism attempts to square itself with these patterns of moral reasoning, either it gives the *wrong* answer as to why some action is right, or, in giving something like the right answer, it appeals to potential disutilities which exist only because most people are not utilitarians. Take, for example, the professional obligation to report grades accurately. Commonsense morality will say that if someone works hard and does well, she deserves the grade she has earned. Utilitarians will say that there is social benefit in reporting grades that accurately reflect performances. Of course, this statement is generally true; but it fails to capture the more fundamental reason underlying this obligation, that concerning fairness and desert. In addition, we know very well that in particular cases a given student might benefit significantly from receiving a higher grade than is deserved. And it may be that this can be accomplished with little risk of discovery or of consequent disutilities for others. In response, the utilitarian can say that while these risks are low, they are not negligible and that the consequences of discovery, or even of strong suspicion on the part of other students, may engender very harmful feelings of indignation and mistrust. This statement also may be true. But the utilitarian cannot legitimately trade on these potential disutilities. For the indignation and mistrust in question are attitudes that derive from people's general commitment to the moral value of accuracy and fairness in grading, regardless of opportunities to benefit a given individual by misrepresentation. In other words, the attitudes to which the utilitarian now appeals themselves are a reflection of moral values and beliefs that people would not have if they were made over in the utilitarian image. (I do not mean to suggest by any of this that there cannot be certain very unusual and especially sympathetic cases that may warrant misrepresentation.)

Classical utilitarianism simply cannot properly recognize that factors of relationship, both personal and professional, as well as of rights and desert radically restrict or qualify the morally single-minded promotion of everyone's interests. Consequently, utilitarianism is blind to many forms of contextual variability in the weight of morally relevant considerations that commonsense morality embodies. If a former paramedic and neighbourhood resident fails to help a known drug dealer who is shot on the street, this situation is not as bad as would be a doctor's refusal to treat this patient when he is brought to the emergency room. Again, the professional requirement to evaluate students honestly and accurately is stricter and more determinate than the similar requirement that a coach in little league evaluate honestly and fairly the performance of the young athletes in her charge. Suppose, for example, that one youngster is much better than all the others but is also cocky and inclined to lord it over the other kids. To counteract this self-conceit and immodesty, as well as its effects on the team, the coach might sometimes employ a double standard in team meetings involving evaluations. She might emphasize or exaggerate the positive aspects of the performance of the less skilled players while, in effect, evaluating the hotshot in terms of higher standards, more relative to the best players in the league. If employed with some subtlety and sensitivity, this strategy might be quite effective and permissible. For similar reasons, it would not be permissible, I think, to use any similar strategy in evaluating student performance in university classes.

In a very different way, deontological theories face an equally daunting problem in accommodating any kind of contextual variability in the force and import of moral principles, precepts, and rules. Deontological reasons for action are commonly thought to owe their primary status as moral reasons to our nature as persons, not to circumstances or particular relationships. Also, most deontological theories, like Ross's system of prima facie duties, require that we weigh and balance competing deontic reasons in reaching all-things-considered judgments about right and wrong. In this case, however, the weight of a deontic principle or reason must be fixed and unvarying across contexts. As Michael Philips argues, if relative weight is not fixed for deontic reasons in a general, context-independent way, it is difficult to see what *weighing* such reasons for and against an action could mean. If relative weight is not fixed in this way, we would be thrown back on intuition to determine these weights in different contexts.[2] And if that were so, why not just say that intuition decides the rightness or wrongness of an act and entirely give up talking about weighing and balancing? Such resort to intuition, however, means abandoning any hope of systematically *explaining* the variable force of moral reasons or of offering any *method* of resolving conflicts about these variations.[3]

Therefore, in order to preserve functional coherence for the idea of weighing moral reasons deontological theories must accept what Philips calls the constancy assumption: If a morally relevant consideration makes a difference of a certain magnitude in two otherwise identical cases, it makes the same degree of difference in *any* two otherwise identical cases. This is precisely what it means for moral considerations to have a fixed relative weight. As a specific and special instance of the constancy assumption, relative to the paradigm theory, it follows that if the principle of autonomy has a certain force and import for A in relation to B, then it must have equivalent force and import for C in relation to B. I shall return to this point in the next section.

We saw above that utilitarianism has difficulty reconciling itself with some commonly recognized forms of contextual variation in the weight of moral rules. We have just seen that deontologism's method of deciding moral issues by weighing deontic reasons either reduces to intuition or requires a fixed relative weight for these reasons. If the latter, deontologism is committed to the denial of all contextual variability of the kind in question. Yet we seem to confront such variability everywhere we look in common moral experience. Contrary to utilitarian impartiality, failing to save family members is worse than failing to save strangers, other things being equal. Contrary to the constancy assumption (as we shall see below) the moral significance of homicide may vary between contexts despite equivalence in the interests of those who die, in the motives and intentions of agents, and in expectable outcomes for the particular case. More generally, standards of truth-telling and disclosure may vary between a competitive business context and that of scientific research, or between the context of international negotiations and that of journalism. Standards of social responsibility are different in important ways within the corporate world than they are within government, and so forth.

Contextualism to the Rescue

By contrast with traditional forms of top-down normative theory, contextualism has no difficulty recognizing and accounting for contextual variation in moral standards and the weight of moral reasons. And, most important, contextualism's recognition of variable weight for moral considerations can be both principled and critical. The kind of contextualism I favour would seek to explain or justify such differences in instrumental terms; in terms, that is, of the basic purpose of given moral rules, or of their purpose in relation to the primary social functions and values that help to define different domains of social life – such as the family, the criminal justice system, the economic system, the medical system, and so on. The prominence of obligations to family, for example, serves in support of the goals and values of family life, especially those of love and intimacy, mutual support, and the provision of a nurturing and protective environment for children. Or again, the point of the general rule requiring truthfulness is to facilitate the exchange of useful information and to support relations of trust. The moral significance of conformity with the rule therefore increases with the importance of the kind of information that is exchanged and with the threat of endangering important forms of trust by its violation. This variability can help to explain the moral difference between deliberate misrepresentation of facts in journalism, for example, and deliberate misrepresentation of the strength of one's desires in certain business deals, especially if it is coupled with reflections on the social functions of journalism and business. Reference to differences in role-related functions between domains also will explain examples like that of the coach and the professor given above.[4]

Regarding basic patterns of contextualist moral criticism, we can note, first, that social functions and purposes that inform practice within a domain may, at times, be subject to critical reformation. Witness the popularity of current reformulations of the primary functions of business, which now incorporate reference to environmental sustainability as constraining the pursuit of prosperity and material progress. Secondly, practices within domains can be criticized as not promoting relevant values or purposes effectively. Both patterns of criticism will typically combine normative and empirical elements.

Until the rise of applied ethics in recent years moral philosophy in this century paid little attention to domain-related moral standards. It was simply assumed, as I said earlier concerning the paradigm theory, that we could generate domain-specific and role-related standards by adapting basic principles to the specific circumstances of any domain, and do so with meaningful results. Following Philips, I have tried to outline some fundamental reasons for thinking that this optimistic, usually unquestioned assumption, is deeply troubled. According to the constancy assumption, deontologism must remain insensitive to any contextual variability in the force of rules resulting from applications of its principles across domains. If it abandons the constancy assumption – surely the better course – it must fall back on intuition in recognizing such variation and yet remain mute regarding its explanation. This dilemma would seem to be a crippling liability attaching to the philosophical assumption in question so far as derivation of domain-related standards from deontological principles is concerned. Even more clearly, classical utilitarianism also betrays the basic presupposition of traditional moral philosophy, that abstract normative theory will somehow provide a foundation from which to generate or explain appropriate domain-related moral standards. Utilitarianism cannot even properly recognize common moral rules concerning rights and desert; nor can it explain contextual variations in the weight of the requirement to give aid, as well as in other moral standards whose weight varies as a function of differences in relationships.

By contrast, contextualism agrees with the view that a fundamental pattern of moral reasoning consists of appeals to moral rules that combine instrumental validity at one level with deontological force at another. What contextualism adds to this perception is the idea that the instrumental justification of rules and standards may be domain sensitive. In consequence, the weight and import of many rules and morally relevant considerations may vary across domains and contexts. In so far as governing purposes and values associated with various domains are reasonable, however, these variations will be essentially systematic and explainable.[5] It is these basic theoretical features of contextualism, together with its thoroughly bottom-up and socially embedded orientation to moral problems themselves, that give this approach considerable power and relevance to applied ethics.

A general conception of social morality from an instrumentalist perspective may help to unify the contextualist approach to moral reasoning as I have outlined it. We can think of social moralities as social instruments for the promotion and maintenance of valuable forms of life. The moral point of view is now essentially focused on how we ought to relate to one another in the service of this general end, as it is embodied in the various primary domains of social life. Although contextualism, as I conceive it, is thus a kind of socially embedded rule utilitarianism, the emphasis on moral rules that guide social interactions and relationships within various social contexts helpfully displaces the traditional utilitarian focus on impartial aggregation over individual utilities. An equally important contrast between contextualism and traditional rule utilitarianism is the fact that contextualism is piecemeal and pragmatic, whereas rule utilitarianism tends to be utopian. The latter is typically utopian in that, like traditional contractarianism, it proposes a wholesale and systematic construction of a set of basic moral rules for a given society. In my estimation, however, ethical theory of this type, often called ideal rule utilitarianism, fails to constitute even a normative theory, properly speaking. It amounts, instead, to an abstract formula for generating a normative theory for a given society. Ideal rule utilitarianism thus defines a project whose product would be a normative theory, if anyone could ever convincingly carry it out.

Concluding Transitions

Returning to my opening remarks about the hegemony of the paradigm theory in bioethics, I see its rise as both fortunate and unfortunate for applied ethics. As mentioned, it secured respect and legitimacy for bioethics and consequently for applied ethics generally. It also tended to establish itself as a model of how to relate the traditions of moral philosophy to other domains of applied ethics, such as business ethics and environmental ethics. Efforts of this kind, however, even though they persist today, have been much less successful than they have with bioethics in integrating summary accounts of our central theoretical traditions in moral philosophy with real issues in these other domains. Nothing even approaches the status of a paradigm theory of business ethics or, certainly, of environmental ethics, to mention two prominent fields that have received a lot of philosophical attention.

In my view, it is an accident in the history of philosophy that the area that first gave rise to genuine interest in applied ethics in this century, viz., medicine, is an area whose basic moral dimensions, both structurally and historically, naturally lent themselves to the kind of treatment they got via the paradigm theory. That is, in medical practice there is a powerful, institutionalized set of closely related professions ministering to the needs of sick and often vulnerable and defenceless people. Naturally the basic moral tensions that arise here concern the potential abuse of individuals, for the greater good of a greater number; the likely dominance of paternalistic authority; possible conflicts of interest, having their basis in the potential for conflict between individual patient interest and professional interest, as in medical research, for example; and so forth. All problems of these kinds lend themselves to generalizing treatments in terms of Kantian and utilitarian ideals and tensions between them. Moreover, recognition of these kinds of moral tension was, of course, already enshrined and variously addressed in the history of medical ethics, in terms of principles of *primum non nocere*, informed consent, non-abandonment, adherence to community treatment standards, and so forth. Although I cannot explore this topic further here, and mean no derogation of the real achievements of the paradigm theory, the situation that moral philosophy faces regarding other areas in applied ethics is simply different, and in many ways much more complex, than the one it has encountered in its association with medicine. This is why general introductory chapters that review main traditions in moral philosophy as a prelude to discussions of moral problems in business and the professions, or concerning the environment, typically seem so curiously dissociated from the problems they are meant to illuminate.

We should also realize that the basic principles of the paradigm theory, while they can claim some association with the main traditions of normative theory, are in no very clear sense *derived* from these traditions. Consider, in particular, the principle of beneficence. By focusing almost exclusively on individual patient benefit, this principle radically departs from classical utilitarianism's defining, impartial concern with the interests of everyone. In fact, as we have already seen, it is precisely because of its maximally embracing and impartial focus on *outcomes* that utilitarianism itself is unable to countenance the very kind of domain specificity that the principle of beneficence represents for the field of medicine. The claim of Kantian heritage for the bioethical principle of autonomy has much greater legitimacy. But for Kant, the autonomous functioning of pure practical reason *was* morality, the whole of it. Any version of the autonomy principle that we find in the paradigm theory has to be weighed in the balance with other principles in various cases of conflict. Neither Kantianism nor most other deontological approaches supply a useful method for doing so. We have seen how deontologism either condemns us to the constancy assumption or abandons us to unguided intuition. Therefore, in so far as the paradigm theory makes some show of having a method here, it tends to do so by resort to the kind of situated, domain-sensitive, instrumental reasoning that is at the heart of contextualism. When it does so, as we shall see in the next section, it leaves its basic principles idling in the background with nothing much to do.

Following Michael Philips's lead, I have so far been at pains to outline contextualism's capacity to explain both domain-specific variability in moral standards as well as patterns of contextual variation in the weight of moral reasons more generally. I believe that the instrumental structure of these explanations, together with the outline of basic strategies for critizing received ideas about the social goals of domains and practices related to those goals, deepens the philosophical attractiveness of contextualism. I have tried also to indicate why contextualism's general, bottom-up approach is likely to be more useful in applied ethics as a whole than will be continued efforts to emulate the model set by the paradigm theory.

These theoretical capacities and attractions of contextualism are, however, of limited further significance in relation to an assessment of the paradigm theory per se. This is so, of course, because that theory is specifically focused on the single domain of medicine. Nevertheless, as I indicated above, there will be occasion early in the next section to mention one way in which the matter of contextual variability in the moral weight of rules is relevant to the paradigm theory. But the main focus of this section will be whether the paradigm theory has the power to guide medical morality effectively at the level of practice.

II. Theory and Practice[6]

As we have seen, the paradigm theory of bioethics exemplifies the applied ethics model of moral reasoning oriented to the field of medicine. My principle concern in this part of the paper is the methodological conflict between this model and contextualism. Before turning in this direction, however, we should consider the prior question of the moral scope of the paradigm theory.

The Question of Scope

The essential content of the paradigm theory is its three basic principles of autonomy, beneficence, and justice. But to whom, exactly, do these principles apply, and on what basis? This is the question of scope. It is a request for some account of what constitutes moral status, of what gives something this sort of standing. Unfortunately, the paradigm theory is silent on the question of moral standing itself – what must something be like in order to qualify as a subject of serious moral concern in its own right? The abortion issue, for instance, has tended to formulate the question of fetal moral status as the question of whether a fetus has a right to life. Perhaps it has been the abortion issue, more than any other, that has dramatized the need for a general account of the conditions for moral standing. By now the general issue itself has cropped up all over the field of bioethics: in connection, for example, with the use of anencephalic babies as organ donors; in regard to the therapeutic transfer of fetal tissue; in respect of research with embryos and their use in some of the new reproductive technologies; in the treatment of the most severely impaired infants and adults; and regarding the recommendation that we include neo-cortical collapse as an additional criterion of death, thus liberalizing the criterion of 'whole brain death.' We should note, also, that moral status, as a fundamental issue, has become a dominant preoccupation of the developing field of environmental ethics, with consequent implications for business ethics.

This omission is a serious limitation of the paradigm theory. It means that the theory is more or less useless in those many areas of bioethical decision-making where the crucial issue is precisely that of moral status. Although this point is obvious, it is none the less important to remind ourselves how critically dependent the paradigm theory is on some supplementary account of moral standing. Our philosophical heritage, moreover, is not particularly helpful on this matter. Anything one is able to infer about moral status from our central traditions in moral theory seems to be either too restrictive, as is the case with Kant, or too vague and indeterminate to guide the discriminations that are called for today.

Contextual Variation concerning Autonomy

As promised in part I, I now return to the topic of contextual variability in the moral significance of principle. As bioethics has developed over the last twenty-five years, the patient's family has been universally acknowledged to have a significant role in treatment decisions for incompetent patients. But since competency is often uncertain, episodic, and otherwise variable, the involvement of family members is expanded. Furthermore, in cases of refusal of treatment by competent patients, families are frequently involved by way of consultation with doctors and other care givers and through interaction with the patient himself. All of this scenario is familiar. What is significant for the present debate, however, is that the legitimate involvement of family, in these familiar ways within the health care setting, creates the potential for the kind of contextual variation in the moral significance of moral precepts and rules, such as respect for autonomy, that I described in part I.

For example, in some instances of refusal of life-sustaining treatment, family members may rightly feel a sense of *obligation* to the one they love to exercise persuasion of various kinds, which may mean engaging doctors in stalling tactics, or using other means to buy time, in an effort to get the patient to change his mind. To the extent that particulars of given family relationships, including shared and failed understandings, values, and established forms of interpersonal communication, may justify these behaviours, as they surely can do sometimes, it would seem to create an explanatory problem for the paradigm theory. According to that theory, the principle of autonomy should speak univocally to all those who are properly involved in treatment decisions for which that principle speaks decisively, or with some definite force. This is, after all, part of what it usually means for principles to determine cases. In a situation like that just described, however, the force and import of the principle of autonomy seems to me to vary significantly between the doctor's situation and that of the family. The principle, in this case, has less decisive weight and is less restrictive for the family than for the doctors. The family may properly engage in many efforts at persuasion, taking many different forms, which in terms of their persistence and their style would be quite inappropriate for the doctor. What 'respecting the autonomy' of the patient *means* for these different agents – the family and the doctor – and its moral weight in these circumstances are not equivalent.

It may be that if she perceives the family as sincere and well intentioned and the patient's situation as not completely hopeless, particularly in the light of the love and care the family wants to provide, the doctor will temporize. Equally, after some reasonable time without success in changing the patient's mind, the family will need, morally need, to acquiesce. But the point remains that to respect autonomy, the doctor must accept the patient's initial decision after only so much counselling and advice giving, offered only in certain professional forms. The principle of respect for autonomy falls much less restrictively, and with much less direct force on the family. That the family, in the end, may have to concede its force changes none of this. The point of theoretical interest here concerns how the paradigm theory is to explain the principle of autonomy's actually having variable moral force and import, from equally legitimate and recognized perspectives, in relation to the same case. For that theory is supposed to be in the business of articulating, for the medical domain, specifications of general principles that are binding on all of us simply as properly involved moral agents.

It might be said that the force of the principle of autonomy applies univocally in the imagined circumstances but that the family, unlike the doctor, is under certain obligations to the patient which, at least temporarily, *override* the respect for autonomy. To be effective, it should be noted, this point must be put in this way – in terms, that is, of one thing overriding another. Nothing can actually make the force of the requirement to respect autonomy for the family weaker than it is for the doctor. Otherwise something will still be wrong with the assumptions of the paradigm theory concerning how principles determine what is right and wrong. In any event, I do not think that this response works. I myself said that the family may *feel* a sense of obligation to the patient born of love and loyalty and in keeping with their family ways. But I do not believe that the family, in such a case as I describe, is ipso facto under any general moral obligation to want to change the patient's mind. This family simply does want to do so; and this patient, being of them, may well understand.

All happy families may be happy in the same way, as Tolstoy says, but no family is always happy. How families deal with situations like the one imagined will rightly vary over some considerable range of possibilities. Granting that there is *some* form of general obligation of concern and care on the part of the family, this state need not oppose, let alone override, respect for autonomy. We are thus thrown back on the explanation I offered above, concerning contextual variation in the force and import of respect for autonomy between the family and the doctor. So far as I can see, the basic assumptions of the paradigm theory and of the applied ethics model of moral reasoning leave no way to recognize, let alone explain or justify, such variations. Sympathetic moral consciousness recognizes this difference; contextualism can explain it.

Wide Reflective Equilibrium

Moral theories are traditionally thought to serve two functions, one intellectual and one practical. They aim to achieve a comprehensive, ordered and systematic understanding of the moral domain or of some significant part of it. They are also supposed to guide moral practice by providing the proper ground for decision making in fundamental principles. My remarks so far, concerning the scope of the paradigm theory and contextual variation in force for the autonomy principle, pertain more or less to its basic structure. This structure is not complete without an account of moral standing. And it is not adequate if, in basic structural terms, it precludes recognition of the kind of variable force for the principle of autonomy that certainly appears to be possible at times between family and health care providers. (It is worthy of note here that recognition of this kind of role-related ambiguity concerning autonomy has been implicit in much recent discussion in practical bioethics regarding conflicts and tensions between family and doctors.) In this section and the next, however, we take up issues of practical methodology. Our primary question is whether the paradigm theory has the power to guide practical moral decisions effectively. To declare myself at the outset, I believe that we would benefit from separating, much more clearly than we do at present, our ideas about the intellectual and educational functions of general theory from ideas about its practical, action-guiding power.

For the intellectual demand for comprehensiveness may simply be at odds with the practical need for domain-sensitive specificity concerning moral rules and values.

I have already alluded to the common charge against the paradigm theory that, even though it is an improvement over straight Kantianism or utilitarianism, its principles are still too abstract to yield definite results. Moral reasoning, even when one is directly seeking principled solutions, is simply not a matter of applying principles in any straightforward way. The whole deductivist approach that characterizes the applied ethics model, and hence the paradigm theory, is too unidirectional and top down in its basic conception. It does not take adequate account of the complexities of interplay between our understanding of practical issues and our understanding of principles.

This criticism of the paradigm theory may have had considerable effect in earlier phases of the history of bioethics. At this point, however, there are very few strict deductivists left in bioethics, and probably none at all who have had any experience with moral problems in clinical settings. In contrast to the unidirectional application of principles in a deductivist fashion, most current work in bioethics appears sensitive to the need for a Rawlsian kind of 'reflective equilibrium' between principles and concrete judgments. The method of wide reflective equilibrium (WRE) seeks coherence among three divisions of moral thought: our considered moral judgments, a set of principles designed to rationalize and order these judgments, and a set of relevant background theories or understandings about subjects such as human nature and psychology, the workings of the law and procedural justice, conditions for social stability and change, and the socio-economic structure of society.[7]

The process of theory building can be said to begin with our most secure considered judgments, which may be either general or particular. Next we develop a set of principles that rationally orders and explains these judgments. This is the first criterion for judging the acceptability of a set of principles: their ability to bring the whole array of our considered judgments into coherent order. Secondly, principles must be judged against the general theories we hold about human psychology, social practicability, the functioning of various institutions, and so forth. This constraint, concerning fit with our background theoretical commitments, is especially important because it is this level of assessment that provides a check against the distortions of self-interest, class bias, and ideology. Equally important, there is no point of definitive, epistemological priority or foundationalism in wide reflective equilibrium theory. Principles may be modified or rejected under the pressure of considered moral judgments. Considered moral judgments remain open to revision under the pressure of theory-based principles. The most we ever achieve is 'provisional fixed points' among our considered moral judgments.[8] The method consists, then, in a process of dialectical interchange among the three main elements of moral thought, adjusting and revising our considered judgments, our principles, and our background theories in an effort to achieve overall congruence or reflective equilibrium. As will become clear below, a critical implication of WRE for our purposes is that the principles of the paradigm theory can override contextually derived moral judgments.

The Unbearable Lightness of Principle

Even when the sophistication of reflective equilibrium theory is included, the applied ethics model in bioethics remains open to the charge of being seriously mistaken. It can be said to leave out of account the very complex processes of *interpretation* that constitute our moral understanding both of cases and of principles. Most important, within the complex realities of practice, it is dominantly the interpretation of cases that informs our understanding of principles rather than principles guiding the resolution of cases. All or most of the real work in actual moral reasoning and decision making is case driven rather than theory driven. Therefore, the criticism would continue, the applied ethics model, even when amended by the methodology of reflective equilibrium, sustains the illusion that bioethics is essentially or primarily a matter of constructing and applying principles, when in fact it is almost anything but this. I shall attempt to develop this argument in the remainder of this section and in the next one.

I have just claimed that, within actual processes of moral reasoning concerning genuine problems, it is more often that moral resolution by case analysis informs our understanding of principles than that principles serve in the resolution of cases. It is largely from a close comparison of relevant cases that we discover, or invent, more determinate meanings for the often conflicting values and principles that give situated moral problems their basic shape. We can exemplify this point by considering the following case. A man with multiple sclerosis is admitted to the hospital for treatment of spinal meningitis with bacterial origin. His past history indicates a very satisfactory adjustment to MS. He has taken an active part in family life, he has had various interests, hobbies, and so forth. Despite this history and the fact that his MS has not worsened, the man refuses antibiotic therapy to treat his meningitis, saying only that he wants to be left alone and allowed to die with dignity. Suppose consultation with the family reveals that the patient has been very withdrawn and depressed lately. It is also learned that the patient has been deprived for some time of the usual attentions and support of other family members because of a prolonged crisis elsewhere in the family. More evidence of the same kind makes it fairly probably that the patient's decision is a product of a sense of self-pity and worthlessness accompanying feelings of isolation and depression. Physicians explain to the patient what they think is happening with him; they inform him decisively that they intend to give him antibiotics to save his life and that family counselling will be provided in due course. The patient is silent. Antibiotics are administered, the man recovers completely, family counselling reveals to the family the importance of this patient's being informed and involved in family affairs, and everything turns out well.

What of the principle of autonomy? It was, in fact, this kind of case that persuaded many people in bioethics that the conditions for the kind of autonomous choice that must be respected in medicine are more complex than they had realized. Particularly when the stakes are high, it is not enough merely to be competent and rational in a legal sense. It can also be critical whether the choice is *authentic*, in the sense of being consonant with – or at least not clearly disconsonant with – one's own most important values and commitments.[9] We all are liable to make distorted, uncharacteristic, and inauthentic decisions under the strain of severe depression, fear, or grief. As a kind of insurance against this liability, therefore, we all benefit from an interpretation of autonomy that allows for some degree of paternalism in the light of clear evidence of inauthenticity, especially within an institutional setting like that of medicine. The very nature of serious illness accentuates the liability in question, and the seriousness of the circumstances makes the cost of honouring inauthenticity very high. Whether one agrees with this sketch of an argument or not, its pattern of reasoning, which has in fact been very influential, illustrates the way in which moral interpretation determines the understanding of principle rather than principle determining the morality of cases.

Can we now go confidently forth with applications of the principle of autonomy under this new, more complex understanding of its essential force in the clinical setting? We cannot. I recently became aware of a case concerning a patient who is paraplegic as a result of a motorcycle accident. The psychological dimensions of this case are endlessly complicated but, on the patient's part, critically turn on a deep, pervasive sense of victimization, coupled with extreme, generalized anger and resentment. After years in hospital, effectively refusing all rehabilitative programs, the patient's present condition makes discharge unthinkable. Most recently the patient has adamantly refused to eat and resisted all offers of and efforts towards help and counselling, while continually abusing health care staff. What makes this situation most disturbing is the way the patient's confused tendency to blame everyone and everything for his condition prevents him from genuinely 'owning' and taking responsibility for his decision not to eat. Yet he is fully competent. Arguably, therefore, we confront here a thoroughly embittered and essentially *inauthentic* refusal of food, threatening the life of the patient. Yet everything indicates that attempting to force-feed this patient would be brutal and without foreseeable end. If force-feeding were attempted, the situation would likely be even worse than what Annas reports – and, in my judgment, rightly condemns – about another case involving the refusal to eat, the Bouvia case in California.[10]

What are we to say now about our previous reflections on the interpretation of autonomy in the clinical setting? What we have to realize, I think, is that it is not an insignificant feature of the former case that, even in the absence of consent and cooperation, it was possible to provide effective therapy, quickly and easily, and without great physical invasiveness or brutality. Although it is not to my purpose to pursue the point at length, I would argue that we need to take into account considerations of physical invasiveness, its forms and likely duration, when qualifying the principle of autonomy in terms of authenticity.

Lessons from the Lightness of Principle

Contrary to the applied-ethics model of moral reasoning, an enormous amount of the real work in bioethics is composed of interpretation and the lateral comparison of cases. Even when principles do come into the picture, they often seem to come, so to speak, from the wrong direction relative to the applied ethics model. True, a developed sense of relatively fundamental values and principles may initially shape the moral contours of cases. Apart from this framing function, however, what is generally characteristic of bioethical reasoning about live issues is a bottom-up illumination of principle through interpretive comparison of cases, rather than a top-down resolution of cases by principles. It is, of course, perfectly consistent with wide reflective equilibrium theory that one should find considered moral judgment forcing modifications and adjustments in our commitments to principle. Nevertheless, what is damaging to WRE, and to the applied-ethics model generally, is the dominance of case-driven methodology in the moral confrontation with real problems. Even so, it may be said in defence of the applied ethics model, that the preceding criticisms concentrate exclusively on problematic and difficult cases. There are easy cases too, in sum total, indefinitely more of them than hard cases. When we reach new refinements of principle, these understandings must carry forward so as to yield moral guidance for many relevantly similar cases. Since such instances are numerous, moral reasoning involves many deductive applications of principle, in bioethics as elsewhere – just as the applied ethics model says it does.

I have no intention of disputing this point. But it is important to remind ourselves that what is really at issue is the relative *importance* of inductive over deductive phases in moral reasoning, rather than relative frequency. It is true, of course, that provisionally fixed understandings of principle will carry over so as to determine relevantly similar cases. But it is equally true, and more relevant to the present debate, that the less obvious the similarity in question, the more must analogical and interpretive reasoning precede 'application' – thus confirming contextualism's claim about what is most important. Alternatively, the more obvious the similarity in question, the less important the new application of principle is for the purposes of understanding what moral reasoning is like in its interesting and progressive phases. Presumably, it is moral reasoning in its practically most significant modes that we want to understand and accurately model. In any case, this is a guiding assumption of contextualism. From this point of view, moral reasoning appears vastly more varied, flexible, complex, and interesting than the applied-ethics model allows for.

III. Modest Work for Moral Philosophy

A crucial question is whether appeals to abstract moral principle ever decisively override considered moral judgment. As this is ultimately a question about the moral psychology of individuals it is hard to know. But the very possibility is difficult to understand if the particular judgment appears to the agent to be well supported by appropriate comparisons, generalizations and so forth. In any case, one may plausibly think that abstract principle virtually never succeeds in overriding well considered moral judgment in this sense. Where appeals to abstract theory fail, however, other forms of philosophical theorizing and reflection can often succeed. What is clearly most helpful in practice is theoretical work that directly addresses and undercuts the reasons that are thought to support a certain position.

Consider the issue of euthanasia, currently perhaps the issue of greatest social importance in bioethics. The paradigm theory offers nothing of any direct usefulness in relation to this issue beyond providing (what one would not have needed anyway) a common terminological framework for stating its main tensions. And to do even this the paradigm theory has to revert to a general principle of social utility to set against that of autonomy, since the basic tension is not between autonomy and beneficence or justice. Indirectly, the most that can be said for the paradigm theory is that it has helped historically to shift the central focus of the debate over euthanasia from an earlier concentration on beneficence – 'they shoot horses, don't they' – to that of autonomy – 'people ought to have a right.' Then this prospective right confronts the argument from social risks.

Significantly, philosophy's greatest contribution to the euthanasia debate has come not from any appeal to normative theory, but from the ongoing discussion of the moral relevance of the distinction between killing and letting die. The dominant tendency in these discussions has been to argue that the bare difference between killing and letting die in itself makes no moral difference. Of course, proving this point would constitute real progress in the euthanasia debate. It would effectively reduce the entire issue to the question of the social risks that might accompany relaxation of the current ban on mercy killing and assistance in suicide. I do not agree with the standard arguments asserting lack of moral relevance for the killing/letting-die distinction. But I agree that the euthanasia debate is properly reducible to the question of social risks. I briefly explain these views in the next section. I see this issue as exemplifying almost perfectly the kind and level of philosophical work that seems to me most useful in bioethics. By exploring it I hope also to illustrate further contextualism's general methodology, especially concerning the explanation of contextual variability in the weight of moral considerations.

The Moral Relevalence of Killing versus Letting Die

There is a voluminous literature in contemporary philosophy concerning the moral relevance of the distinction between killing and letting die. Although much of this debate is interesting and worthy of study, it is also possible to discuss the issue in question by getting above a lot of the detail of this debate. I propose to do this by summarizing the structure of the two most powerful arguments intended to show that the killing/letting-die distinction lacks intrinsic moral relevance.

The 'Number-of-Ways' Analysis
Roughly, one kills by doing something that directly causes death; one lets die by refraining from doing something that would have prevented death in these circumstances. In a famous paper Jonathan Bennett argued that this distinction must be morally neutral because it is reducible to an essentially numerical comparison between two contrasting ratios concerning movements and results.[11] When A kills B, there are some few movements A could make in the circumstances that would result in B's death, as against many movements that would not have this result, and A makes one of these few movements. When A lets B die, there are many movements A could make in the circumstances that would result in B's death, as against some few movements that would avoid this result, and A makes one of these many movements. Call this the 'number-of-ways' analysis of the killing/letting-die distinction. Again, Bennett's point is that there is something preposterous in the idea that this sort of numerical difference in itself could be morally relevant.

The Equivalence Thesis

More recently, James Rachels has also argued that the killing/letting-die distinction is, in itself, morally inert.[12] He attempts to establish this claim by generalizing from a crucial comparison of cases. In the first case, the cousin of a small boy, who stands to gain from the boy's death, enters the bathroom where the boy is bathing and drowns him by holding his head under the water. He then arranges things to look like an accident. The second case is exactly the same except that as the cousin enters the bathroom with murder in his heart the boy slips, hits his head, and slides unconscious beneath the surface. Although he could easily save the boy, the cousin watches him until he drowns, remaining ready all the while to force the boy's head back under water should he begin to revive on his own. Call this the case of the 'two cousins.'

Taking these cases to involve the same intention (to secure the death of the boy), the same motive (greed), and the same expectable outcome (the death), we are to recognize that moral responsibility is equivalent between them. Hence we are to accept the generalization that whenever these factors of motive, intention, and certainty of outcome are equivalent, or symmetrical, there can be no moral difference between killing and letting die. This is Rachels's equivalence thesis. And his strategy appears to be based on the constancy assumption in that it appears to be taken for granted that if this distinction makes no moral difference in this pair of cases, it makes no moral difference in any pair of otherwise identical cases.

Some Counter-Examples

Both Bennett's 'number-of-ways' analysis and Rachels's equivalence thesis are vulnerable to counter-example. Sikora counters Bennett's analysis with the following case.[13] Their boat having just sunk, A and B are alone in the water, miles from land. One small life-preserver floats nearby. If A does not get it he will drown; ditto for B. A gets the life-preserver and leaves B to drown. In securing the life-preserver for himself, A, in this case, moves in one of the relatively few ways he could move in the circumstances that would result in B's death. But contra the 'number-of-ways' analysis, he does not kill B; he lets B die.

Philippa Foot, among others, has rejected Rachels's equivalence thesis.[14] She provides cases in which we encounter rights not to be killed (even though death be a benefit) but do not encounter rights to be saved from death (where that would jeopardize some greater good). In these situations, intentions, motives, and outcomes might be comparable, yet the distinction between killing and letting die still registers a morally important difference. For example, suppose a fleeing army must leave behind two mortally wounded soldiers in a barren land. One of these soldiers requests a merciful bullet in the head; the other declines.

Suppose the commander has certain medical supplies that, if left, would preserve this soldier's life for a while. If these supplies are needed by the retreating army, this fact may cancel any obligation to assist in this way. So the soldier may be left to die. On the other hand, it would be wrong in the circumstances to kill this soldier, even if death would be a benefit to him.

I have never found Foot's cases to be telling against the equivalence thesis, because that thesis takes it for granted that the attitude towards death, on the part of the one who dies, is also to be held constant in any comparisons. Imagine instead the following sort of case. Ché and Judas were former comrades in some revolutionary struggle. On good but not conclusive grounds, Ché comes to believe, near the time of the event, that Judas betrayed their cause in a way that led to an ambush in which many of their compatriots were killed. The revolution is eventually suppressed. Now, years later, Ché learns of the whereabouts of Judas. He plans to kill him, to knock on his door and shoot him down in the moment of recognition. Judas has a weak heart. Confronting Ché on his porch he immediately collapses with a heart attack. Ché knows CPR; he could save Judas's life. Instead, he watches him die at his feet.[15] If your intuitions agree with mine, it will seem that Ché letting Judas die is less bad, more easily justified or excused, than would be his killing him.

Looking for Explanations

The initial power and attractiveness of both the 'number-of-ways' analysis and especially the equivalence thesis, combined with these apparently effective but piecemeal responses, create a situation that cries out for a more comprehensive philosophical perspective that will explain these conflicts. I believe we can begin to construct such a perspective by going back to the obvious first question: why is killing *generally* worse than letting die? First, it is simply more important, for everyone's protection, that people be prohibited from killing others compared with their being disposed or required to save lives. But beyond this, the obligation to give aid generally, and to prevent deaths in particular, is necessarily an imperfect obligation in a roughly Kantian sense. If letting die is leaving things undone the doing of which would save somebody's life somewhere, then we all are letting people die all of the time. Given the facts of poverty, disease, and endangerment in our world, it is unthinkable, practically speaking, that there should be an obligation even to minimize the number of people one lets die. For to save even a significant fraction of the lives one theoretically *could* save would leave one time for little else. From an abstract perspective, the obligation to give aid is therefore imperfect, which is to say vague and indeterminate, in terms of both its relative strength and its scope. By contrast, of course, the obligation not to kill is very powerful, extends its protection towards everyone, and admits of only few and generally acknowledged exceptions.

For any world like ours, then, a moral rule against killing will be more powerful in the abstract than a rule requiring aid. It will be more powerful because the protection it affords is vastly greater; and because what it normally requires (the *avoidance* of certain actions) is much clearer and much more easily complied with than what would normally be required (the *performance* of certain actions) in order to save lives. Concerning the ethical aspects of the distinction between killing and letting die, therefore, we have all the explanation we need of why it is *normally* worse to kill than to let die.[16]

It is consistent with this explanation, however, that various factors can conspire in particular circumstances to make letting die morally equivalent to killing. These factors will concern the nature of motives and intentions, considerations of the ease with which life-saving assistance might be provided, and perhaps also the force of social norms associated with personal, familial, and professional relationships. In this way, and with an eye on the protective functions of morality, we can easily accommodate examples of moral equivalence like Rachels's case of the 'two cousins.' What is more difficult is to explain why Rachels's equivalence thesis does not hold in general, as the case of Ché and Judas appears to establish. Why, that is, do we find moral variability in the significance of killing versus letting die even when motives, intentions and the certainty of outcomes are held constant?

In my view, the explanation of why Ché's letting Judas die is less bad than his actually killing him has to do with the differential force of certain, somewhat vague, norms affecting the notions of revenge and the private pursuit of justice. Once sees that Judas is beyond the reach of the law; one understands, or sympathizes with, Ché's desire to avenge his comrades; perhaps one feels that some sort of confrontation is necessary, even that Judas's death may be just, supposing that Judas really is guilty. On the other hand, for Ché, convinced but not actually certain of Judas's guilt, to take matters fully into his own hands, for him summarily to assassinate Judas, is taking on too much in the circumstances. Viewing morality instrumentally, society can afford to tolerate actions of letting someone die that are motivated as Ché's action is; it cannot endorse or condone murder, even in cases like his, although stories like his may evoke leniency.

The effect of cases like 'Ché and Judas' (and there are others) is to show that the moral relevance of the killing/letting-die distinction may be sensitive to context in ways not recognized by the equivalence thesis. Between different contexts, this distinction may gain or lose moral relevance because of its relation to various moral norms appropriate to those contexts, even while intentions, motives, and outcomes remain constant between killing and letting die.

Implications for Euthanasia

As we have just seen, the moral significance of the killing/letting-die distinction, understood as a difference in the form of causal involvement in death, can vary from zero to gigantic. It is zero between Rachels's 'two cousins' and gigantic in the comparison between, say, killing several innocent Bangladeshis and allowing several to die by going about one's business as an art therapist in Nebraska. We have found that the variation in moral relevance that this distinction may reflect is more sensitive to normative considerations associated with context than any specific enumeration of conditions of equivalence is likely to capture. Most important, however, the general difference in moral relevance between killing and letting die, as well as occasional equivalence and contextual variation, all are explained in *instrumental* terms. It is the greater general utility of a rule against killing that explains why it is normally worse to kill than to let die; and it is the general utility of allowing the duty to save and the duty not to kill to speak with the same force, in certain special circumstances, that explains the cases of equivalence; again, it is the variable contextual relevance of certain norms reflecting more subtle considerations of general utility that explains failures of equivalence despite symmetry in intention and outcome.

If the preceding analysis is correct, or even roughly correct, then the entire debate over assistance in suicide and euthanasia must resolve itself into the question of social consequences. The question of the social risks and benefits of legalization of these practices, under certain safeguards and restrictions, is the only question there can be. There is simply no room for any sort of deontological claim that killing is somehow inherently or intrinsically worse than letting die. According to the above argument, all differences in moral significance or relevance for this distinction are *given* to it by instrumental considerations.

Contextualism versus Applied Ethics

The dispute between contextualism and the applied ethics model[17] is essentially a disagreement over the nature of moral reasoning and justification. Traditional moral philosophy has virtually identified the possibility of genuine moral knowledge with the possibility of universally valid ethical theory. Accordingly, it has supposed that all acceptable moral standards, of every time and place, can be rationally ordered and explained by reference to some set of fundamental principles. A corollary of this conception of moral knowledge has been the view that moral reasoning is essentially a matter of deductively applying basic principles to cases.

Contextualism, by contrast, is sceptical about the very possibility of any complete, universally valid ethical theory that is even remotely adequate to the moral life. This scepticism springs from the sense that whatever appearance of universality is achieved by general normative theory is necessarily purchased at the price of separating thought about morality from the historical and sociological realities, traditions, and practices of particular cultures. The result of this separation is a level of abstraction and ahistoricism that makes traditional ethical theory virtually useless in guiding moral decision-making about real problems in specific social settings. This is the fundamental reason for contextualism's claim that we would do well to separate our thoughts about the intellectual ambitions of normative theory, having to do with systematic, ordered, synoptic, but inevitably oversimplified understandings of the complex phenomenon of social morality, from thoughts about the practical usefulness of its constructions.

As an example of applied ethics in the classic sense, the paradigm theory of bioethics departs from the traditional aspirations of moral philosophy only by restricting its focus to the domain of medicine and by accepting the coherentist methodology of WRE theory. Notwithstanding the real value of this focus and this methodological refinement, the basic problems of uncertain relevance and abstraction remain acute even at this level of theory. The paradigm theory's most explicit principle is that of autonomy. Yet we saw how this principle continues to undergo case-driven qualification and reinterpretation. Moreover, the paradigm theory seems unable to accommodate or explain contextual variability in the force and import of this principle, which appears to occur sometimes between family on the one hand and health care professionals on the other. The principle of beneficence is, in itself, very vague, although it has received greater determinateness through subsidiary elaboration of precepts employing the concept of best interests of the patient. But again, for problematic cases, which always abound, one can never rely simply on the force and applicability of any current formulation of a best-interest standard. Concerning the principle of justice in bioethics, matters are even worse, since the meaning of this principle remains mostly a mystery.

In consequence of these general difficulties with application, it becomes extremely difficult to conceive of any realistic circumstances in which the principles of the paradigm theory could be supposed to have the morally decisive power, over contextually justified considered judgments, that the applied ethics model seems to require of them. That is, even within the anti-foundationalist concessions of WRE theory, reference to principle is supposed to retain some significant tendency to override considered judgment. Regarding the basic principles of the paradigm theory, this seems virtually never to be the case.

On the contrary, as I hoped to illustrate via the discussion of killing versus letting die, what typically does overcome considered judgment is theoretical reflection that addresses and undercuts the reasons that explain why such judgment has taken the course and form that it has. This point is obvious, yet it opens onto a whole world of work for moral philosophy. There are countless examples of issues of immediate relevance to moral practice that require philosophical examination, from the issue of moral standing itself to the nature of unjust discrimination. Take the current debate in the United States over the rights of gays and lesbians to serve in the military. Suppose we say that justifiable difference in treatment of individuals can never depend solely on status (gender, race, disability, etc.) as opposed to conduct or performance. But then, can merely *declaring* oneself to be homosexual count as conduct in the relevant sense? Suppose one sees no way to prove that it cannot. Can we then prove that conduct that actually justifies difference of treatment can never gain its justifying character solely from the attitudes or prejudices of others? What if, on the basis of arguments concerning its typical conditions of cohabitation, the military is held to be a singular exception?

IV. Summing Up

At this point, exponents of the applied ethics model of moral reasoning can reply that, however much their application is conditioned by inductive processes and the heuristics of moral interpretation, and however much we encounter contextual variability in their application, abstract principles must ultimately be seen to have *normative force* in moral reasoning and understanding. For in order to criticize moral judgments and practices effectively, and in order to work towards uniformity among our judgments, moral principle in some form must be capable of shaping and reforming our moral deliberations and decisions. This argument is unobjectionable and it poses no threat to contextualism.

As we have seen, at least in outline, contextualism incorporates and emphasizes strategies for criticizing moral values and judgments. Certainly, too, the results of critical reflection on issues like that of the meaning of unjustified discrimination, the moral relevance of killing versus letting die, and so forth, all have potential moral significance and normative power. More to the present point, however, contextualism does not deny the normative force of moral principle, even of the most abstract kind. It is more a question of how and when we know what this force actually is. For, to repeat, we sometimes read from a given situation the morally most reasonable thing to do. Here certain well-established values or principles can be seen evidently to apply. Secondly, concerning the kind of cases that are methodologically interesting – the genuinely problematic cases – it will still be the tensional structure of values and principles that shapes the nature of the problem itself. This structure also reveals the normative force of principle. Finally, after interpretation, comparative case analysis, further reasoning about consequences, and the rest have issued in a reasonable, well-justified moral view, we can always construct a deductive syllogism that derives our moral conclusion from the principle we then see it as upholding. Relative to such a construction, we shall say that it is conformity with the major premise of the syllogism that makes the particular case, described in the minor premise, right or wrong. This agreement gives the reason why it, and all relevantly similar cases, have the moral quality they have. In the same vein, we can say that conformity with the stated principle explains the morality of the case; or we can say that the relation between the principle and the facts of the case, as revealed in the syllogism, justifies the moral conclusion. In fact, how can we resist saying any of these things? These three considerations certainly uphold the normative force of moral principle. It is also easy to see, in outline anyway, how such provisional fixed points in the moral landscape (as justified considered judgment permits) could be interconnected in various ways, both inductive and deductive, to chart potent moral campaigns. These considerations, too, are consistent with contextualism.

All that contextualism need insist upon is our recognizing that, in confrontation with real moral problems, the deductive construction of moral explanation and justification is retrospective. In a far more important, essential, and primary sense, justification is a *process*. It is the process, in all of its interpretive and analogical complexity, of arriving at a considered moral judgment and defending it as a reasonable alternative within the context of the problem. Leaving aside the question of the viability of the conception of normative theory that lies behind it, and any consequent problem in accounting for contextual variation in the weight of moral reasons, the difficulties with the applied ethics model are twofold. It has tended to confuse the deductive explanatory pattern that is a product of moral reasoning with the inductive process that is its essential method. To the extent that it acknowledges inductive processes in moral reasoning, it also ignores their greater relative importance, over procedures of deductive application, for moral progress.

Notes

As indicated, I am indebted to Michael Philips for several important ideas and leading suggestions that I have made use of in this paper. I want also to thank my colleagues Howard Jackson and Peter Remnant for helpful discussion and painstaking editorial advice.

1 T.L. Beauchamp and T.F. Childress, *Principles of Biomedical Ethics* (New York: Oxford University Press, 1994) p. x.

2 I should point out that Ross himself does see his prima facie duties as arising from relationships of various kinds. He also treats the balancing or 'weighing' of prima facie reasons as essentially a matter of intuition. This is exactly why his theory gives so little guidance concerning what we actually should do when the answer is not already obvious to commonsense. See W.D. Ross, *The Right and the Good* (Oxford: Clarendon Press, 1930).

3 See M. Philips, 'Weighing Moral Reasons,' *Mind*, vol. 96 (1987) pp. 367–75. In my statement of this difficulty for deontologism and of the constancy assumption in the next paragraph I paraphrase rather freely from Philips.

4 For a fuller sketch of a similar view of contextual variability in moral standards, to which my entire summary is indebted, see M. Philips, 'How to Think Systematically about Business Ethics,' in E.R. Winkler and J.R. Coombs (eds), *Applied Ethics: A Reader* (Oxford: Blackwell Publishers, 1993) pp. 185–200.

5 Again I acknowledge my indebtedness to Philips in connection with this point concerning the systematic nature of variations in the weight of moral reasons. See 'Weighing Moral Reasons,' p. 373.

6 Some of my discussion in this section borrows from my previous work, especially that concerning the significance of moral interpretation. See 'From Kantianism to Contextualism: The Rise and Fall of the Paradigm Theory in Bioethics,' in Winkler and Coombs, *Applied Ethics*, pp. 343–65.

7 Rawls's original idea of reflective equilibrium in theory construction is further developed and defended by Norman Daniels in his 'Wide Reflective Equilibrium and Theory Acceptance in Ethics,' *Journal of Philosophy*, vol. 76 (1979) pp. 256–82. My sketch of wide reflective equilibrium owes a lot to Daniels's article and to John Arras's discussion of the way this method is reflected in work in bioethics. See Arras, 'Methodology in Bioethics: Applied Ethics vs. the New Casuistry,' unpublished manuscript, presented at a conference on 'Bioethics as an Intellectual Field,' Institute of the Medical Humanities, Galveston, Texas, 1986.

8 Daniels, 'Wide Reflective Theory,' p. 267.

9 For a defence of this view, see B. Miller, 'Autonomy and Refusing Life Saving Treatment,' *Hastings Center Report*, vol. 11 (1981) pp. 22–8.

10 G. Annas, 'When Suicide Prevention Becomes Brutality: The Case of Elizabeth Bouvia,' *Hastings Center Report*, vol. 14 (1984) pp. 20–2; idem, 'Elizabeth Bouvia: Whose Space Is This Anyway?' *Hastings Center Report*, vol. 16 (1986) pp. 24–5.

11 J. Bennett, 'Whatever the Consequences,' *Analysis*, vol. 26 (1966).

12 J. Rachels, 'Active and Passive Euthanasia,' *New England Journal of Medicine*, vol. 292 (1975) pp. 78–80.

13 R.I. Silora, 'Rule Utilitarianism and Applied Ethics,' in Winkler and Coombs, *Applied Ethics*, pp. 91–2.

14 P. Foot, 'Euthanasia,' *Philosophy and Public Affairs*, vol. 6 (1987) pp. 85–112.

15 This is a similar case to one provided by Philips in 'Weighing Moral Reasons,'
    p. 370.
16 Sikora offers a similar explanation of why killing is normally worse than letting die,
    although he links his explanation to the *approximate* accuracy of Bennett's 'number-
    of-ways' analysis. See 'Rule Utilitarianism and Applied Ethics,' pp. 92–3.
17 Again, this section repeats several points I have argued in 'From Kantianism to Con-
    textualism.'

The Role of Principles in Practical Ethics

TOM L. BEAUCHAMP

Recent moral philosophy and practical ethics have produced a variety of misgivings about the role of principles in moral reasoning, and especially about their value for professional ethics and practical decisionmaking. These qualms motivate the analysis below.

I. The Opposition to Principles

Reservations about principles have been expressed by representatives of virtue theory, casuistry, impartial rule theory, the ethics of care, and several other types of theory. I begin with a brief sample of their criticisms.

Virtue Theory

First, the language of principles, some claim, descends from evaluations we make of the character and motives of persons.[1] To speak of a morally good or virtuous *action* done from principle is elliptical for an evaluation of the motive or virtue of the *actor*.[2] Others in virtue theory point to the ways in which we use, follow, or emulate models of the moral person without resort to principles.[3] Various writers in practical ethics have also argued that the attempt in a principle-based account to make obligations, codes, or procedures paradigmatic will not improve decisionmaking and conduct in the professions, because the only reliable protection against unacceptable ethical behavior is good character.[4]

Casuistry

Second, contemporary casuists have been at the forefront of the critique of principles. Casuists regard ethics as neither a science nor a theory. Rather, ethics is based on seasoned practices that need not rely on principles. Moral reasoning turns on paradigm cases, analogies, models, classification schemes, and even immediate intuition and discerning insight about particulars.[5] Some casuists find principles 'tyrannical,' because they obstruct compromise and the resolution of moral problems by generating a gridlock of conflicting principled positions, rendering moral debate hostile and intemperate.[6]

Impartial Rule Accounts

Third, the self-styled Dartmouth Descriptivists – K. Danner Clouser, Bernard Gert, and Ronald Green – coined the expression 'principlism' to denigrate theories containing a plural body of principles, which they see as 'in fact not guides to action' and as little more than checklists of values without deep moral substance. Such principles lack systematic order and rely on an underlying philosophical theory that is too weak to guide action or to handle conflicts among principles.[7]

Ethics of Care and Partialist Theories

Fourth, many other contemporary writers find principles generally irrelevant, unproductive, ineffectual, or overly constrictive. They note that our moral responses rely on our emotions, our capacity for sympathy, our sense of friendship, and our models and knowledge of how caring people behave. They remark, in particular, how difficult it is to capture contextual responsibilities through universal principles and rules, which are not sufficiently subtle or nuanced to guide us from one case to the next.[8]

I believe that a misunderstanding of principles and a misleading account of the theories that are under attack appear in many of these criticisms. At the same time, I acknowledge that many who promote these views have produced persuasive arguments and penetrating criticisms of principles. Before assessing these criticisms, I shall describe the type of principles and the correlative assumptions that I shall defend and the kind I shall reject. One of my hypotheses is that critics typically have directed their arguments at only a narrow range of principles that deserves to be rejected, and then they have generalized their rejection of principles to other types of principles that should be retained.

The Nature of Principles

I begin with the relevant general sense of 'principle.' A principle is a fundamental standard of conduct on which many other moral standards and judgments depend. A principle is an essential norm in a system of thought or belief, forming a basis of moral reasoning in that system. We expect all persons of good moral character to have learned principles and to have them firmly built into their belief structure and to reflect these beliefs in their patterns of moral thinking.

Using this generic meaning of 'moral principle,' I shall now examine two different and more detailed senses of 'moral principle.' The first I shall call the *robust* sense. After rejecting this account, I shall consider a more defensible account, which I shall call the prima facie sense.

The Robust Conception of Principles

Various philosophers in the history of modern ethics seem to assume roughly the robust sense. Although it is debatable that any philosopher ever has defended precisely the conditions of this view that I shall offer, assorted representatives of utilitarianism, Kantianism, ethical egoism, and divine command theories provide plausible examples.[9] In this robust account, X is a moral principle if and only if it is

1. *General*
2. *Normative*
3. *Substantive*
4A. *Unexceptionable*
5A. *Foundational*
6. *Theory-summarizing.*

To qualify as a principle in the robust sense, all six conditions must be satisfied. I shall briefly explain each condition.

1. General: A principle is applicable to (governs) a broad range of circumstances, and in this regard contrasts with specific propositions. As the territory governed by a norm is narrowed (the conditions becoming more specific – for example, shifting from 'all persons' to 'all adult persons'), it becomes increasingly less likely that the norm can qualify as a principle. For example, a principle of respect for autonomy ideally should apply to all autonomous persons and autonomous actions. By contrast, a norm of respecting informed refusals that applies only to circumstances of informed refusal in medicine will be too narrow to qualify as a moral principle. A principle, then, must be of severely limited specificity (and in this respect, I shall later say, a principle by its nature is not yet specified, and its generality consists in this feature). There are practical reasons for keeping principles at such a high level of generality. They must be learned by all persons so that they can give guidance about what should be done in the usual range of cases. If principles were very specific, it would be difficult to remember and absorb the resulting large number of principles.

2. *Normative:* A principle is a standard of right, good, or obligatory action, and in this capacity it directs actions and provides a basis for the critical evaluation of action. We can *act on* the basis of a principle, *breach* a principle, *critically evaluate* by appeal to a principle, etc. Descriptive statements therefore cannot be principles, and social practices and conventions may or may not be normative in the relevant sense. For example, taking lunch at noon can be a practice without being a normative requirement. Even a practice like seeking the consent of patients need not be normative. Such practices and conventions are often *made* normative, however, as occurs when practices are turned into professional codes of ethics.

3. *Substantive:* A principle is a substantive requirement, not merely a formal requirement. Principles express moral content, not the form such content must take. Consider, for example, the conditions of generality and normativity – (1) and (2) above. These requirements are conceptual conditions of principles that do not themselves qualify as principles. Similarly, requirements of *universal form* (as in 'A moral judgment is universalizable'), *categoricalness* (as in 'A principle is a categorical imperative'), *supremacy* (acceptance of a norm as supreme, final, or overriding), *simplicity*, and *prescriptivity* (taking the form of action-guiding imperatives) may be meta-conditions or perhaps principles in a theory or in meta-ethics; but they are not moral principles in the relevant sense.

Philosophers who have assumed that the above three conditions are necessary conditions of a moral principle have rarely supposed that they are jointly sufficient conditions. At least three other (more controversial) conditions also seem to be considered necessary in some works in order to constitute a set of sufficient conditions.

4A. *Unexceptionable:* A moral principle has no exceptions, even if it conflicts with other principles. If a theory advances more than one principle, it gives an ambiguous directive as to which principle has priority *unless* the theory designates what John Stuart Mill called 'a determinate order of precedence' (or lexical ordering) among its principles.[10] If exceptions were permitted, the principle would require another principle to account for the exception. There can therefore be only one supreme moral principle or one canonical precedence for principles. This structure constitutes the authority empowered to override any apparent moral conflict.

5A. *Foundational:* A moral principle provides a foundation on which other moral rules or judgments are supported and justified. A principle does not receive *its* support, validity, or justification from any other principle. Moral principles are therefore necessary for the justification of all other justified norms.

6. Theory-summarizing: A moral principle represents and incorporates an underlying theory that serves to justify the principle. The principle summarizes the normative force of the theory, or some vital aspect of it.

Twenty-five years ago, Jerry Schneewind argued that conditions roughly like these six are so 'widely accepted' in moral philosophy that they 'constitute a sort of orthodoxy' about principles and justification. Schneewind held that the acceptance of such (foundational or first) principles is tied to related assumptions in moral epistemology – in particular that moral knowledge requires these first principles, because without them (i) we could not reason about moral problems, (ii) a moral system would not be coherent and rational, and (iii) justification would not be possible.[11]

Whether Schneewind was right about the landscape of moral philosophy in 1968 is not a matter I can explore here, but his provocative thesis would surely be incorrect if applied to contemporary moral theory. Beliefs of the sort he found constituted a pervasive orthodoxy are now widely rejected, largely because conditions 4A–6 are now widely rejected. This sociology of moral philosophy is not important, of course. The immediate question is whether ethical theory must or should understand principles in terms of conditions 4A–6.

The Prima Facie Conception of Principles

I shall simply assume (though Schneewind did not) that those who, like myself, reject conditions 4A–6 need not for this reason reject *principles*. There is an alternative conception of principles, which I shall call the prima facie conception as a tribute to the pioneering work of W.D. Ross.[12] The prima facie conception jettisons conditions 4A–6, substituting conditions 4B and 5B below while retaining conditions 1–3.[13] Thus, X is a principle *only if* (but perhaps not *if*) it is

1. *General*
2. *Normative*
3. *Substantive*
4B. *Exceptionable (prima facie)*
5B. *Nonfoundational*

In this conception a moral principle may, but also may not represent and incorporate an underlying moral theory that justifies one or more principles. One may accept principles while advocating an anti-theory position, which is precisely what some casuists seem to recommend. Therefore, there is no requirement parallel to condition 6. (I would want to modify condition 1, as 1B, allowing this account to utilize degrees or levels of generality among principles – but I shall not attempt to fill out this detail here.)

4B. Exceptionable: A moral principle can be overridden if it encounters a contingent conflict. There are exceptions to all principles, each of which is merely prima facie. When principles contingently conflict, no supreme principle is available to determine an overriding obligation. There will not always be a bridging principle available to resolve conflicts among principles.

5B. Nonfoundational: No principle or set of ordered principles provides the sole foundation on the basis of which all other rules or judgments are supported and receive their justification. A principle need not be underived and itself may receive support from what John Rawls has called our *considered judgments* – that is, those moral convictions that inspire the highest confidence and can be safely presumed to have the lowest level of bias, such as judgments that racial discrimination, religious intolerance, and political favoritism are morally improper and prohibited. These considered judgments themselves are 'foundational' only in the weak sense that they are justified without argumentative support and are the proper starting points for moral thinking.

How considered judgments serve as 'foundations' (in the weak sense) is a fascinating topic in its own right. Here I shall only propose the following as necessary conditions of a considered judgment: (1) a moral *judgment* occurs; (2) *impartiality* is maintained; (3) the person making the judgment is *competent* to make it; (4) the judgment is *generalizable* to apply to all cases relevantly similar to those originally judged.[14] In addition, coherence is a vital background consideration for status as a considered judgment. Widespread and recalcitrant contigent conflict among norms would discredit them as considered judgments. Considered judgments, then, typically will have a rich history of adaptation in moral experience and reliability over time that underlies our belief that they are credible and trustworthy.

When generalized to relevantly similar cases, these judgments may or may not qualify as principles or rules (see the above five conditions), but a proper theoretical ideal is to make principles and the relevant features of considered judgments *coincide*, perhaps through a process of mutual adjustment (see 'reflective equilibrium,' below). This procedure encourages us to start at any level of generality (including at the bottom, with judgments about cases) and move up, then descend again to cases after a rise to the top – or the converse, if one starts at a high level. In this conception, the considered judgments with which we begin constructing an ethical theory themselves can be at any level of generality and may be expressed as principles, rules, maxims, ideals, models, and even as normative judgments about cases.[15] If these considered judgments occur at a lower level of generality than principles, they support principles bottom up, rather than being supported by principles top down. For example, if considered judgments appear in the form 'Socrates is a model of integrity' or

'Juries must not be (nonjudicially) influenced during their deliberations,' these considered judgments in turn can be used to support principles; they are not merely judgments that stand in need of support *by* principles.

Once we acknowledge that principles are exceptionable and nonfoundational, we are free to view every moral conclusion supported by a principle and every principle itself as subject to rejoinder, refutation, and reformulation. Obviously this position represents a sharp departure from the model of robust principles and secure derivative conclusions.

Reasons for Dispatching the Robust Conception

What is wrong with the robust conception and why does it need to be displaced by the prima facie conception? Many problems render the robust conception doubtful, but I will confine my discussion to two.

Distance from Common Morality
Philosophers who have tried to defend robust principles have produced rather splendid failures because they oversimplify and attempt to reduce considered judgments in one part of morality (e.g., beliefs about justice) to other beliefs in some other part of morality (e.g., beliefs about utility). This reductionist program of simplification and unification is the heart of the problem. The reductions proposed are less plausible than the initial considered judgments and create more problems and doubts than those judgments themselves create. Although philosophical ingenuity is not lacking in these writings, close contact is often lost with the widely shared, core premises in that body of norms of conduct from which philosophical thinking about ethics begins (but does not end). In this domain I can find no principle that conforms to the model of robust principles. The principles we cite and rely on invariably follow the prima facie model; they include principles of promise keeping, truth telling, confidentiality, not causing harm, the distribution of social resources by need, and so forth. The model of robust principles, then, seems imposed on the considered judgments of ordinary morality, rather than drawn from those judgments.

Problems in Deductivism
A second problem is that robust principles are theoretically linked to a deductivist model of reasoning and justification, which requires the application of a preexisting principle or rule to a case falling under the principle or rule. In this conception, reasoning and justification occur only if general principles (and rules), together with the relevant facts of a situation, support inferences to correct or justified judgments. One apparent deductivist, Alan Donagan, describes his

'simple deductive' account in the following terms: 'The structure consisting of fundamental principle, derived precepts, and specificatory premises is strictly deductive; for every derived precept is strictly deduced, by way of some specificatory premise, either from the fundamental principle or from some precept already derived ... [S]ome concept either in the fundamental principle or in a derived precept is applied to some new species of case.'[16]

Deductivism has recently been characterized by critics of principles as a top-down 'application' of principles or rules (a conception that motivated use of the term 'applied ethics'). The deductive form is the following:

1. All acts of description A are obligatory.
2. Act b is of description A.
   Therefore,
3. Act b is obligatory.

The following example conforms to this model:

1′. All policies that maximize social utility are obligatory.
2′. The policy of keeping patients' records confidential maximizes social utility.
    Therefore,
3′. The policy of keeping patients' records confidential is obligatory.

A particular judgment or belief is justified in this model by subsuming it under one or more general norms, which themselves are justified by bringing them under a principle.

Although the robust model of principles apparently presumes deductivism, the prima facie model does not do so (despite the accusations of some critics of prima facie principles). The reason for the unbreakable bond between the robust conception and deductivism is the following. Only unexceptionable principles permit one to know whether one's conclusions are *justified*. It is not enough to know that a conclusion *follows logically* from a prima facie principle (exceptionability transfers). On the prima facie model one could know premises with certainty (say, 1′ and 2′), make a correct deduction, and still not know whether the conclusion is justified (say, 3′). *Irrefutable, decisive, or categorical reasons* for moral conclusions come only from robust principles, thus supplying a direct link between deductivism and robust principles. A robust principle is particularly attractive if as a single principle in a monistic system it both unifies a theory and expresses the core of morality as a coherent whole.

Critics of all uses of principles in ethics have sometimes incorrectly implied that any theory deeply committed to *principles* must be deductivist. This criticism is profoundly mistaken. A prima facie conception is the enemy, not the friend, of deductivism. It is not the function of prima facie principles to be instruments for *deducing* unexceptionable rules or judgments. On the prima facie model, the rightness or permissibility of an action cannot in any situation of contigent conflict be derived directly from principles or rules and is always dependent on moral thinking in the circumstances of conflict. A nondeductivist account of moral thinking therefore must supplement any moral theory committed to prima facie principles or rules.

For example, suppose that the principle of nonmaleficence ('Avoid causing harm to others' – or, more elaborately, 'One ought not to inflict evil or harm') supports a rule against killing ('Do not kill'), and that this rule in turn supports a policy against physician-assisted euthanasia ('Do not engage in physician-assisted euthanasia'). Even if the rule follows deductively from the principle, the rule will not disallow exceptions (the principle is prima facie, and killing is not necessarily harmful or wrongful). The policy also may follow deductively from the rule but will not disallow exceptions (the rule is prima facie, and physician-assisted euthanasia is not necessarily harmful or wrongful). Qualifications will in this manner be introduced on any prima facie norm.

Because of the many potential conflicts between rules against killing and rules of respecting autonomy and relieving pain and suffering, one has not got very far in tracing some direct line of descent from the principle of nonmaleficence to policies against physician-assisted euthanasia. Only rebuttable conclusions are achieved. For example, although it is (prima facie) wrong to bring about someone's death, it is not always morally wrong, on balance, to cause someone's death. What makes it wrong, when it is wrong, is that a person is harmed – that is, suffers a setback to interests that the person otherwise would not have experienced. In particular, one is caused the loss of the capacity to plan and choose a future, together with a deprivation of expectable goods – both harming and wronging a person. If a person desires death rather than life's more typical goods and projects, however, then causing that person's death at his or her autonomous request does not either harm or wrong the person (though it might still harm others – or society – by setting back their interests, which might be a reason against a policy or *practice*). To the contrary, not to help such persons in their dying sometimes frustrates their plans and causes them a loss, thereby harming them. Therefore, by appealing to a principle of nonmaleficence – here bolstered by a principle of respect for autonomy – we might come to support policies favoring voluntary euthanasia as easily as policies disfavoring it.

Of course, *if* lines of descent in premises and conclusions were straightforward (in the way suggested by 1–3), one could layer out the logic of the moral life in terms of principles as top-down elements of reasoning and then pretend that even in the prima facie conception deductive subsumption captures the form of our reasoning. This model is more misleading than serviceable, however, because the lines of descent in our moral thinking are much more complicated (both bottom up and top down) than this linear model of deductive subsumption can capture, whether or not principles are involved. When we deliberate about and reach difficult moral judgments, we almost never move to a conclusion from one or two principles or even from one or two considered judgments at any level. Several norms often join together in practical judgment. Not some linear descent of argument, but several persuasive and often loosely related considerations support our conclusions.

To take a typical example, when the U.S. Supreme Court in 1991 decided the employers cannot legitimately adopt fetal protection policies that exclude women of childbearing age from a hazardous workplace because such policies involve illegal sex discrimination, far more was at work in the court's reasoning than some principle of nondiscrimination. The court rightly drew from multiple and diverse considerations of the risk of prenatal injuries, the moral status of the fetus, the status of legally valid waivers and legal liability for injury, the relevance or irrelevance of highly toxic environments, the limits of corporate responsibility to ensure a safe workplace, etc. As Mr Justice White made clear in his interesting dissent in this case, even a slight movement in one's assessment of any one of these factors (for him it was highly toxic environments) could lead either to a different conclusion or to a qualification of one's conclusion.[17]

Among the problems with the hypothesis of a linear order or dependence among propositions (so that a lower-level judgment or rule always depends on a higher-level, foundational principle) is its presumption that any justified judgment depends on a more general principle and that this ordering cannot be reversed so that the more general depends on the less general. This account envisions a unilateral descent from principles to cases, rather than bilateral influence. But whether a moral proposition is *dependent upon* other propositions, is known *independent of* other propositions, or is a source of support that other moral propositions *are dependent upon* cannot be decided by either the content of the proposition or its degree of generality (or its satisfaction of conditions similar to 1–5B). Whether a general action-guide – say, a requirement of equal treatment – depends for its justification and use on particular considered judgments, such as the desirability of prohibiting sexual discrimination in the workplace or rather the general on the particular, is a matter of what is known and can be inferred with warrant in specific settings (so-called inferential support as a matter of epistemic context).

This analysis can be used to illustrate why contemporary casuists who have resisted principles – without differentiating the type of principle that forms their target – misunderstand how similar their methods are to those involved in a principle-oriented theory that accepts only prima facie principles. Prima facie principles, merged with the methods I am proposing, are entirely compatible with casuistry. If one substitutes the casuists' term 'paradigm case' for 'considered judgment,' the methodology I am outlining need not differ in significant respects from the methods proposed by casuists.[18] Paradigm cases become paradigms because of prior commitments to central values that are preserved from one case to the next case; for the casuist to move constructively from case to case, a norm of moral relevance must connect the cases. Rules of relevant features across cases themselves will be, not a part of the case, but a way of interpreting and linking cases. To recognize a case as a *paradigm* case is implicitly to accept whatever 'principles' or 'rules' allow the paradigms to be extended to other cases. Think of it this way: Whatever we learn from a case and then transport to another case cannot be entirely specific to the first case; some degree of generality must be present in order to lead us to the next case. The greater the level of generality, the closer we come to a principle. The process is that of isolating and lifting general features of the case that we anticipate being repeated in other cases.

If norms can be accepted as justified without argument either at or near the bottom (from the paradigm case, which is identical to the more particular considered judgment) and at the top (principles), the casuist must accept prima facie principles and the principlist must accept paradigm cases. Moreover, it seems unlikely that we shall encounter *a pure case* of being either at the top or at the bottom, because beliefs at the top affect beliefs at the bottom, and viceversa. The paradigm cases of the casuists are theory laden, and a theory is fueled by paradigm cases. The currently popular division of types of moral theory into top down and bottom up thus may be more misleading than helpful.

The Recurrent Complaint of Abstractness and Indeterminacy

Nonetheless, despite this accommodating analysis, a complaint heard repeatedly by critics of principles, including the casuists, still must be faced. The criticism is that principles are indeterminate and lacking in moral guidance. To address this problem of indeterminacy, I begin with an acceptance of Henry Richardson's arguments that principles must be specified for many circumstances of practical decisionmaking and formulation of policy, especially when principles are in conflict. Richardson notes that we sometimes *apply* norms directly to cases or successfully *balance* conflicting norms. But in managing complex or problematic cases involving contingent conflicts, the first line of attack should be to specify norms and thereby to eradicate the conflicts. Of course, many already specified norms will need further specification to handle new circumstances of indeterminateness or conflict. Progressive specification will be needed to handle further problems, gradually reducing the circumstances of contingent conflict (that abstract principles have insufficient content to resolve) to more manageable dimensions.[19]

The following is a typical example. Research data and conclusions generated by private corporations that produce commercial health-care products and services are often valuable to the health community at large. Yet the information is proprietary to the corporation, and the interests of stockholders must be protected. Publishing research that is valuable to the public's health is a moral obligation, but so is protecting the stockholder's interests. Corporate officers therefore must carefully balance duties to stockholders with duties to society and professional colleagues. The first order of business for a corporation attempting to devise an adequate set of moral guidelines to govern these responsibilities will be to state the conditions under which the methods, techniques, and findings of its research and product development will be shared and the conditions under which the data will be kept confidential. In so acting, corporate officers will be engaged in a process of specifying (prima facie) principles and rendering them coherent, thereby replacing initial incoherence. For example, the corporate officers in this health information example might specify as follows: (1) 'Disclose *all* available information about (a) *epidemiologic research* regarding workplace safety and (b) *research on product risks and safety*; disseminate all findings, so that the widest possible community benefits from the research.' (2) 'Disseminate *no* findings of research pertaining to (a) product development and (b) consumer preferences.' Although contingent conflicts are still possible among even these rules (e.g., between rule 1b and rule 2a), incoherence, the possibilities for contingent conflict, and subjective balancing all are substantially reduced by these specifications.

To specify a principle is sometimes merely to augment its spare content by constructing a more specific rule. For example, principles of self-determination can be made more specific in the form of rules of privacy, rules of confidentiality, rules of informed consent, and the like. Usually, however, new specifications or rules have a more complicated origin. They rely on more than a single principle and they alter practices that are already in place. Creativity in both design and content emerge. Because we inventively create rather than simply discover such rules, John Mackie rightly argues that ethics is 'invented.'[20] We do not invent the *considered* judgments with which we begin, but we do invent many rules and policies that specify commitments in those judgments. For example, since approximately 1966 we have been inventing rules and policies in the United States to protect human subjects of biomedical and behavioral research; these rules extend well beyond the content of any pre-existing principles and practices relevant to the development of these rules (and now the latest Department of Energy cases of radiation experiments).

However, justification is, of course, an indispensable constraint on such specification and invention. One who specifies and invents a new rule must show that the proposed specification fits coherently with other norms in the pre-existing system of norms. Specification as a method must, then, be coupled with a larger model of coherence that appeals to considered judgments and to the overall coherence introduced by a proposed specification. So understood, specification holds out the possibility of a continually expanding normative viewpoint that, although novel and creative, is nonetheless faithful to initial norms (which are not renounced unless found to be incoherent). It also tightens rather than weakens coherence among the full range of accepted norms. In short, this general model for theory involves a careful selection of considered judgments (one's axioms), faithful specification, and probes for coherence by way of what Rawls has called reflective equilibrium.[21] From this perspective, specification is one arm of a larger method of coherence.

We cannot reasonably expect that the strategy of specification will function as a cure-all for our deepest problems of moral conflict. Specification will not eliminate competing proposals for the resolution of contingent conflicts, and in a problematic or dilemmatic case, several specifications will emerge that are well-defended proposals for resolution, thereby reintroducing the conflict and lack of resolution that kindled the need for specification in the first place. If one believes, as I do, that some contingent moral conflict is inevitable and ineliminable by even the best methods of ethics, then specification will be of assistance only in those contexts in which it has a reasonable prospect of success. We shall not always be able to spot those contexts in advance, however, and a circumstance in which rival specifications are allowed to compete is, on the whole, likely to serve us better than a circumstance that impedes this marketplace of ideas.

On Closing the Gap between Principles and Practice

Critics of principles may at this point persist with the question, 'Do principles, *even when carefully specified* and made into rules and policies, enable us to reach practical judgments, or are they still far too indeterminate? If so, is there not a massive gap between principles and practice?' It seems that any specification needs a further specification and every significant term in a specification requires additional interpretation. Critics of principles have therefore suggested that we never get very far in practical decisionmaking if we are equipped only with considered judgments and principles.[22]

One proposal now of increasing popularity in the attempt to escape these problems while reducing the gap between principles and practice is the following. *In professional ethics* we should embed principles and rules in the professional ethics intrinsic to the traditions and practices of the profession(s) in question. In biomedical ethics, for example, traditional health care contexts supply their own versions of morality for medicine; the culture of medicine supplies considered judgments through its acknowledged role responsibilities and professional goals. These traditions internally present understandings of obligations and virtues that have been adapted over decades or centuries for professional practice.

Although I am as eager as those who celebrate practices and those who are engaged in clinical ethics to see traditional norms in medical ethics fused with the model of principles I have been supporting, we should be very cautious about relying on professional practice standards as more than a source for considered judgments that generate *starting points* in professional ethics – just as they do in ethical theory more generally. The methodology, then, should be similar for professional ethics and general normative ethics. Whether a customary standard exists within the relevant fields of practice is often questionable, and negligent care might be perpetuated if professionals have only inferior traditions and practices to offer (whether through ignorance, as a genuine conviction, for reasons of professional solidarity, or for reasons of financial interest and freedom from outside interference). For example, inferior standards for the use of children, prisoners, and animals in medical experimentation may have become a part of the tradition. In general, it is doubtful that many of the most important questions in contemporary biomedical ethics can be adequately addressed exclusively by the traditions and practices of the health care professions – even if they were carefully reconstructed.

I believe that internal shared moralities in professions stand to make their strongest contribution if they are engaged in reflective encounter with external perspectives that do not wholly rely on tradition. In this way norms that have traditionally been overlooked can come to affect and even be embedded in the practices of the professions. Consider, for example, conflicts of obligation that emerge from the dual roles of research scientist and clinical practitioner. As an investigator, the physician has an obligation to generate scientific knowledge that will benefit *future* patients. As a clinical practitioner, the physician has obligations of care that require acting in the best interests of *present* patients. The very notion of a physician-as-scientist suggests two roles that can pull in different directions, each role having its own specifiable set of obligations rife with the potential for contingent conflict. Considerable thought has been given to these role obligations in biomedical traditions, which form proper starting points. However, relatively little interest in or thought about conflict of interest is found in these traditions. To make these various obligations more precise, specific, and conflict free will require moving beyond the traditional practices and role responsibilities of health care institutions by bringing our best reflections on conflict of interest into the picture, wherever those reflections may originate.

Some years ago, John Rawls argued that moral theory involves the investigation of 'the substantive moral conceptions that people hold, or would hold, under suitably defined conditions. In order to do this, one tries to find *a scheme of principles* that match people's considered judgments and general convictions in reflective equilibrium. This scheme of principles represents their moral conception and characterizes their moral sensibility.'[23] It seems to me that this characterization has it just about right. The identification of principles helps us both to locate and to refine our moral values. It is one way, and perhaps the best way, to capture the heart and the soul of morality. If this is right, then principles have both a practical value for practical ethics and an intellectual value in ethical theory.

Notes

1 See Philippa Foot, *Virtues and Vices* (Oxford: Basil Blackwell, 1978); Gregory Tianosky, 'Supererogation, Wrongdoing, and Vice,' *Journal of Philosophy* 83 (1986): 26–40; G.E.M. Anscombe, 'Modern Moral Philosophy,' *Philosophy* 33 (1958): 1–19.

2 Cf. Alasdair MacIntyre, *After Virtue: A Study in Moral Theory*, 2d ed. (Notre Dame, IN: University of Notre Dame Press, 1984), esp. pp. 175–80, 225ff; Dorothy Emmet, *Rules, Roles, and Relations* (New York: St Martin's Press, 1966); David Hume, *A Treatise of Human Nature*, second edition, ed. L.A. Selby-Bigge and P.H. Nidditch (Oxford: Clarendon Press, 1978), p. 478; and Martin Benjamin, *Splitting the Difference: Compromise and Integrity in Ethics and Politics* (Lawrence: University Press of Kansas, 1990), pp. 59–72.

3 See Lawrence A. Blum, 'Moral Exemplars,' *Midwest Studies in Philosophy* 13 (1988); and Edith Wyschogrod, *Saints and Postmodernism: Revisioning Moral Philosophy* (Chicago: University of Chicago Press, 1990), p. xxiii.

4 A classic treatment is H.K. Beecher, 'Ethics and Clinical Research,' *New England Journal of Medicine* 274 (1966): 1354–60. See also Gregory Pence, *Ethical Options in Medicine* (Oradell, NJ: Medical Economics Co., 1980), p. 177.

5 Albert Jonsen and Stephen Toulmin, *The Abuse of Casuistry* (Berkeley and Los Angeles: University of California Press, 1988), pp. 11–19, 66–7, 251–4, 296–9; A. Jonsen, 'Casuistry as Methodology in Clinical Ethics,' *Theoretical Medicine* 12 (1991): 299–302; John D. Arras, 'Getting Down to Cases: The Revival of Casuistry in Bioethics,' *Journal of Medicine and Philosophy* 16 (1991): 31–3; A. Jonsen, 'Casuistry and Clinical Ethics,' *Theoretical Medicine* 7 (1986): 67–71; idem, 'Practice versus Theory,' *Hastings Center Report* 20 (July/August 1990): 32–4. Although some casuists are critical of theory, others encourage principles and theory construction. See Baruch Brody, *Life and Death Decision Making* (New York: Oxford University Press, 1988), p. 13.

6 Stephen Toulmin, 'The Tyranny of Principles,' *Hastings Center Report* 11 (December 1981): 31–9. Toulmin several times indicates that his target is 'the cult of absolute principles' (p. 37); principles that can be overridden therefore do not seem to fall within the scope of his critique.

7 See K. Danner Clouser and Bernard Gert, 'A Critique of Principlism,' *Journal of Medicine and Philosophy* 15 (1990): 219–36; and Ronald M. Green, Gert, and Clouser, 'The Method of Public Morality versus the Method of Principlism,' *Journal of Medicine and Philosophy* 18 (1993): 477–89.

8 See Nel Noddings, *Caring: A Feminine Approach to Ethics and Moral Education* (Berkeley: University of California Press, 1984); Martha Nussbaum, *Love's Knowledge* (Oxford: Oxford University Press, 1990); Alisa L. Carse, 'The "Voice of Care,"' *Journal of Medicine and Philosophy* 16 (1991): 5–28; and Annette Baier, 'Trust and Antitrust,' *Ethics* 96 (1986): 231–60.

9 This sense constitutes what has often been called a *first principle:* a primary proposition that is considered self-evident and upon which further reasoning or belief is based. Berkeley, in *Alciphron*, III.1, makes these principles analogous to 'fundamental theorems.' See also Locke, *Essay Concerning Human Understanding*, I.i.10; Reid, *Essays on the Intellectual Powers of Man*, VI.6.

10 Mill, *Utilitarianism*, in vol. 10 of *The Collected Works of John Stuart Mill* (Toronto: University of Toronto Press, 1969), ch. 1, third paragraph. In utilitarianism only the principle of utility is a principle in the relevant sense.

11 J.B. Schneewind, 'Moral Knowledge and Moral Principles' (1968), as reprinted in *Revisions: Changing Perspectives in Moral Philosophy*, ed. Stanley Hauerwas and Alasdair MacIntyre (Notre Dame, IN: University of Notre Dame Press, 1983), pp. 113, 118–20.

12 'Prima facie duty' is Ross's term. It indicates that an obligation must be fulfilled unless it conflicts on a particular occasion with an equal or stronger obligation. A prima facie obligation is always binding unless overridden or outweighed by competing moral obligations. See Ross, *The Right and the Good* (Oxford: Clarendon Press, 1930), pp. 19–36; idem, *The Foundations of Ethics* (Oxford: Clarendon Press, 1939).

13 A proponent of this view need not rule out, a priori, the possibility of foundational principles. A proponent would *argue* that this conception is preferable to others and in so doing would defend 4B and 5B in ways that are only outlined, not defended, below.

14 On condition 4, cf. R.M. Hare, 'Principles,' in *Essays in Ethical Theory* (Oxford: Clarendon Press, 1989), p. 55. I am indebted to John Rawls for some suggestions about these four conditions (made in private conversation).

15 John Rawls, *A Theory of Justice* (Cambridge, MA: Harvard University Press), pp. 47–51; and 'The Independence of Moral Theory,' *Proceedings and Addresses of the American Philosophical Association* 48 (1974–5): 8.

16 Alan Donagan, *The Theory of Morality* (Chicago: University of Chicago Press, 1977), pp. 71–2; see also pp. 18ff, 24.

17 *Auto Workers v. Johnson Controls, Inc.*, Slip opinion. Argued October 10, 1990 – Decided March 20, 1991.

18 Cf. Toulmin, 'Tyranny of Principles,' p. 37: 'Starting from the paradigm cases that we do understand – what in the simplest situations harm is, and fairness, and cruelty, and generosity – we must simply work our way, one step at a time, to the more complex and perplexing cases in which extremely delicate balances may have to be struck.' David DeGrazia has reminded me that casuists typically have not suggested ways to protect against bias that approximate the protections suggested by those who defend considered judgments.

19 Henry S. Richardson, 'Specifying Norms as a Way to Resolve Concrete Ethical Problems,' *Philosophy and Public Affairs* 19 (Fall 1990): 279–310. See also David DeGrazia's reflections on specification in 'Moving Forward in Biothetical Theory: Theories, Cases, and Specified Principlism,' *Journal of Medicine and Philosophy* 17 (1992): 511–39.

20 J.L. Mackie, *Ethics: Inventing Right and Wrong* (New York: Penguin Books, 1977), esp. pp. 30–7, 106–10, 120–4. Mackie does not mean that individuals create personal moral policies, but that 'intersubjective standards' are built up over time through communal agreements and decisionmaking. What is morally demanded, enforced, and condemned is not merely a matter of what we discover in already available basic principles, but is in addition a matter of what we decide by reference to and in the use and development of those principles.

21 Rawls, *A Theory of Justice*, pp. 20ff, 46–51, 577–80.

22 John Arras has reached this conclusion in several articles.

23 Rawls, 'Independence of Moral Theory,' p. 7 (italics added).

Wide Reflective Equilibrium in Practice

NORMAN DANIELS

Recently, when I was a Fellow in the Program in Ethics and the Professions at Harvard, I was quite astounded to learn from other Fellows that the field of bioethics was in a state of methodological upheaval, fractured along many fault lines, much like Los Angeles but without the sunny climate. They portrayed an intellectual war zone, reminiscent of evolutionary theory or paleontology, where there are many bones to pick. When I expressed my surprise, I was chided. How 'out of it' could I be? Had I had not heard that 'principlism' (a position held by Beauchamp and Childress[1]) had been routed 'from above,' by advocates of 'theory' (like Clouser and Gert[2] and Green[3]) and, more effectively, ambushed 'from below,' by contextualists (like Hoffmaster[4]) and their allies, the casuists (like Jonsen and Toulmin[5])? Had I not heard that 'theory' was out, that 'deductivism' and other 'top-down' approaches were defeated in favour of 'bottom up' ones? The battle was so advanced that new rescue efforts for old fortifications had already been mounted, like Richardson's 'specifying norms'[6] or DeGrazia's 'specified principlism.'[7] I was abashed. I had not noticed that I was working in a war zone and that defending or applying a moral principle put me at risk of taking a sniper's bullet.

Though I am loath to make excuses for not being with it, let me offer three to start with. One is really a confession: I do not read the bioethics literature as widely as I should, except for what bears most directly on the problems I am working on. More important, I thought 'doing ethics' involved familiarity with all these methodological weapons, not just one or some of them. I also thought that we do ethics to solve many different kinds of problems, and that the methods we use plausibly vary with the problems we want to solve and the interests we have in solving them. So much for my naïvete, though I shall defend its charm below. Nevertheless, my morbid interest was stimulated – perhaps I was simply shamed – into taking a closer look at the war zone. The battle reports promised to be at least as interesting as the *New York Times* and might rival *USA Today* or CNN News, but that's pushing it.

A Brief Report from the Battle Zone in the Land of Bioethics

Occupying the Middle Kingdom, a series of fortified hills, are the forces of the 'principlists.' Overlooking the Middle Kingdom there is a more etherial high ground that is occupied by roving bands of Uplanders who are often dubbed 'theorists.' Down in the valley are the Lowlanders, 'contextualists' and 'casuists' and various others, who distrust high places and like the feel of each blade of grass between their bare toes. Somewhat prophetically, the original topographical map for this land was sketched by Beauchamp and Childress.[8] It looked like this:

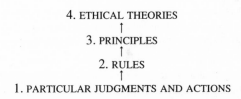

4. ETHICAL THEORIES
↑
3. PRINCIPLES
↑
2. RULES
↑
1. PARTICULAR JUDGMENTS AND ACTIONS

The upward-ascending arrows in the original diagram originally may have indicated only *height*, since it was merely a crude topographical map. The problems arise when Beauchamp and Childress say that justification flows downward, in a direction opposite to their arrows. Thus we would justify particular judgments by subsuming them under rules, and rules by subsuming them under principles, and so on. The current battle, as I understand it, interprets the arrows to mean *priority* or *dominance:* do theories or principles govern the terrain of ethics, or do particular judgments do so in context? The fight is about what directions the arrows should point.

The principlists who occupy the Middle Kingdom include some of the earliest settlers of this land, and they played a very active role in recruiting others to toil and live here as well. Their doctrine was consolidated in an early training manual for such recruits,[9] and this has caused considerable mischief. (The manual has been substantially revised, and its most recent edition is reasonably eclectic.) It is easy for recruits to elevate the kind of simplified instruction involved in a training manual into dogma, much like cadets in a military academy. Some years later its central principles – autonomy, beneficence, nonmaleficence, and justice – have been contemptuously referred to as the 'Georgetown mantra.' In any case large numbers of cadre toil in the vineyards surrounding the Middle Kingdom; their missives and other communications often invoke the mantra.

There is considerable dispute about how we should interpret these principles and their role in governing the land. Like most leaders and prophets, Beauchamp and Childress have said things about them that can be interpreted in various ways. (Ambiguity allows you to be right more often.) Despite the directional arrows in the original map, and despite the claim that justification flows downward from the heights, Beauchamp[10] also insists that theory plays a role at all levels of work in bioethics, and that theory arises not in a vacuum, but out of myriad cases. Had the arrows been bi-directional from the start, allowing each level to influence but not to govern the others and capturing more accurately the nature of justification in ethics, much of the current bloodshed could have been avoided.

More confusing is Beauchamp and Childress's view (in early editions of the manual) that their principles are really neutral between various theories and that bioethicists can (sometimes? often? always?) start working their way downward from the principles, ignoring the greater heights occupied by competing ethical theories. As might be expected, this claim is sharply disputed by Uplanders like Clouser and Gert.[11] Beauchamp and Childress are misleading here; we need work in ethical theory to resolve disputes about priorities among principles as well as about their limits and scope (the point is clarified in the new edition of the manual). Clouser and Gert complain that a smorgasbord or 'anthology' approach to theory is adopted, and that no effort is made to resolve theoretical disputes so that one dominant theory can then be used to resolve disputes about principles, rules, and cases. There is no doubt that Gert has Gert's theory in mind for that role.

A more charitable gloss on what Beauchamp and Childress are saying is that sometimes we can agree on mid-level principles and rules, even while we disagree about theory, and given the pressure to produce practical judgments in real time, not seeking more agreement than we need is good practical advice. A training manual ought to be explicit, however, about whether it is giving tactical or strategic advice. In any case, we should not confuse the pragmatics of good tactical advice with an account of the legitimacy, in this case, of the authority of principles. Here I lodge a complaint against both the Uplanders and the principlists: the appeal to ethical theory is valuable even when it is not one dominant theory we are drawing on but the systematic consideration of issues that bear on the selection of principles and evaluation of cases. This topic is discussed further below.

I have already noted one line of attack made by the Uplander theorists, but they have focused their mortars on other Middle Kingdom targets as well, close to the heart of the mantra. Clouser and Gert[12] argue that 'principles' intoned in the mantra are not really general moral principles, but are 'chapter headings' for a 'discussion of some concepts which are often only superficially related to each other.' Their point is most persuasive in the case of the 'principle' of justice cited by Beauchamp and Childress. No single principle is really articulated; we get a checklist of considerations. These chapter headings cannot generate specific rules for guiding action in particular cases, and resolving disputes about how concerns about autonomy and beneficence conflict, for example, necessarily engages us in appeals to theory. Green[13] makes similar points, decrying the lack of interest in theoretical issues spawned by the prominence within the field of 'principlism.'

More strenuous and varied than the attacks on principlism by the Uplanders is the multi-front campaign launched by the Lowlanders. Lowlanders find their bearings best, they insist, by reading the trail signs in front of them, not by looking to high and distant landmarks. They are much better at finding their way through the trees than at surveying whole forests. They complain that advocates of rules or principles or theories ignore the details and texture of real cases. We should not, they insist, force cases to fit the rubric of simple principles. The real moral terrain is much more finely textured. A careful diagnosis of the pitfalls, rough brush, and swamps is needed before we can reliably find our way in bioethics. Principles – and theories – are of necessity highly idealized and simplified, and, when we pay attention to them, we become impatient of providing truly close diagnosis of a problem. When Middle Kingdomers, invoking their mantra, cast the simple white beam of principle on the ground from on high, attempting to illuminate our path, they cast shadows that hide crucial complexities and may even blind us to the roots and snarls in our way.

The Lowlanders' campaign attacks the appeal to principles at a vulnerable point. To show that a particular principle ought to govern a particular case may require showing that the morally salient features of that case fall under that principle. But careful examination of many aspects of the situation may be needed to decide what the morally salient features are. The problem is compounded when a case seems to fall under conflicting principles. It seems that there is some basis for alliance between the Uplanders and the Lowlanders, but the battle lines are more complex. (In the most recent edition of their manual, Beauchamp and Childress concede ground, agreeing that the original diagram applies only in the simplest cases, when there are no conflicting principles.[14])

The Lowlanders may be right that sometimes close examination of cases can produce agreement about what counts as right action. But this close examination must employ some views about how to convert details or 'data' into real evidence for a conclusion. We do insist on reasons. We want to treat relevantly similar cases in similar ways. We need some way of determining what counts as similar in the relevant ways. We need to know when to discount differences and when to rest weight on them. We need, in effect, more systematic accounts of what we are doing. But that is exactly what reason-giving, appeals to principle, and the development of moral theory were supposed to do: provide us with a basis for converting observations into evidence for a view. The hard work of ethics lies not only in its observations and diagnosis of the particular case, but in figuring out what count as relevant moral reasons for treating situations the way we should.

To one degree or another the Lowlanders' emphasis on context and case feeds an anti-theory inclination, not simply an anti-principlist stance. They are no doubt right that sometimes, after deliberation, we may agree on what to do about particular cases when we are far from seeing how appeals to ethical theory or even to principles can help. They then suggest that by accumulating agreement around cases we can reason our way 'analogically' toward some modest principles. Arras[15] notes that this causistical approach may not be so theory free as it claims, that it may quite conventionally, in unnoticed ways, accept without question important features of our social institutions and practices. Unnoticed theory is still theory, but unnoticed, it is unexamined. Unexamined assumptions underlying our agreement may not, after all, be justifiable.

It is not surprising then that the two-front attack on principlism is not a coordinated one after all. The Uplanders may welcome the assault by the Lowlanders on the Middle Kingdom, but the Lowlanders are just as suspicious of the theorists as they are of the principlists. Like the principlists, the Lowlanders fear that theory turns idle wheels and does not contribute to moral decisions in real time. So the Uplanders, too, have little patience with and offer no true alliance with the Lowlanders, whatever tribe of contextualists or casuist they belong to.

A Peace Proposal

Is there a Nobel Peace Prize in the offing here? Can peace be brought to this land? Are there points of agreement that we could use to leverage further agreements? Is there a basis for cooperation? Could there be a division of moral labor that would allow all to cooperate in a joint endeavor, or at least to live in peace, pursuing their own efforts and contributing individually to our knowing better what we ought to do?

One proposal that aims at bridging the gap between principlists and contextualists is Richardson's[16] suggestion that the real work of practical ethics lies in 'specifying norms.' Acknowledging the point of careful diagnosis of a situation and sensitivity to context, while at the same time insisting that norms or principles must provide us with a bridge between cases, Richardson describes how we must successively qualify our principles or 'specify' the norms we use so that they better fit or apply to particular cases. We must work back and forth between case or cases and principles, carrying out this refinement of the principle. We get proper specification when we arrive at an equilibrium between the texture of the case and our moral beliefs about it and the qualifications we need on the principle or principles we had thought should apply to it. This is a version of what has been called narrow reflective equilibrium – we revise our principles and judgments about cases until we achieve an equilibrium. DeGrazia[17] endorses this approach, calling it 'specified principlism,' adding the suggestion, perhaps in an appeal to the Uplanders, that we construe ethical theory as the various branching specifications of principles that result when we carry out this process extensively. There is merit in this Richardson-DeGrazia proposal, but I think the picture of theory it presents is still impoverished. I believe work in ethics must seek a very wide reflective equilibrium that erodes many of the distinctions about the levels of terrain in the kingdom of bioethics.

Justification in ethics rests, I have long thought, on a broad coherentist approach involving beliefs at many levels.[18] Though we may be committed quite firmly to some views, no beliefs are beyond revision. It is very important that we see how diverse these types of beliefs are. I include here our beliefs about particular cases; about rules and principles and virtues and how to apply or act on them; about the right-making properties of actions, policies, and institutions; about the conflict between consequentialist and deontological views; about partiality and impartiality and the moral point of view; about motivation, moral development, strains of moral commitment, and the limits of ethics; about the nature of persons; about the role or function of ethics in our lives; about the implications of game theory, decision theory and accounts of rationality for morality; about the ways we should reply to moral skepticism and moral disagreement; and about moral justification itself. As is evident from this broad and encompassing list, the elements of moral theory are diverse.

When I suggest that 'theory' must be appealed to, I do not mean some particular comprehensive view, such as that of Kant or Mill, that takes a particular stand on some of these areas, though some might accept such theories. I mean our appeal to some or all of these elements involved in the process of giving a systematic account of moral beliefs and practices. These elements are involved in the effort to achieve *wide reflective equilibrium*, the coherence of our beliefs about many of these matters. Wide reflective equilibrium is actually endorsed as an account of justification by various of the disputants, including Beauchamp, DeGrazia, and Green; key elements in it are appealed to by Hoffmaster and to some extent by Jonsen and Toulmin. This suggests that there may be some common ground after all, provided it can be used and shared appropriately.

'Doing ethics' involves trying to solve very different kinds of problems answering to rather different interests we may have, some quite practical, others more theoretical. Sometimes we want to know what to do in this case, or in developing this policy or designing this institution. Sometimes our problem is in understanding the relationship between this case, policy, or institution and others and making sure we adopt an approach consistent with what we are convinced we ought to do elsewhere. Sometimes our problem is to provide a systematic account of some salient element in our approach to thinking about cases, for example, an account of the nature of rights or virtues or consequences. We can sometimes presume considerable agreement on some aspects of the problem but not on others; so the practical problem may be how to leverage agreement we already have to reduce areas of disagreement. *There is no one thing we do that is always central to solving an ethical problem, for there is no one paradigmatic ethical problem.*

Putting the point about justification together with this claim that there are many types of ethical problems, I conclude that doing ethics may require doing many different kinds of things. Sometimes it may require doing many of them at once. Sometimes we can narrow our effort.

Much of the methodological dispute comes from ignoring the first and second points. It comes from looking at one kind of problem and one kind of effort and insisting it is the primary problem or effort and that other methodologies are wrong not to see its primacy. My peace proposal thus constitutes a kind of plea for toleration. It is an effort to see the kernel of truth in many approaches, while I refuse to treat the kernel as the whole ear of corn. Ethics, or bioethics, should not be top down or bottom up. Or rather, how bottom up or top down it should be may depend on the problem and our purpose in solving it. My comments in what follows will be an attempt to illustrate this plea with examples. I use examples from my own work not because I think it is the best work, or because it is even the best illustration of my point, but only because I am most familiar with it and confident about the motivation behind it. (Remember, I earlier confessed to not reading widely enough.)

Like many of the disputants in battle zone, I shall decry the division between 'practical ethics' and 'ethical theory.' I thus join ranks with disputants from every camp, including Beauchamp, Green, Hoffmaster, and others. Specifically, I believe that the 'purism' that pervades many of the best Ph.D programs is unjustifiable and damaging. Good work in ethics tests theory and forces its development by trying to solve practical problems and showing what guidance theory can give. So too, efforts to solve practical problems often can make little progress without some guidance from theory. Ideally, people who do ethics should have rigorous training in both areas of problem solving. Unfortunately, 'mainstream' purists often do not want to get their hands dirty with practical problems, preferring the more tractable, idealized thought experiments of 'philosophers.' Too many people in bioethics and other areas of practical ethics do not want to fill their heads with 'theory' that may seem to turn no wheels, at least for their purposes, or that does not interest clinicians or policy makers. Given the diverse disciplines that lead people into bioethics – law, theology, medicine, philosophy – it is not surprising that many have little training in ethical theory and find it difficult to acquire. My plea for toleration is coupled with a plea for rigor and comprehensiveness in training in ethics. Nevertheless, with a judicious focus on problems, good work can often result even without the kind of rigorous, comprehensive training that is ideal. There is plenty of room for a division of moral labor.

I doubt these remarks provide the basis for a Nobel Peace Prize, but I do want to illustrate why I think there is common ground that the different combatants must learn to till together. The illustrations that follow highlight kernels of truth that can be culled from the positions defended by various disputants. The suggestion is that they help delineate that common ground.

Landmarks in the Peaceable Kingdom

1. We do not have to agree about everything to solve moral problems

In an early paper Jonsen and Butler[19] introduced the phrase 'public ethics' to delimit a type of problem facing bioethics, the application of normative ethics to public policy. Public ethics deals with making particular public moral decisions about specific matters that are pressing and that do not involve profound structural changes in the social order.[20] Because the matters of policy do not involve fundamental changes, some agreement on relevant principles can be expected. By articulating these principles, clarifying policy options in the light of them, and then ranking the moral options for policy choices, public ethics has a reasonably specific agenda that can yield results without forcing us to engage in the most abstract philosophical ethics. Indeed, Jonsen and Butler[21] introduce the neologism 'infraethics' to describe this level of ethical inquiry and to distinguish it from the more theoretical or 'metaethical' inquiry they say is characteristic of normative ethics more generally.

The work of public ethics is modest: it does not seek to challenge or justify more fundamental moral principles, as it might have to do if more fundamental social change were at issue, and so theory plays a modest role. Under the pressure to solve a practical problem in real time, we engage only in as much abstraction as we need to solve the problem. Still, public ethics requires sensitivity to context; for the implications of different policy options and their moral consequences relative to the principles must be made explicit. This characterization of the method involved in public ethics is *problem driven*. It does not purport to be a methodological description of the whole domain of bioethics or of ethics more generally. In that regard it differs from the 'principlism' attributed to Beauchamp and Childress.

I want to describe a recent example of public ethics in which I was involved. Dan Brock[22] has described the work we did together on the principles and values underlying Clinton's health care reform proposal.[23] The Ethics Working Group was a diverse group of academics including philosophers, lawyers, doctors, and theologians. We were diverse in our philosophical training and beliefs – for example, some were communitarians who thought in a very religious framework ('stewardship' was their term for resource allocation) and others were quite secular proponents of various views about justice. Had we sought agreement on philosophical fundamentals, we would never have got anyplace. Instead, we were able to agree on some fourteen basic 'principles and values' that we thought ought to govern health care reform, including the Clinton proposal. We intended them to serve as a test of the Clinton proposal and alternatives. What we are calling principles here would not pass muster as such in Clouser's or Gert's view; but neither are they 'chapter headings'. I think of them as 'design principles' that capture morally desirable features of health care institutions.[24]

Agreeing on principles and values without deeper agreement on the underlying theory of justice has its risks and limitations. Specifically, it leaves us less able to resolve disputes that arise when the principles conflict. Can we trade comprehensiveness of benefits in order to secure universality of access? Developing a framework of such principles, however, does give a matrix within which features of institutional design can be assessed for the moral implications relative to the principles. Thus we can note that a long-term phase-in of universal access, especially if it is made contingent on savings generated by reform, constitutes a serious violation of the principles. Similarly, if a reform plan makes the content of their benefit package shrink when savings are inadequate to fund subsidies to low-income individuals, then recasting this constraint on subsidies as a clear sacrifice of the principle assuring comprehensive benefits shows what is morally at stake. Further argument is then needed to resolve disputes about priorities, and some disputes may not be resolved at all if they reflect more fundamental disagreements.

I believe there is value to the ethical work involved in articulating these principles underlying health care reform, even though my own work much more specifically ties such principles to a specific theory of justice for health care. There is a need for a reasonable division of moral labor; an ethics working group constituted to reflect diversity in the field and in the society as a whole cannot be expected to arrive at complete agreement on underlying theory within the real-time limits set by the task force. Our solution reflects the problem we were set: we had to understand the context well, see the implications of institutional design, and find some framework of principles and values that let us improve areas of agreement where possible.

2. Most problems resist either straightforward 'top-down' or 'bottom-up' approaches

The HIV epidemic raised two problems that derive from the risk of transmission in medical settings (nosocomial risks). Do physicians have a duty to treat HIV+ patients despite the risks they impose? Do patients have a right to know the HIV status of their physicians, at least for invasive procedures? I think these problems illustrate the futility of thinking that their ethical resolution could rely solely on a top-down appeal to principle or a bottom-up careful examination of context and case.

In the late 1980s it was common in the United States to hear some physicians, even through their professional associations, assert that they would not treat AIDS patients. They insisted they had no 'duty to treat.' They insisted they had never agreed to face those risks, did not want to, and were not obliged to. In effect, they insisted they had not ever consented to take those particular risks, and it did not matter that some other physicians had consented or would consent. Some professional associations, such as the AMA, disagreed, at least by 1987. The AMA insisted that physicians were obliged to treat 'without regard to risks,' that they had a tradition of acting virtuously in the face of epidemics, at least in recent history, and that refusing to treat in the case of HIV patients was 'invidious discrimination.'

A careful examination of the context revealed that the risks of transmission to physicians were very low but were not risks that could be ignored. In fact, the estimated risks could vary considerably with the type of medical activity and the incidence of HIV in the local patient population. An obligation to face any risk whatsoever, such as that asserted by the AMA, was indefensible. But even if obligations to take risks in general arose out of voluntary acts, such as undergoing the training and identifying with the role of being a physician, then how could we accommodate the variability of this risk? The solution to the problem is to claim that physicians undertake a package of obligations when they enter that professional role, including an obligation to face some standard level of risk. Obligations to take much greater risks would require further, more specific consent. Refusal to face standard risks – and HIV risks seemed standard if HVB risks did – would then seem like invidious discrimination, if directed only against HIV patients. Role-based obligations come in clusters or packages, and individuals adopting these roles and assuming these obligations are not free to choose and custom-design their consent and thus their obligations.[25]

This proposal has some resemblance to the Richardson-DeGrazia view about specifying norms. I had modified the principles about consent and about physician obligations to respond to the specifics of risk taking in these situations. But the analysis of professional obligations that facilitated the modification (or clarification) involved doing a piece of theoretical work, not 'theory' in the sense of invoking some overarching general theory, such as that of Kant or of Mill, but a careful analysis of the nature of obligations, facilitated by interesting work by others developing a virtue-based account of professional obligations.[26]

A second example which makes the same point, involves the conflicting-right claims that HIV-infected health care workers and patients can make. The issue came to public attention in the glare of the discovery that a Florida dentist had infected (perhaps deliberately, we may now suspect) five or six patients. A campaign was launched by one victim to require physician disclosure of HIV status, following compulsory testing, and the removal of infected practitioners. The AMA argued that physicians must 'Do no harm!' and inferred that this meant they should disclose their status to patients or remove themselves from invasive procedures. The centers for disease control passed regulations that seemed to capitulate to the public fears: the regulations, still in place, called for infected practitioners to refrain from engaging in 'exposure-prone' procedures. On the other side, advocates for infected health care workers insisted these workers had rights, like all handicapped workers, to be allowed to work unless they imposed 'significant' risks on fellow workers or patients. Since the risks of transmission were minuscule – between 1 in 40,000 and 1 in 400,000 from a known infected surgeon, and only 1 in 20,000,000 from any surgeon – these did not constitute significant risks.

Which right claim should be given priority? Doesn't context help? What context? Knowing these levels of risks does not help us in the way we might think. Although it might seem irrational to worry about these risks when we routinely ignore greater ones in medical contexts, it is not really irrational for a patient to want to find out a surgeon's status and to switch surgeons at no cost to herself. Nor should we follow the AMA in thinking that 'Do no harm!' means that these physicians have abandoned the protection of the rights of handicapped workers. Presumably, physicians should avoid imposing harms not worth the risk of imposing, keeping the benefits in mind. So these right claims seem intractably juxtaposed, and it is not at all obvious, simply working back and forth between principle and case, how we should 'specify the norm' or modify the principles in narrow reflective equilibrium. Nor is it obvious that protecting equality of opportunity or protecting patient autonomy should be given priority over the other.

The solution comes from involving both a piece of theory and a careful diagnosis of the details of the case.[27] The unconstrained exercise of patient rights here has the effect, on plausible assumptions about the costs and effects of different strategies of risk-reduction, of setting up a many-person prisoners' dilemma. Each person is made less safe by a system that gives full reign to patients' rights to know and to switch, since the resources needed to carry out the strategy, rational from each patient's point of view, are an ineffective way of reducing transmission risks. An analysis and proposed solution like this one require both careful diagnosis of the context and appropriate invocation of a piece of theory.

3. The standard model of 'applied ethics' – plugging facts into principles –
does not work in the peaceable kingdom

Nearly all disputants agree that the term 'applied ethics' is misleading. It suggests that there is a supply of ready-to-hand general moral theories or principles and that the task of finding out what to do in particular cases consists of specifying the 'facts' that would connect the general principle to a specific case. No doubt this picture may have been influenced by positivist views about scientific laws: in order to get predictions from laws we simply need to specify the relevant observations. In the philosophy of science we long ago rejected this view, acknowledging among other things that an extensive body of auxiliary theories must be brought to bear before we can decide just what 'data' will count as evidence for a theory or as predictions that follow from it. We do not simply plug data points into formulae. Similarly in ethics, we need a much more sophisticated view of the relationship between general principles and particular cases. How general principles really can guide action is much more complicated than the 'applied ethics' picture allows. I illustrate the point with two examples.

When I began thinking about justice and health care delivery, having spent much of the 1970s working on problems in the general theory of justice, I thought it should be easy to 'apply' principles like those argued for by Rawls to health care. I was in the grip of a false picture of 'applied ethics.' Rawls's principles, I was aware, were developed under a special, idealizing assumption: that fully functional people should specify principles of fair cooperation. No one was ill or disabled. I was immediately stymied.[28] Should health care be governed by a principle aimed at making maximally well off those who were worst off? Or did Rawls's theory need to add a new primary social good: health care? Or would some other principle do the job? Looking from the theory 'down' to the system of delivery, it was quite unclear what 'applying' the principles really meant.

I had to reverse directions to make any progress.[29] I began to think directly about health care and the different kinds of things it does for us. I had to answer questions about why we might think some of those functions had special moral importance. I had to think about cases in which we felt that assisting people with medical services was an obligation and when we thought assisting them was not. Gradually, I focused on the generalization that disease and disability impair the range of opportunities open to us, whereas health care services that we think we are obliged to offer to people protects that range of opportunities. What emerged was the claim that a general principle assuring fair equality of opportunity should govern the design of health care systems. But even here the account of fair equality of opportunity had to be broadened from its focus on access to jobs and offices. Extending Rawls's theory meant not simply plugging in the facts, but modifying the theory in modest and reasonable ways. My procedure required development of an account of what health care does for us and its importance that was sensitive to the wide variety of health care functions and captured many of our intuitive judgments and practices, for example, regarding insurance coverage. Only then did it become clear how to connect general principles – appropriately modified – to the world of institutions.

My second example shows that these lessons do not sink in quickly. Once I had developed an account of justice for health care that appealed to the fair equality of opportunity principle, I thought that principle would actually be able to guide us in some detail in designing institutions that allocated health care resources equitably. I thought it would tell us how, under resource constraints, we should limit access to beneficial services. I have since concluded that the gap between principle and guidance in institutional design is quite wide and that we do not yet know how to fill it. Again, it was by examining actual cases of rationing decisions that it became apparent general principles fell short of offering adequate guidance. Let me explain briefly.

The fair equality of opportunity principle gives some guidance about rationing. Quite generally, it implies that under resource constraints, we should use our resources in ways that most effectively protect the range of opportunities open to us, focusing on services that maintain normal functioning. More specifically, it supports a distinction between treatment and enhancement, though that is a more complicated story to which I shall return shortly. It also supports a distinction between proven and unproven treatments, though just how the line should be drawn is another issue. But how much priority should we give to treating those whose opportunities are most impaired by disease or disability? How much 'opportunity cost' should we impose on those who are less ill in order to help those most ill or disabled? Giving full priority – maximizing benefits for the worst off – seems implausible; so does giving no priority to them. Is there a principled position in between? We have no philosophical account of one, and the equal opportunity principle fails to guide us. Similarly, how much weight should we give to getting the best outcomes, measured in health benefits, from resources? Giving full priority to achieving best outcomes may mean that we deny some people equal or fair chances at some benefits. Here, too, either extreme seems implausible: we intuitively reject always going for best outcomes or always going for equal chances at some benefit; but we have no principled way of determining an intermediary policy.

These 'unsolved' rationing problems show just how indeterminate the equal opportunity principle is.[30] It fails to guide our action at a crucial point, where we must design institutions and policies to embody general principles under resource constraints. The problem is general. The same issue arises outside health care, for example, when we try to allocate educational resources or legal aid services. We encounter the same unsolved rationing problems.

One way out is to try to appeal to fair procedures for making the relevant choices about institutional design, but we have given little attention to what counts as a fair procedure for solving this kind of problem.[31] The implication of this analysis is that we must revise considerably our view about the nature of general distributive principles; they cannot guide action as we might have hoped. It could be that the general lesson is that many general principles must fall short of guiding action without an acceptable process for making determinate choices that fall within a class of outcomes acceptable in the light of the general principles. This is a feature of general theory ignored in the literature.

One lesson from these examples is that work in ethical theory is enriched in very deep ways by forcing the question of how the theory guides action into very specific areas of practice. It is much too easy for 'pure' theory to think it offers guidance when it does not. We discover the problem only when we test the theory against practice. To put the point contentiously, 'applied ethics' makes an essential contribution to 'ethical theory.' Stated more clearly, we fail to do our best work at either level if we do not see them as part of the same project.

4. Impatience with the limits of theory should not drive us to think that an examination of context alone can guide us

Several years ago, James Sabin and I began examining how clinicians made decisions about what is 'medically necessary' mental health care. We asked clinicians to describe what they found to be 'hard cases' in their own practices. We found a clear tension in the judgments made by different practitioners – sometimes the tension was strongly felt within a single practitioner.[32] Some 'hard-line' clinicians strongly held the view that their services were aimed at treating diagnosable disorders; more 'expansive' clinicians were inclined to use their skills to reduce any kind of unhappiness they encountered. They arrived at quite different judgments about what was 'medically necessary,' moving in quite different ways on many particular cases. When they disagreed about particular cases, it was not so much about the 'facts' of the case, though 'expansive' clinicians were often inclined to broaden diagnostic categories to try to fit their inclinations about particular patients, and 'hard-line' clinicians were somewhat more inclined to hold patients 'responsible' for attitudes and behaviors that expansive clinicians tended to view as symptoms of an underlying disorder.

Our analysis suggests that different clinicians have internalized somewhat different views about the goals and limits of medicine. These views can be connected to rather different theoretical stances or 'glosses' on the notion of equality of opportunity. For example, the 'hard-line' clinicians make judgments that fit quite well the view that there is a reasonably sharp line that we can draw between treatment and enhancement and that our obligations in health care are to restore people to some notion of 'normal functioning.' The 'expansive' clinicians seem to think that any limitation on functioning, even if it is part of a normal range, can impose disadvantages on people, and it is the task of medicine to provide people with equal capabilities to be or achieve whatever they want in life. What this finding suggested to us is that considerable disagreement in practice actually reflected this deeper underlying disagreement at the level of theory about the demands of equality.[33]

It seems impossible, simply by comparing cases, to resolve the dispute among these clinicians about what should be viewed as medically necessary treatment. To resolve the dispute, we must give some arguments that show why it is preferable to adopt one view of the demands of equality and the goals of medicine rather than the other. We must raise our heads above the level of 'context' and 'case' to see where to go in this matter. Thinking we can avoid an appeal to theory if we can agree at least on cases, after careful diagnosis, is not helpful if there are systematic disagreements on cases that reflect related disagreements in theory. Conversely, to repeat a point made earlier, considering the cases involved here can lead to clarification and modification of the underlying theory.[34]

5. There is moral surprise in the peaceable kingdom

The process of ethical inquiry can lead us to change our minds about what we think is right. We may begin with a view about what is right in a particular case or type of case and discover that we cannot sustain that view on more careful consideration of other cases and relevant theory. We may begin with a piece of theory that we can no longer support. Surprise can occur at any level. We are surprised because we discover even our firmly held views are revisable. I mention briefly three examples, two of which I have already noted.

When I first began thinking about health hazard regulation in the workplace, I believed it should be easy to defend the criterion underlying standards in U.S. law, specifically, the requirement that exposure to harmful toxins should be reduced 'to the extent it is technologically feasible' to do so. Deep in my heart, I was for worker safety and health and had few compunctions about government regulation, even if it imposed significant costs on employers. When I asked myself, however, just why it was reasonable to restrict the options of workers to take some risks for hazard pay, I found it more difficult to explain my initial view.[35] Suppose we provide workers with adequate information about the risks they faced and suppose we internalize the costs of the health risks we impose on these workers. Suppose we can approximate the costs of internalization by cleaning up the workplace to the point that it is cost beneficial to do so. Cleaning it up further costs more than we save in health care costs. Why not let workers negotiate for hazard-pay extra costs between a cost-benefit standard and the technological feasibility criterion? Is insisting on the higher level of health protection unjustifiably paternalistic?

I was able to justify the higher standard, after considering in some detail the context, only under the following condition. The array of choices open to typical workers facing such hazard pay negotiation would have to be an unfairly restricted set of choices. That situation might well be true in the United States, though it is unlikely that the U.S. Congress would admit it as a reason for its legislating such a stiff criterion. In a more just society, if these workers had a fair or just range of choices open to them, then the strict criterion would seem unjustifiably paternalistic. This outcome surprised me.

I have already indicated two other examples of surprise. In the controversy about HIV-infected professionals, I found my view shifted twice.[36] At first, I thought the risks were so low – so 'insignificant' – that any restriction on infected workers was a violation of their rights as handicapped workers. Yet after I persuaded myself that it was indeed rational for individuals to avoid even small risks if they could do so at no cost to themselves by finding out their physician's HIV status and switching if necessary, I could not see how to avoid the force of the AMA or CDC positions. My view has now returned to opposing restrictions, but for very different reasons from those I originally had. Am I morally indecisive? Overly intellectual? The surprise to me is that the shift in what I believed to be right in these cases was dramatic and based on reasoned deliberation.

A final surprise to me was the discovery that general distributive principles could fall so short of guiding decisions about institutional design, as my discussion about rationing suggests. I have been forced quite dramatically to rethink what kinds of moral arguments must be brought to bear on questions of rationing and institutional design. I now think we must pay much more attention to problems of fair process and to refinements of democratic theory.

Peace in Our Times?

My point in developing these examples is to highlight why the strife we now see seems so pointless and avoidable. Let me conclude by indicating the points I think form a basis for a cooperative division of moral labor in ethics.

1. There is not one kind of ethical problem but there are many kinds, and different problems require somewhat different approaches.
2. Because there are many types of problems and a division of moral labor is reasonable, many people from many different disciplines and training backgrounds can expect to make import contributions in bioethics.
3. As contextualists, casuists, and other Lowlanders argue, it is essential to develop a careful diagnosis of a moral issue and to be wary of forcing it prematurely into the mold provided by ready-to-hand principles.
4. As principlists and theorists of various clans insist, we must provide reasons for our moral views that allow us to see relationships among cases and begin to assure ourselves we have consistent approaches and coherent accounts of what we are doing.
5. Most ethical problem solving cannot, therefore, be either top down or bottom up but must be multifaceted and responsive to the demands of both context and theory.
6. The diverse appeals to theoretical considerations we need to make in solving problems should not be confused with the adoption of some particular comprehensive moral view; some may accept such views, but most people have much more eclectic and diverse conceptions of theory.
7. Though we begin with firm views on some issues and matters of theory, we must hold all our views to be revisable in the light of good arguments and in an effort to seek the widest coherence in our beliefs.
8. Reasonable people can end up disagreeing on moral matters; disagreement is not a sign of ignorance, evil, or irrationality. We have no infallible faculty or method for resolving disagreements or arriving at moral truths, and moral

progress depends on our having respect for the sources of disagreements and a commitment to finding arguments that prove persuasive.

No doubt there are other elements that should be included but those listed are necessary elements in any peace settlement.

Notes

1 Tom L. Beauchamp and James F. Childress, *Principles of Biomedical Ethics* (New York: Oxford University Press, 1979; 1983; 1989; 1994).

2 K. Danner Clouser and Bernard Gert, 'A Critique of Principlism,' *Journal of Medicine and Philosophy* 15 (1990): 219–36.

3 R.M. Green, 'Method in Bioethics: A Troubled Assessment,' *Journal of Medicine and Philosophy* 15 (1990): 179–97.

4 Barry Hoffmaster, 'The Theory and Practice of Applied Ethics,' *Dialogue* 30 (1991): 213–34.

5 Albert R. Jonsen and Stephen Toulmin, *The Abuse of Casuistry: A History of Moral Reasoning* (Berkeley: University of California Press, 1988).

6 Henry Richardson, 'Specifying Norms as a Way to Resolve Concrete Ethical Problems,' *Philosophy and Public Affairs* 19:4 (Fall 1990): 279–310.

7 David DeGrazia, 'Moving Forward in Bioethical Theory: Theories, Cases, and Specified Principlism,' *Journal of Medicine and Philosophy* 17 (1992): 511–39.

8 Beauchamp and Childress, *Principles of Biomedical Ethics*, p. 5 (1979); p. 15 (1994).

9 Beauchamp and Childress, *Principles of Biomedical Ethics* (1979).

10 Tom L. Beauchamp, 'On eliminating the Distinction between Applied Ethics and Ethical Theory,' *Monist* 67 (1984): 515–31.

11 Clouser and Gert, 'A Critique of Principlism,' p. 231.

12 Ibid., p. 221.

13 Green, 'Method in Bioethics,' pp. 188ff.

14 Beauchamp and Childress, *Principles of Bioethics* (1994), p. 16.

15 John Arras, 'Getting Down to Cases: The Revival of Casuistry in Bioethics,' *Journal of Medicine and Philosophy* 16 (1991): 29–51, p. 39.

16 Richardson, 'Specifying Norms,' pp. 280ff.

17 DeGrazia, 'Moving Forward,' p. 512.

18 Norman Daniels, 'Wide Reflective Equilibrium and Theory Acceptance in Ethics,' *Journal of Philosophy* 76:5 (May 1979): 256–82; idem, 'Reflective Equilibrium and Archimedean Points,' *Canadian Journal of Philosophy*, 10:1 (March 1980): 83–103; see also idem, *Justice and Justification: Reflective Equilibrium in Theory and Practice* (New York: Cambridge University Press) (1996).

19 Albert R. Jonsen and Lewis H. Butler, 'Public Ethics and Policy Making,' *Hastings Center Report* 5 (August 1975): 19–31.

20 Ibid., p. 22; they cite Daniel Callahan, *Abortion: Law, Choice and Morality* (New York: Macmillan, 1970), p. 341, for introducing the related notion, 'moral policy.'

21 Jonsen and Butler, 'Public Ethics,' p. 24.

22 See this volume, pp. 271–96

23 White House Domestic Policy Council, *The President's Health Security Plan* (New York: Times Books, 1993), and Dan Brock and Norman Daniels, 'Ethical Foundations of the Clinton Administration's Proposed Health Care System,' *JAMA*, 271: 15 (1994): 1189–96.

24 See Norman Daniels, *Seeking Fair Treatment: From the AIDS Epidemic to National Health Care Reform* (New York: Oxford, 1995), ch. 8.

25 Norman, Daniels, 'Duty to Treat or Right to Refuse?' *Hastings Center Report* 21:2 (March–April 1991): 36–46; see also idem, *Seeking Fair Treatment*, ch 2.

26 See A. Zuger and S.M. Miles, 'Physicians, AIDS, and Occupational Risk,' *JAMA* 258:14 (1987): 1924–8; and J. Arras, 'The Fragile Web of Responsibility: AIDS and the Duty to Treat,' *Hastings Center Report* 18 (suppl., 1988): 10–20.

27 Norman Daniels, 'HIV-Infected Health Care Professionals: Public Threat or Public Sacrifice?' *Milbank Quarterly* 70:1 (1992): 3–42; idem, 'HIV-Infected Professionals, Patient Rights, and the Switching Dilemma,' *JAMA* 267:10 (1992): 1368–71; idem, *Seeking Fair Treatment*, ch. 3.

28 Norman Daniels, 'Rights to Health Care and Distributive Justice: Programmatic Worries,' *Journal of Medicine and Philosophy* 4:2 (1979): 174–91.

29 See idem, *Just Health Care* (New York: Cambridge University Press, 1985).

30 See idem, 'Rationing Fairly: Programmatic Considerations,' *Bioethics* 7:2–3: 224–33.

31 See 'Fair Procedures and Just Rationing,' in idem, *Justice and Justification*.

32 J. Sabin and N. Daniels, 'Determining "Medical Necessity" in Mental Health Practice: A Study of Clinical Reasoning and a Proposal for Insurance Policy,' *Hastings Center Report* 24:6 (November–December 1994): 5–13.

33 A. Sen, 'Justice: Means versus Freedoms,' *Philosophy and Public Affairs* 19 (Spring 1990): 111–21; idem, *Inequality Reexamined* (Cambridge MA: Harvard University Press, 1992); G.A. Cohen, 'On the Currency of Egalitarian Justice,' *Ethics* 99:4 (1989): 906–44; R. Arneson, 'Equality and Equality of Opportunity for Welfare,' *Philosophical Studies* 54 (1988): 79–95; and N. Daniels, 'Equality of What? Welfare, Resources, or Capabilities?' *Philosophy and Phenomenological Research* 50 (suppl. Fall 1990): 273–96; J. Rawls, *Political Liberalism* (New York: Columbia University Press, 1993).

34 See Rawls, *Political Liberalism*, pp. 182–5, and Daniels, 'Equality of What?'

35 Daniels, *Just Health Care*, ch. 7.

36 Daniels, *Seeking Fair Treatment*, ch. 3.

Bioethics through the Back Door: Phenomenology, Narratives, and Insights into Infertility

LAURA SHANNER

Much of the debate within philosophical bioethics has centred on a classic theoretical problem: are ethical problems best solved by appeal to 'top-down' approaches – those that emphasize principles or theories that may be applied, sometimes deductively, to specific problems in medical ethics – or by 'bottom-up' approaches, which start from the context or particularities of a case and work up to paradigms and principles? Norman Daniels has characterized this debate in this volume as a civil war among the Uplanders (serious theorists), principlists (principles advocates), and Lowlanders (context or case-based approaches). He suggests that both top-down and bottom-up types of reasoning are needed to solve ethical problems, and has offered reflective equilibrium as a way to negotiate a peace treaty. This negotiation strategy strikes me as far more promising than opting to join any of the competing camps; having been raised on the Georgetown principles, I now find myself coming of age in context-dependent feminism, and resolving the tension between top-down and bottom-up approaches has become not just a theoretical exercise but an attempt to integrate equally compelling aspects of the problems at hand.

Although Daniels's metaphor of war among the theorists, principlists, and casuists may not be too far from the truth of activity in bioethics, what interests me more is understanding what exactly it is that we are fighting over. That is, how do we define the problem at hand to which the assorted theorists battle for prominence in offering resolutions? On my cynical days, it seems that the battles in philosophical bioethics are over little more than the rewards of academia; we want our pet theories to be published in repeated editions and become standard reference points, even when they risk being caricatured. On better days, however, I remember that we are struggling to resolve difficult problems that are deeply important to the people whose bodies and lives are affected by medical interventions. The disagreement is really over the best approach to take in solving the problem; my question now is: How do we go about deciding what the problem *is* that needs to be solved?

Whatever theoretical tools you have in your bag, whether they involve top-down or bottom-up approaches, applying those tools to the wrong question often leads to an answer that is not particularly useful. There is an old adage that says 'when all you have is a hammer, everything looks like a nail.' Trying to drive a screw with a hammer does not work well, and using a hammer to remove a splinter from your thumb is disastrous. Academic philosophers tend to have a specific and limited set of tools – a theory or a set of principles – and we often try to apply them equally in courtrooms, boardrooms, hospital rooms, private rooms, and everywhere else we go. Often these tools work well across the range of settings, but sometimes they seem to miss the point, and sometimes they compound the dilemmas and confuse us even further. Approaching a complex, real-life situation with a theoretical framework in mind sometimes allows us to answer a theoretical question that was asked, but fails to respond adequately to the more difficult practical problem. This is the heart of criticisms that philosophers inhabit ivory towers and know not of what they speak – for a philosopher attempting to work in applied areas like bioethics, such a criticism is damning indeed.

I suggest, therefore, that we try to find a different point of entry – a back door – into bioethical problems. Instead of starting from a theoretical construct and looking to see which elements of a medical decision fit our existing categories, I suggest that philosophers start by attempting truly to understand the problem they are seeking to resolve. One mechanism for doing this is to reflect phenomenologically on our own lived experiences, or to offer a reflective narrative of the situation from our perspective within it. For situations that lie outside our personal experience, we may elicit narratives and descriptions that others can offer of their experiences and integrate these reports reflectively into a new narrative account of the phenomenon we are trying to understand. In both cases, we try to give an account of what it is like to have this experience. As an example, I shall focus in this paper on infertility and the use of new reproductive technologies (NRTs), such as in vitro fertilization (IVF), as a form of relief. Several ways of framing questions about IVF have led to interesting debates about embryo status, rights to reproduce, and whether infertility deserves a high ranking among our medical priorities, but both the treatments and the debates about them seem largely to have failed to provide much genuine relief for infertility. If we explore infertility as a lived experience, blending individual patient narratives into a narrative of the phenomenon, we can begin to see a different set of practical problems, different sorts of solutions for those problems, and new ethical issues to be addressed. Perhaps with this new understanding of the problem, our ethical discussions about infertility treatment may become less constrained by the walls of the ivory tower and more helpful to the patients.

At the end of the paper, another problem that haunts theoretical bioethics will be revisited: is bioethics merely ethical theory applied to a biomedical setting, or is it in some way *sui generis*? Taking a position different from that implied by several authors in this collection, I shall conclude that bioethics is a unique enterprise, and that it simply will not be sufficient for philosophers to wander into the hospital with no new tools other than those they have used in general ethical discussions.

Phenomenology and Narrative Bioethics

The attempt to describe the meaning of lived experience is known as *phenomenology*. Although the term is most often associated with the writings of Edmund Husserl and his followers in the early twentieth century, I need to emphasize that I make no claim whatsoever to interpret Continental texts; my approach has been inspired more by contemporary feminist writers who attempt to give voice to women's experiences that have been inaccurately or incompletely described by predominantly male philosophers and physicians.[1] The language of phenomenological reflection therefore may involve attempts to describe 'being-in-the-world' in a Continental sense, or it may simply report in less abstract terms *what it is like* to be male or female, to have an illness, or, for this paper, to be infertile. We should observe that illnesses, disabilities, and medical interventions have vastly more often than not been described, treated, and regulated by healthy, able-bodied health care providers and theorists. We should therefore challenge not just the institutional and political structures in which these experiences are embedded, but our very understanding of the experiences themselves.

Although few mainstream bioethicists have consciously adopted a phenomenological approach, variations on the methodology are emerging in attempts to understand the meanings of medical interactions, pain, illness, and confrontations with death as lived experiences. Richard Zaner, Howard Brody, and Warren Reich can be classified as early phenomenologists in bioethics,[2] and projects like Eric Cassell's *The Nature of Suffering* and S. Kay Toombs's *The Meaning of Illness*[3] deepen the tradition. Toombs, for example, describes phenomenology in Husserlian terms as a reflective enterprise in which 'the phenomenologist is committed to the effort to begin with what is given in immediate experience, to turn to the essential features of what presents itself as it presents itself to consciousness, and thereby to clarify the constitutive activity of consciousness and the sense-structure of experiencing.'[4] In less jargon-laden terms, phenomenologists focus on a lived experience, but do not become wrapped up in living it;

instead, they distance themselves from (or 'bracket') the experience in order to reflect upon it. Essential components of the experience itself, and also of what it is like to be experiencing it, are identified and described. Our goal, therefore, is to interpret the experience *as it is experienced*. An important aspect of phenomenological, as opposed to analytical, approaches is the attempt to disregard a priori categories, assumptions, and preconceptions about the experience. In Toombs's words again, 'in the phenomenological attitude, one places in abeyance one's taken-for-granted presuppositions about the nature of "reality," one's commitments to certain habitual ways of interpreting the world.'[5] Benjamin Crabtree and William Miller describe how one does this: 'Phenomenology seeks to understand the lived experience of individuals and their intentions within their 'lifeworld.' It answers the question, What is it like to have a certain experience? To accomplish this, investigators must 'bracket' their own preconceptions and enter into the individual's lifeworld and use the self as an experiencing interpreter. Paradigm cases and theories are frequently identified, and the experience is presented as descriptive narrative.'[6]

While paradigm cases have been referred to in this definition, phenomenological and narrative approaches are not a standard case presentation; bioethics cases are usually chosen or constructed to illustrate pre-existing categories, such as medical diagnoses and a priori ethical principles. Even in casuistry, cases are usually developed with paradigms in mind rather than taken as phenomenal, lived experiences. Rarely is a case presented as an opportunity to live an experience of illness or treatment vicariously, or to reflect upon the meaning of the condition or interaction for the persons most intimately affected by it.

A brief example may clarify the distinctions between the phenomenological approach and the theoretical, principle-based, casuist, and political feminist approaches discussed by other authors in this collection. How would you describe what is happening as you read this paper? From an abstract theoretical approach, we quickly observe that this is a philosophy paper rather than, say, one in physics or medieval history; from there, we can break the paper down into its component arguments and identify examples of philosophical reasoning. This seems to be the method used by R.M. Hare, who approaches bioethics from his brand of utilitarianism, which he distinguishes from a care, virtue, or situation ethic. A principles approach, like the autonomy-beneficence-justice triad popularized by Tom Beauchamp, suggests a series of rules or protocols that ought generally to be observed: in philosophy papers, for example, autonomy allows me to write (and you to read) about the topics of our choosing; beneficence requires that I write concise and interesting prose to avoid boring the reader, and that reviewers be kind even when critical; justice entails that each contributor be compensated equally for her/his contributions. A casuist like Al Jonsen would observe that after reading several philosophy papers, we begin to identify paradigms of good paper structure, argumentation, and insight, and then we may classify this paper as 'good' or 'bad' depending upon the relationship between its unique factors and the paradigms. A different form of context-based assessment, more in line with the work of Laura Purdy, Christine Overall, Sue Sherwin, and Kathryn Morgan, would focus on the social and political context in which this paper is presented. A feminist, for example, would note that I am one of few women represented in this volume and in philosophy generally, and that the academic institutions that support this type of work are strongly heirarchical.

A phenomenological approach is different. Reflect for a moment on what it is like for you to be experiencing this paper right now. Anyone could make several category assessments about what is happening, but that person does not really know what it is like for you to be reading this paper. Since you have been busy thinking about my words, *you* may not even be aware of what it is like for you to be here. You might have forgotten that you are an embodied being: How does the weight of your body feel against the chair – are you aware of where you stop and the furniture begins? How quickly are you breathing? (A Continentalist who thinks my interpretation of phenomenology is mangled might be hyperventilating.) More important, what meaning does this paper have for you? Is it something you are supposed to read for a course or review, or is it a show of personal support for me to share my work even though you do not really understand or care what the paper is about, or is this a paper that you selected in the hope that it would contribute to your understanding of bioethics? At a specific level, are you profiting from this paper, and at a more general level, is reading academic papers a worthwhile activity? We need to avoid being too absorbed in the moment, however, and instead bracket the experience to reflect on its essence. Whether you are hungry or sleepy today is an interesting fact about you, but it does not offer much insight into this paper or papers generally. We seek shared meaning, not merely unreflective perceptions about the process of reading.

The phenomenology or lived experience of reading this paper is probably different for me than it is for you; I am less likely than you to be surprised by anything contained in the text because, after all, I wrote it. When you read this paper in its printed form, and especially when I present it to you at a conference or seminar, I am more likely than you to be concerned that it is well received. Even if you and I were in the same room as my ideas were conveyed from the page to your mind, our lived experiences of this process would be quite different. Thus, a seemingly ordinary academic paper, *as it is experienced by the author, readers, and listeners*, may turn out to be a complex phenomenon.

Imagine, therefore, how different the perceptions of what is happening might be when the event is not an academic discusussion, but a confrontation with disability or death. Kay Toombs subtitled her book, 'A phenomenological account of the different perspectives of physician and patient,' indicating the complexity of medical phenomena as lived by the key players. Doctors are trained to identify and treat physical ailments, and when all you have is a hammer, everything starts looking like a nail. Bioethicists should therefore be wary of a priori assumptions about medical conditions and treatments and should not accept medical accounts of a case as the whole or even the primary story, because much more is likely to be happening at levels that we often ignore. What else is going on in the medical crisis beyond the diagnosis, especially for the ones whose lives and bodies are most profoundly affected? *What is it like* to be in the situation being considered?

Once we move beyond superficial descriptions and seriously try to understand what it means to have an illness or treat it, or even to write or read academic papers, we are in a much better position to refine theories, to develop principles or rules of behaviour, to look for paradigms of good and bad examples, and to challenge the phenomenon's socio-political context. In other words, all of the top-down and bottom-up methodologies come back into play, and they can even continue their civil war over how the final judgments are made. Before we can apply those theories, however, we must first be attentive to the nature of the phenomenon that we are attempting to address.

Narratives

The phenomenological approach involves paying attention to lived experience and reflecting upon what it is like to be living it. This is usually not easy. Husserl focused on 'being-in-the-world,' a condition that applies to all of us but upon which we rarely reflect; this basic and obvious experience is thus astoundingly difficult to articulate. When the phenomenologist is attempting to describe *someone else's* more specific lived experience, however, additional avenues of inquiry are required. I have no personal experience with infertility, for example, and I needed a way to 'enter the lifeworld' and 'use [myself] as an experiencing interpreter' of infertility patients. Indeed, most bioethicists do not have chronic debilitating diseases or injuries, life-threatening illnesses, or excruciating physical pain; Kay Toombs's phenomenology of illness and Sue Wendell's writings on disability[7] are rare exceptions motivated by their own lived experiences. The majority of bioethics literature on pregnancy and abortion has been written by men, none of whom to my knowledge have first-hand, lived experience of being pregnant. In short, most bioethicists are writing a lot about things of which we know very little.

One option to remedy this lack of phenomenological understanding is to force philosophers to suffer a variety of inconvenient to downright dreadful experiences in order to write knowledgeably about them. This option is clearly unacceptable, however, for both ethical and practical reasons. A better mechanism for coming to understand what we are talking about is to draw upon the narratives of an experience as told by people who have lived it; that is, to allow patients to talk in their own ways about infertility, pregnancy, illness, disability, or confrontations with death. The phenomenological attitude does not allow us to settle for pre-reflective descriptions of experience, however, but guides us to identify and describe the constituent elements of the experience and to reflect upon what it is like to be living it.

Experience regarding a phenomenon is thus not necessarily restricted to the one who is immediately or most intensely connected to it; experience may also be understood as any genuine insight into the reality. Writing about nursing practice, Patricia Benner links phenomenology, experience, and narratives: "'Experience,'' defined from a phenomenological perspective, refers to the turning around, the adding of nuance, the amending or changing of preconceived notions or perceptions of the situation ... Experience occurs when one encounters a practical situation in such a way that one's understanding of the situation is altered. Experience then is considered the active history of a tradition ... that can be captured in narratives of the practice.'[8]

Narratives may take several forms in medicine and medical ethics. One approach, as described in a recent paper by Jan Marta,[9] is to employ an individual patient's narrative of life experiences in differential diagnosis to resolve a physical condition that turned out to have psychosomatic roots. Rita Kielstein and Hans-Martin Sass suggest in a recent article that doctors employ case scenarios to elicit narrative accounts of a patient's values in developing an advance directive.[10] A different approach is to explore literary images of medicine and illness conveyed by the voices of narrators and fictional characters; for example, Leo Tolstoy's *The Death of Ivan Illych* offers a moving example of a once-powerful man's confrontation with illness, dependence, and death.

The variation on narratives that I shall pursue involves integrating multiple stories and perspectives on a topic to construct a narrative of a phenomenon or practice that extends beyond individuals. In short, it emphasizes listening to the people who are living the experience about which we are trying to develop policies, so that we can understand what it is like for them to be having that experience. While each individual is likely to have unique perceptions, conflicts, and meanings associated with reproduction, embodiment, health, illness, and death, and even different perceptions of the same disease or condition, we may nevertheless develop useful understandings of a shared human condition that arises in response to common circumstances. Further, while an individual's story may guide us to specific case resolutions, often we also need to establish policies that transcend individual cases. What is at stake for people in a given situation, and how can we best help them? Common themes in the individual narratives often converge, allowing us to convey a nuanced and altered understanding in a new composite narrative of practices and shared phenomena.

Methodology

Philosophers are often wary of field research or empirical data, but I think that applied ethicists need to look beyond our home department. If nothing else, practitioners are generally not as amused as we are by energetic abstract discussions, and they quite reasonably ignore our suggestions if they think we are ignorant of the realities of their work. More important, however, I think philosophy can take us only so far by itself; the walls of the ivory tower really do exist, and they sometimes impede our progress in applied ethics.

Crabtree and Miller classify philosophy as one of several types of qualitative research, serving as 'a generator and clarifier for ... other research styles.'[11] The philosophical approach generates the key questions that I believe we need to ask in any bioethical situation: What is important here? What is at stake for the patient(s)? (In Crabtree and Miller's scheme, these are questions of identification.) What is it like to have this condition and to undergo treatment? What meanings and practices occur in lived experience (description, qualitative)? What assumptions have we made about the condition and the options for responding to it? What value do we place on life, comfort, fertility, or other types of functioning (description, normative)? Are our assumptions coherent with the phenomenon as a lived experience? What patterns exist in the phenomenon, and how do they correlate to other social, medical, linguistic, and ethical phenomena (explanation generation / association)?

Finding answers to questions like these would seem to require extensive familiarity with the phenomenon in question. *Experience* of the lived clinical realities is required as fodder for accurate bioethical reflection; in other words, philosophy must be supplemented with *field research*, for which Crabtree and Miller provide another useful definition: 'The field researcher is directly and personally engaged in an interpretive focus on the human field of activity with the goal of generating holistic and realistic descriptions and/or explanations ... [F]ield research has no prepackaged research designs. Rather, specific data collection methods, sampling procedures, and analysis styles are used to create unique, question-specific designs that evolve throughout the research process. These qualitative or field designs take the form of either a case study or a topical study.'[12] Case studies, of course, have been a mainstay of bioethics since the inception of the discipline. A topical study focuses not on a case, but on a limited sphere of activities or meanings for a defined group; for example, in this volume I am focusing on infertility patients who seek IVF, Kathryn Morgan discusses the biopolitics of elective cosmetic surgery, and Christine Overall approaches pediatrics with an ethic of child care.

Several criticisms of the narrative method and field research in philosophy become apparent at this point, although I believe the narrative approach can be defended against them. Since there is no prepackaged research design, the first problem is to prevent the qualitative researcher from imposing his or her subjective biases on the description, or from allowing anecdotes and squeaky wheels to skew the interpretation. Although philosophers tend to shun empirical and statistical data, challenges to the validity of a phenomenological description are usually quantitative in nature: What percentage of people actually experience it this way? If relevant quantitative information is available, it should certainly be incorporated into the argument to defend the strength of the claims being made. In the absence of such data, the phenomenological bioethicist should acknowledge the lack of statistical information (and thereby suggest that researchers in other disciplines do the needed work), grant the range and variety of human experiences, but then refocus our attention on understanding the phenomenon as it is experienced by whatever number of people happen to experience it. That a phenomenon exists at all, especially when it raises identifiable moral and practical concerns, justifies exploring the nature of the phenomenon without first quantifying it. In other words, while we ought to be quite active in protesting an avoidable harm that comes to 80 per cent of a patient group, we ought not dismiss an avoidable harm just because only 5 per cent of the group perceive it as a problem; members of the 5 per cent minority deserve to be heard and to be defended.

Quantifying thus allows us to specify the scope of a problem and to compare one problem with others, perhaps to decide which should receive the fastest or most focused investment of resources, but quantifying may also distract us from the more basic ethical issues at stake. As Howard Brody has observed, a quantitative description of experiences and normative concepts may become 'a classic case of the measurable driving out the important.'[13] Part of the work of philosophical bioethics (along with many other philosophical specialties) is to challenge the epistemological assumptions underlying mechanisms to measure complex human phenomena; for example, IQ tests do not reliably measure intelligence as a richly understood functional capacity, and EEGs do not conclusively measure the presence of consciousness, the existence of souls, or the exact moment of death.

All of us exist in the world, and yet Husserl initiated an enormously complex project in trying to articulate what it means to be as being is experienced; taking a sidewalk survey of people's attitudes about existence is unlikely to uncover philosophically significant or useful truths. In addition, persons facing a serious illness or injury are often too busy coping with the problem to engage in extended philosophical reflection. A statistical survey to identify the percentage of average patients who would describe their experience in a particular way is therefore quite unlikely to uncover the deeper *meanings* of the experience, although these mechanisms clearly can offer us both guiding insights and indications that our theories are inconsistent with their experiences. Thus, while we need to listen to the narratives of those having the experience, we should not automatically conclude that their pre-reflective reports tell the full story. We must distinguish reflective from non-reflective accounts and interpret the narratives through further work of phenomenological reflection.

This task raises a second problem: whose definitions or descriptions are preferred? Is the patient, a doctor, a psychologist, a philosopher, or indeed anyone in a privileged position to interpret the patient's narrative? This is, of course, an epistemological and value problem common to competency analysis, psychotherapy, and many autonomy/beneficence conflicts. On the one hand, we need to recognize the limitations that most of us encounter in reflecting upon our experiences, which may be compounded in medical settings by denial, exhaustion, fear, pain, and compromised mental alertness; on the other hand, we do not want to impose yet another distanced and inaccurate interpretation of the patient's lived reality, just as medicalized versions of 'best interests' and males' descriptions of pregnancy have so often failed to capture patients' experience. This conflict does not invalidate the method of narrative phenomenology, but it constantly forces us to recognize the limits of the approach and to challenge and bracket our presuppositions. More often than not, this bracketing of presuppositions makes the narrative seem more complex and sometimes paradoxical.

We should observe that all uses of cases in top-down and bottom-up theoretical approaches also require the case constructor to assume a privileged position in defining the 'important' aspects of the case and therefore to face the same challenge. These other approaches usually do not call attention to this problem and they often prevent us from asking about it, because challenging the categories makes the case too complicated to illustrate effectively a principle or paradigm. The phenomenological attitude thus provides a built-in complacency check that the other theories do not offer: we should leave our principles and preconceptions at the door, and get over our fear of complexity. Real life can be messy, complicated, and full of ambiguity, but real life – not a sanitized, abstracted version of it – is what poses our most compelling ethical problems.

Luckily, there are several mechanisms to prevent our being led astray by anecdotes and squeaky wheels who misrepresent a phenomenon. The most important is *triangulation*, or the use and cross-checking of multiple data sources, methods, records, and even theoretical perspectives, to identify points of coherence in the topic being studied. Sources with different perspectives on the phenomenon may give different descriptions, so we would be most justified in looking for the 'truth' in the areas where the perspectives overlap and cohere. Brody contrasts triangulation with the Cartesian, analytic, deductivist model of logical reasoning: when one step follows indubitably from another, there is no need for triangulation and coherence. A more pragmatic approach to complex subjects that cannot be reduced to simple, indubitable theorems, however, requires a hypothesis or theory to cohere with a range of ideas and perspectives. Triangulation, then, is a particular application of Daniels's wide reflective equilibrium.[14]

A newcomer to a topic in bioethics should therefore listen without preconceptions to a range of the people involved: especially patients, but also nurses, physicians and counsellors who work with this patient group; health policy analysts and economists who situate a particular clinical condition or treatment into a larger construction of a health care system; and members of the variety of religious and social groups who emphasize non-medical and non-economic values. While many people will give pre-reflective or even self-serving accounts rather than insightful narratives, themes and categories gradually emerge through repetition. As the researcher becomes aware of these emerging themes, more specific questions can be directed to the sources for confirmation or disconfirmation. The clearer the themes become, the easier it is to identify *key informants*, those reflective individuals who can provide the insights that fill a particular researcher's conceptual gaps. *Member checks* can then be done, which is the process of 'recycling [the] analysis back to key informants.'[15]

I suggest that bioethics field research of this sort is crucial for comparing one condition or treatment with others, as must occur in resource allocation and health policy discussions. Clarifying and comparing values also requires this deep understanding of the kinds of problems to be addressed. It is simply not enough, for example, to assume that death, illness, and physical pain are merely 'bad' – what sort of bad? How bad? When forced to choose one or another, how can we compare types of badness? Subtle, taken-for-granted elements of a condition or treatment that raise new ethical issues are often invisible to those who do not go into the field; for example, many people are surprised to learn that infertility clinics routinely supply soft-core pornography to assist men to provide sperm samples. Field researchers are also more likely to observe unexpected behaviours and statements that reveal a reality suppressed in more formal interviews, surveys, or literature generated by the professionals and patients being observed. In other words, genuinely helpful philosophical reflection on a practice or institution requires that it be examined *as it is lived and experienced*, not as it is presupposed or as it is packaged.

Insights into Infertility

I started writing about infertility by trying to assign it to a category: is it a disease or disability that should be treated medically, or is it a mere desire frustration that earns a low priority for research and funding? IVF is usually debated on grounds of its acceptability as if it existed in isolation from the meaning of pregnancy, parenting, and infertility in human life; the most attention has been devoted to whether embryos are persons who should not be experimented upon, manipulated, frozen, donated, or thrown away, and the Vatican challenged the separation of conception and intercourse as violating the 'dignity of procreation' through intercourse[16] while reiterating its own contributions to social norms for marriage and parenting that cause so much of infertility's distress. Infertile persons are often lumped with other people in larger theoretical agendas: many feminist critics challenge IVF as one more of a series of male-dominated medical intrusions into women's bodies and reproductive processes, while the mainstream debate emphasizes rights to reproduce and rights to have access to infertility treatments. In short, IVF raised the same old bioethics dilemmas: what are the limits of autonomy in the face of risks for others (the embryos and offspring), the risks of the treatments for patients, and the usual vexing problems of resource allocation?

I began to wonder whether IVF was just another new treatment, or whether infertility presents any unique insights and problems as a life experience of the patients who seek treatment for it. Very little philosophical attention has been paid to what I call the child-wish, yet it is a rich and resonant human experience. The philosophical (as well as political and clinical) discourse on IVF has been much like a debate on euthanasia policy without a consideration of the meaning of death. I wondered if we could better understand what was at stake for infertility patients – and thus better categorize infertility – by talking to patients directly and articulating a phenomenology of infertility. The attempt proved to be a genuine experience in Benner's sense: I came away from it with an altered and nuanced perception of the situation and eventually abandoned my original set of categories as irrelevant.

Most of my field research was conducted in clinical centres throughout Australia.[17] My triangulated sources for the phenomenology of infertility include patients, former patients, psychologists, social workers, nurses, clinical researchers, physicians, and governmental health policy analysts in the United States, Australia, Canada, and Great Britain. Their perspectives were conveyed in published writings, unpublished papers and addresses, interviews, responses to a survey I distributed to patients, and contributions to patient support-group newsletters. Although limited quantitative psychological and sociological research has been done with infertility patients,[18] there is nevertheless a wide consensus on the stages of grief and coping with infertility; descriptions of shame, emptiness, failure, and similar feelings; the roller-coaster of emotions entailed by IVF protocols; and the social pressures typically brought to bear on childless adults. While individual stories may vary, the following narrative of the phenomenon of infertility is a composite sketch of hundreds of patients' stories told to me directly, related by counsellors, and published in various formats.

A Narrative of Infertility as a Phenomenon

John and Mary had always assumed their fertility, and even feared it; for years they carefully used contraceptives and practised birth control, but finally they were ready to begin planning their family in earnest. After several months of trying to initiate a pregnancy, nothing was happening. They were surprised by this turn of events and experienced some denial even after undergoing clinical work-ups.[19] Both were generally healthy and free of pain. Certainly the tests were mistaken!

As the realization of their infertility sank in, they became angry. They were angry at the injustice of their infertility when babies are born to neglectful or abusive parents, at the inability of physicians to solve the problem, at a desire that cannot be fulfilled, at the lack of understanding in society, at the spouse who does not meet expectations of fertility or support, and at their own inability to cope better with the situation. They were angry about the choices being denied to them, and about the nosiness of other people. 'I get so angry at the feminists who tell us that we don't really want to have children, like we're too stupid to know that we're being manipulated,' Mary said. 'Just because *they* don't want children doesn't mean that we don't genuinely want them.'[20] They felt out of control,[21] their bodies refusing to control birth as they were supposed to, which made them feel more angry and afraid: 'I've earned university degrees, achieved success in my career, and have a happy marriage. I really believe that if you work hard enough, you can get what you want. Except for a baby. I am doing everything, and I still can't have one.'[22]

The anger and frustration began to mix with guilt about past behaviours that they secretly believed might have contributed to the infertility: contraceptives and delayed childbearing to develop their careers were central to the guilt, as

were previous affairs and possible unnoticed infections. Were they being pun-
ished for a previous abortion, giving a child up for adoption, or abandoning a
child he did not even realize he had fathered? Was God mocking them for masturbation, homosexual thoughts, or even sexual pleasure? They felt guilty not
only for their own infertility, but for their inability to support each other and for
disappointing their relatives who wanted grandchildren.

Guilt turned into *shame*, 'the distressed apprehension of the self as inadequate or diminished: it requires if not an actual audience before whom my defi-
ciencies are paraded, then an internalized audience with the capacity to judge
me, hence internalized standards of judgment. Further, shame requires the recognition that I *am*, in some important sense, as I am seen to be.'[23] It was not just
a feeling that they had *done* something wrong, but that their *essential selves*
were inadequate, diminished, and unworthy. 'I feel like a failure,' both said
repeatedly; 'I feel a big, black, gaping emptiness inside me,' she said.[24] 'Maybe
my partner should trade me in for a better model.' Their self-esteem and self-
image were frequently battered in the ongoing struggle with infertility. Old
memories of shameful hurts – being too short to play basketball, being the last
girl to wear a bra, being painfully shy as a child – were brought to the surface;
any doubts about their bodies or their competence were reactivated and confirmed by their inability to produce a child.[25] The embarrassing and invasive
medical exams and procedures, along with the constant intervention with their
sexual behaviours, intensified feelings of shame related to sexual taboos.

Thus, dealing with the disappointment of infertility would have been hard
enough on its own, but many deeper psychological issues that had been
repressed or ignored surfaced. The guilt resulted from unresolved feelings about
previous behaviours, and other unresolved feelings of inadequacy, low self-
esteem, poor body image, discomfort with being an adult, problems with their
parents, and gender identity (masculinity/femininity) sometimes re-emerged.
We often try to settle unresolved childhood problems by 'doing it right this
time' with our own children, but infertile people are denied that opportunity.
The greater the unresolved problems, the greater the need to have a child.

Mary and John began to feel intense isolation both from others who did not
understand the nature of the infertility crisis, and also from each other. They felt
left out of their peer group and wanted to be like their friends and siblings who
were having children. Their families pressured them to produce grandchildren,
nieces, and nephews. Meanwhile, it hurt to be around children, or people with
children: 'I used to play with my nieces and make things with them, but I want
to do this with my own little girl. It hurts too much to be with them, so no more
sewing projects.'[26] Infertility was quickly becoming a social disease.

Infertility is often labelled a 'disease of couples,'[27] largely because both partners are required for normal reproduction, which distinguishes it from other medical maladies; she had had an accident once and required his care for a lengthy convalescence that disrupted both their lives, but that wasn't a 'disease of couples.' Infertility is essentially social because it affects not just the ill or injured body, but the formation of new family relationships. Couples, extended families, and social groups – as well as individuals – are deprived of the opportunity to have and raise a child. Having children is also the usual way of moving from the generation of children to the generation of parents/adults, leaving infertile persons in a dilemma about how to accomplish the transition. Studies show that people tend to judge adults without children as selfish, immature, unreliable, and hedonistic;[28] John and Mary did not need studies to tell them that.

If their own feelings and imaginations did not provide enough fuel for the flames of guilt and shame, other people did. Constant questions ('So, when are you two going to settle down and have some kids?') reminded them of their inability to do so. She overheard neighbours describe her as cold, fussy, uptight, career oriented, materialistic, and too interested in keeping the house tidy to be a good mother. His colleagues joked about impotence and latent homosexuality; perhaps one of them should demonstrate how a 'real' man makes a baby?[29] Sexuality is multi-faceted, but many people link fertility with both gender identity (attractiveness) and potency (libido); it is not uncommon for men to develop impotence after a diagnosis of a low sperm count,[30] and both partners may feel increasingly unattractive, unresponsive, and inadequate. She said, 'I grew up expecting to develop curves and have babies. I have the curves, but not the babies. I don't feel like a real woman' and 'I've always expected I'd be a mommy. If I'm not a mother, then what am I?'[31] The inability to inseminate or conceive can trigger a massive identity crisis by calling into question one's entire sense of self and finding it lacking.

They felt grief, but there was no support for it. We do not hold funerals for miscarried pregnancies, let alone for unconceived ones. She lost the experiences of pregnancy and childbirth, and they both lost the continuity of future generations, the experiences and social role of parenting, and their self-images as parents. Infertility seemed to be a type of death, a 'genetic death' in which they were prevented from contributing to the biological diversity and future of the human species. As he commented, 'Who will carry on the family name? I'm the last. All my ancestors are made nothing by my sterility.' 'You tell me it's not the end of the world not having children. No - but it's the end of my bit in the world, isn't it?'[32] Without children, their own deaths loomed as more final.

The most painful loss was the wanted child itself, who existed as a 'dreamchild' who began in their imaginations when they themselves were small; she actively imagined her future children while playing with dolls, and he did so to a lesser extent.[33] The dream-child has not been fully lost, although every menstrual period feels like another death, and the dream-child is unable to satisfy their longing for a living, real child. Grieving for infertility is therefore a lot like grieving for a soldier missing in action rather than for one who has been killed in battle.[34] This emotional limbo of hope and grief presents a therapeutic dilemma: relief could come either through pregnancy, which may require medical treatment, or through difficult emotional griefwork (often with a counsellor or psychotherapist), but it is quite difficult to do both at the same time. Adoption social workers usually will not place a child with a couple who have unresolved grief regarding their infertility, and continued medical treatment is usually interpreted as an indication that the couple are not yet ready to accept an adopted child for his or her own sake. Thus infertile people face the further dilemma of giving up their last hope of having a genetically related child if they hope to be eligible to adopt a child.

Unable to give up hope, and seeking a way to regain control of this horrible situation, they turned to the infertility clinic. Paradoxically, they lost control. The doctors started to examine, poke, probe, and embarrass them; to monitor, direct, and time their sexual activities (it felt like the doctors were always there in the bedroom with them); and even to create the desired pregnancy through technological processes that the patients only vaguely understood. She felt physically and emotionally devastated by the hormone injections, and the doctors could not provide good evidence or straight answers to her questions about her risks for cancer or other complications in the future; such studies have never been done. She felt physically invaded and embarrassed by the many gynecological interventions and sometimes experienced the interventions as akin to a sexual assault that she had brought upon herself.[35] IVF fails to initiate a pregnancy in at least 80 per cent of treatment cycles, and at least 20 per cent of the pregnancies are later lost in miscarriages. The loss of a confirmed and much-wanted pregnancy was devastating – there had been grief at the loss of the dream-child in monthly menstruation, and the loss of an actual pregnancy vastly exceeded the loss of a merely imagined and desired pregnancy.

Despite the inadequate evidence of safety and efficacy of infertility treatments[36] and the low published success rates even at the best of clinics, the clinical team is usually upbeat and hopeful. There is always a new variation – a new drug, a new technique, different timing. One never knows what will work; some patients get pregnant on their tenth or fourteenth attempt, and the waiting room walls were covered with photos of smiling babies and their parents. John and Mary had stepped on a medical treadmill, and it was getting harder to jump off.

The technological treadmill is a common phenomenon in western medicine, as is perhaps most easily noticed in intensive care and lifesaving technologies. As a society, we often seem to follow an imperative to 'do anything' to achieve a medical goal, no matter how painful, how expensive, or how unrealistic the aim. The medical treadmill also has more personal gears. Some counsellors suggest that painful and intrusive medical procedures may often serve as a form of atonement, and that 'the patient who is eager to "do anything" to achieve a pregnancy, or who volunteers for experimental or dangerous procedures, should be suspected of wishing to assuage guilt.'[37] Some patients feel that ending treatment amounts to voluntary childlessness; as long as they are seeking treatment, the infertility is 'not their fault.' As a result, some patients return for as many as a dozen treatment cycles over a decade or longer, or attend infertility support group meetings not to sort out their options, but to attempt 'to get strong enough to try again' after serious complications.[38] John and Mary had been through painful, expensive, and potentially risky treatments, and IVF hadn't worked. They were still infertile, they had no baby, and few people seemed willing to accept them – and to help them accept themselves – as they were.

This scenario reflects, for many people, what it is like to be infertile.

Implications

It is commonly assumed that infertility is essentially a physical problem of producing children, and that assisting people's bodies to bear or beget children resolves the problem; IVF is therefore a reasonable intervention within a fairly mechanical model of medicine. Metaphorically, IVF is a heavy hammer in the medical toolbox, so infertility is most helpfully depicted as a nail that this tool can work upon. The phenomenology of infertility, however, indicates that this common assumption and the conclusions derived from it are wrong. Most people who are infertile have been that way for a while without recognizing it, and people who do not want children (e.g., celibate clergy) would not be greatly inconvenienced by a diagnosis. Some people adapt fairly easily to a deeply disappointing change in their life plans. For the people who experience infertility as a crisis, and who therefore make the strongest claim to use IVF, the problem clearly is not solely or even primarily physical, although it involves bodily processes. The pain is social and psychological in origin, and treating the body usually cannot relieve these forms of suffering.

When such deep psychological aspects of self, gender identity, maturity, normalcy, and control are called into question, the words of a patient in Melbourne ring true: 'a child is not the cure for infertility.'[39] When high-tech medical assistance is required to provide the child, shameful concerns about one's reproductive or physical inadequacy are hardly relieved. Casting infertility as the absence of a child also does not explain the problem of 'secondary infertility,' which is the inability to bear or beget a second or later child after at least one has been born. Even worse, IVF fails for the vast majority of patients who attempt it, and we offer little if any comfort to those who go home alone. We are therefore falling far short of our goal of relieving infertility when we emphasize the medical initiation of pregnancy as the solution.

Procreation, and the inability to accomplish it implied by infertility, are much more than physical phenomena: they challenge self-images and social roles and in their essence involve a social context. This complex phenomenon cannot be captured adequately in an emphasis on physical functioning or in principles of autonomy to reproduce or to pursue life plans. In the light of the variety of physical and personal circumstances represented in the population, infertile persons need to have a range of treatment options available that genuinely address their concerns rather than mask them or, worse yet, make them feel even more abnormal and out of control.

Supportive counselling or psychotherapy to help individuals accept themselves with limitations is far more effective than surgery for many patients, especially when their forms of distress are not resolved even when the treatment succeeds in producing a child. This recommendation does not preclude the continued availability of medical treatments for infertility, nor does it imply that infertility patients are mentally ill, but it suggests that invasive and largely unsuccessful medical technology ought to be used sparingly and as a last resort rather than as the first suggestion. Whatever type of assistance is employed, the goal should be to help the infertile person to reach a stage of acceptance and to resume plans for the future. This involves resolution of the previous stages of denial, grief, guilt, and isolation – although the feelings are never fully exhausted, they will return with less frequency and intensity over time – and redevelopment of self-esteem, sexuality, and self-image. People at this stage are ready to resume their lives as child free, or they may act on alternatives such as adoption, foster-parenting, or creativity and generativity in projects not involving children. It is no accident that one of the largest infertility patient support groups, with members in several countries, is called RESOLVE. A former IVF patient in Melbourne described her resolution in terms of the layers of issues that had not been apparent to her at first: 'I sought therapy to sort out why I so desperately wanted a child – [it] enabled me to understand the inner conflict and resolve the emotional problem, so I decided to discontinue IVF. [I h]ave accepted my inability to have children, and now feel I do not *need* to (even though it still hurts at times) ... [Now] I channel my energy in a different direction.'[40]

A broader normative implication concerns the role of women in society. Infertility is generally far more damaging to women than to men, both as patients who bear the brunt of drugs and surgery even to treat male infertility, and as infertile persons in a society in which men have far more options than women to achieve success and social status outside parenting roles. When social norms and attitudes about maturity, parenting, and gender identity are explored and revised, especially in regard to the roles and images of women, a person's self-image might be constructed according to more reasonable and attainable ideals. The fact of physical infertility then may lose some of its sting. There will still be deep disappointment and grief for many people, but it may be possible to avoid the deep sense of shame and failure that accompanies the failure to meet entrenched social expectations. Arguing about the right of individuals to seek treatments in order to meet those norms, however, ignores the psychosocial roots of infertility's distress, and does nothing to end the perpetuation of unrealistic, shame-inducing norms and the harms that they cause.

Framing infertility as a psychosocial phenomenon rather than a medical problem also frees us from the interminable debate about whether infertility is a disease or preference frustration, and therefore whether infertility treatment is a legitimate medical need. Infertility causes significant suffering for many people, and beneficence dictates that we attempt to relieve it without causing greater harm with our interventions. A child is often not the cure for infertility, and medicine does not cure the frustrated child-wish. New reproductive technologies may be one option, and may therefore be desired in some cases, but genuine relief for many patients will have to come from primarily non-medical sources. It is less important to classify infertility within our categories of preference and disease than it is to address the multi-faceted suffering on its own terms.

Bioethics as Sui Generis

I promised at the beginning to explain why I think bioethics is a unique enterprise, often quite different not just from philosophical ethics but also from other fields of applied ethics, such as business, legal, or environmental ethics. This is neither an important difference of top-down or bottom-up methodology for problem solving nor a superficial difference in setting, but a reflection of the different types of profound problems raised by bioethics.

An unknown wit stated it perfectly: 'In theory, theory and practice are the same thing. In practice, they're not.' I have already given several reasons for applied philosophers to step out of the department and explore the field to which their theories are meant to apply: as a practical matter, practitioners in a field have greater confidence in people who understand the details and realities of the job, and they are therefore more likely to adopt our recommendations. Subtle interactions and beliefs that raise ethical red flags may be invisible to people who observe only from a distance. As the phenomenology of infertility showed, not truly understanding the nature of the problem to be addressed but accepting the professionals' definition of the situation may prompt interesting but misguided philosophical debates.

Philosophers can offer far more than just the technical services of clarifying definitions and cranking out logical implications. With a good general ethical theory or set of principles, or with a feminist commitment to uncovering and dismantling oppressive contexts, philosophers are able to walk into a variety of settings and offer helpful diagnoses of problems and options for resolution. For example, in legal ethics we observe that attorneys must balance confidentiality to their clients with the interests of those who stand to be harmed by the clients' illegal behaviour. In business ethics, a Fortune 500 company executive must manage confidential information about potential buyouts that might upset the stock market. In journalistic ethics, the philosopher correctly identifies the confidentiality/third-party conflict involved in a reporter's refusal to reveal a source. By the time we get to the hospital, a doctor's conflict over telling a patient's spouse about the patient's positive HIV test sounds routine. With a good theory in hand, the philosopher can enter any setting and identify interesting and important moral issues and may be able to offer advice for resolving the dilemmas.

This consistent theoretical application is a good thing in so far as it keeps our moral practices coherent, but our devotion to a particular framework or theory often blinds us to other possibilities and unique elements of the setting. We can make even more valuable contributions to the understanding of important phenomena if we first gain experience with our topic. Gaining this experience frequently involves leaving philosophy to dabble in empirical data and practical situations, however, and thus applied ethics requires different methodologies than theoretical ethics.

Bioethics also differs from other areas of applied ethics that focus on the ways in which professionals and institutions affect our interests. The key issues in medicine involve more than standard ethical issues, such as disclosure, loyalties, virtues, liberties, or notions of the good, although they are of course critical. Encounters with health care professionals also routinely affect our bodies – *our very selves* with which we interact with the world. Our money, property, social status, career options, relationships, and all sorts of things are obviously extremely important to us, but none of these things *is* us. Drawing upon phenomenology – here in a more straightforwardly Husserlian sense – we observe that no matter what other interests we have, we are embodied beings. Everything we know about the world we encounter through our bodily receptors; everything that we do in the world is done by our bodies; and everything that we know about each other comes through seeing, hearing, touching or otherwise sensing each other (or reading or hearing our forms of communication). When our bodies fail, as the phenomenology of infertility shows, *we* are often perceived as failures and we shamefully perceive ourselves to be inadequate.

Understanding the phenomenology of our embodiment and bodily functions, and thus how we experience alterations in the shape, functioning, feeling, or very existence of our bodies, is required before we start trying to structure medical interactions with rules, principles, paradigms, or theories. I suggest that philosophers should not simply contribute a bag of problem-solving tricks to bioethics, but they should instead lead the effort to untangle and understand what it *means* for us to confront death, birth, illness, technology, and body-changing interventions in the many guises that contemporary medicine provides. Philosophers are particularly well suited to unravel such complicated issues, and there are no more profound or interesting philosophical questions than the meaning of life and the meaning of death; it is unfortunate that so many of us shy away from the search for deep meaning and focus instead on isolated problems.

A Different Metaphor

I would like to close by offering a new metaphor for philosophical contributions to bioethics. While Daniels's war metaphor isn't entirely inappropriate to describe some professional carrying-on, I think we ethicists might be able to structure our work around a more positive image.

Imagine, if you will, a house with doors in the front and back. When you open the front door, what is the first room you see? In most houses, the front door leads to a formal foyer or a living-room; most often, this is where the nicest furniture is kept, the exotic trinkets are on display, and the kids and dogs are forbidden. The front room is the place where company is entertained and formal parties are staged. Strangers knock at the front door; salespeople, canvassers, and religious missionaries present their scripted pitches here. The front door is the formal entry, allowing those who enter to see the orderly, carefully organized front room, often at some distance from the reality of life in the rest of the busy household. It is a beautiful room with colour-coordinated accessories, elegant lines, and a crisp coherence.

Now imagine the back door. It usually opens into the kitchen – busier, messier, and often downright chaotic. The back door is the one through which the household lives and functions, since it connects to the driveway or garage for unloading groceries or carpools and is the door through which muddy children and pets are allowed to enter. The kitchen itself shows the signs of life and sustenance: food is prepared here, the dirty dishes might pile up, and there is a garbage bin under the sink. (You would not normally keep garbage in the living room.) Strangers do not come to the back door; the only people supposed to knock there are friends and neighbours. People who come to the back door are more likely than strangers at the front to have a cup of tea at the breakfast table, to nibble on the leftover dessert, and to have an informal chat with the resident. Having a chat in the kitchen is not at all the same thing as entertaining company in the formal living-room; it is the long and personal sharing of information in a relationship, not merely the passage of time in witty small talk or strained politeness. The back door symbolizes not just informality, but intimacy; in comparison, the front door feels formal and cold.

Now, what does any of this have to do with bioethics? I suggest that there are metaphorical front and back doors into understanding life experiences and medical interventions. We typically approach discussions in bioethics by using formal principles and a priori concepts like autonomy, beneficence, justice, and utility. Such principles might be considered the 'front door' approach: the discussion is formal and orderly, seeking tidy policies and clean resolutions to problems. Elegance and coherence, whether in a theory or in the tasteful decoration of the living-room, are both useful and delightful.

However, some people get carried away with coherence and elegance. Some interior designers, for example, have a signature 'look' and will transform your living room into a unique but unmistakable example of their work. While the final result may be unarguably beautiful, you may have felt frustrated when the family pictures were removed and a painting that you dislike was hung over the sofa because it made a statement. Too bad that it wasn't your statement. I think some philosophers are guilty of the same overexuberance. Rather than identifying the unique values and experiences at stake in a particular setting – distinguishing infertility from cancer, or medicine from journalism – they breeze in with their theoretical sample books, make the place over, and construct the solutions in their own image. While wonderful for their portfolios, and not uninteresting for the rest of us to study, the final result may nevertheless miss the critical elements of the problem for which they were consulted. When someone's life is at stake, such conceit is clearly inappropriate.

Rather than emphasizing treatment categories and a priori principles, perhaps we ought to listen to patients' stories, reflect on the meaning of their situation, and respond with care to their underlying needs. Bioethics routinely confronts highly personal and philosophically profound questions about the meanings of life, death, and embodiment. Such basic questions are not easily captured in formal principles or categories, and they require time to take shape in description and understanding. While principles can tell us how to manage a technology, for example, the narrative gives far better insight into whether a technology addresses the problem in the first place. In other words, rather than stiffly admiring the formal elegance near the front door, or worse yet redecorating someone's living room to suit our own image, we ought to go to the back door and sit down with the patients over a cup of tea long enough to learn what actually is at stake for them.

I do not intend the metaphorical house to represent a theory, a theorist, or any other particular element of moral reasoning. Instead, think of it simply as a setting that establishes an attitude and the degree of honesty and perception with which we conduct our ethical deliberations. In the hospital setting, these attitudes are reflected in different characterizations of a bioethicist as a clinical stranger who has no idea what goes in medical settings, an intrusive academic who rearranges the hospital beds to group patients according to theoretical problem categories, and a philosophically reflective person who sits at the patient's bedside to listen, explore, and reflect upon various points of view before offering an ethical recommendation.

I advocate going through the back door not simply as a metaphor, but as a practical strategy: my best interview with an infertility patient lasted for over three hours while we sat – you guessed it – in her kitchen. Occasionally we were interrupted by her two-year-old son, a product of IVF. It was she who first explained to me in painful, honest, and reflective detail what it was like to have a wonderful child who still could not relieve the sting of her infertility. At the time, she was in the first trimester of a spontaneous pregnancy, and after years of infertility treatments and involvement in patient support groups, she had only recently realized how important 'doing it herself' was to her feeling normal, healthy, and truly womanly. My studied but inexperienced theoretical categories began to fade into the background as the changed and nuanced perceptions of greater experience accumulated. I realized that the moral status of embryos, rights to use IVF, and allocation decisions prompted extremely interesting bioethical debates that entirely missed the point of this woman's problem. Her child from IVF, as wonderful as he was, could not provide the cure she needed; meanwhile, few other avenues of support or understanding were available to her and are not available for most infertile people now. Beneficence requires us to respond to suffering, but the technological response to infertility that we have chosen to emphasize is inadequate; most of us are too busy debating IVF policy, however, to recognize this failing or to look for alternatives.

Perhaps it is time for bioethicists to defect from the war of high and low theorists; philosophers argue enough as it is. Perhaps instead we should open the back door, put on the kettle, and *listen* to the stories of the people whose bodies we are fighting over.

Notes

1 For example, definitions of 'femininity' usually exclude hairy legs, menstruation, and even the endurance and strength of labour and delivery – all decidedly womanly traits that are familiar to most women. Describing the lived reality of being female shows the limitations of definitions generated by mere observation by outsiders, who in this case are males. Works that have been especially influential for me in this regard have been Emily Martin, *The Woman in the Body: A Cultural Analysis of Reproduction* (Boston: Beacon Press, 1987), which contrasts women's descriptions of bodily experiences such as menstruation, pregnancy, labour, and menopause with descriptions found in medical texts; Dale Spender *Man-Made Language*, 2nd ed. (NY: Routledge and Kegan Paul, 1985) for examples of femininity and other male-female terminology differences; and commentary on Spender by Jean Grimshaw, *Philosophy and Feminist Thinking* (Minneapolis: University of Minnesota Press, 1986), especially chapter 3, 'Experience and Reality,' pp. 75–103.
2 See, for example, Richard Zaner, *Ethics and the Clinical Encounter* (Englewood Cliffs NJ: Prentice Hall, 1988); Howard Brody, *Stories of Sickness* (New Haven, CT: Yale University Press, 1987), and Warren T. Reich, 'The Case of the White Oaks Boy,' *Seminars in Perinatology* Special Issue: *Caring for Life in the First of It: Moral Paradigms for Perinatal and Neonatal Ethics* Vol. 11, No. 3, pp. 279–87.
3 Eric J. Cassell, *The Nature of Suffering and the Goals of Medicine* (NY: Oxford, 1991); S. Kay Toombs, *The Meaning of Illness: A Phenomenological Account of the Different Perspectives of Physician and Patient* (Boston: Kluwer, 1993). See also Elaine Scarry, *The Body in Pain: The Making and Unmaking of the World* (New York: Oxford, 1985), which describes pain as an element of torture.
4 Toombs, *Meaning of Illness*, p. xi.
5 Ibid., p. xii.
6 Benjamin F. Crabtree and William L. Miller, 'Primary Care Research: A Multimethod Typology and Qualitative Road Map,' in Crabtree and Miller (ed), *Doing Qualitative Research* (Newbury Park, CA: Sage, 1992), pp. 24–5. The edited volume is directed towards primary care physicians, who tend to do quantitative rather than qualitative research.
7 See, for example, Sue Wendell, 'Toward a Feminist Theory of Disability,' in Helen Bequaert Holmes and Laura Purdy (eds), *Feminist Perspectives in Medical Ethics* (Bloomington: Indiana University Press, 1992), pp. 63–81.

8 Patricia Benner, 'The Role of Experience, Narrative, and Community in Skilled Ethical Comportment,' *Advances in Nursing Science* Vol. 14, No. 2 (1991), p. 2.

9 Jan Marta, 'Narrative Approaches to Bioethics: An Overview,' unpublished paper.

10 Rita Kielstein and Hans-Martin Sass, 'Using Stories to Assess Values and Establish Medical Directives,' *Kennedy Institute of Ethics Journal* Vol. 3, No. 3 (September 1993), pp. 303–25.

11 Crabtree and Miller, *Doing Qualitative Research* pp. 5–6. Four other methods are field research, document-historical, survey, and experiment. Survey and experiment are primarily quantitative, field research is primarily qualitative, and document-historical is mixed.

12 Ibid., p. 5.

13 Howard Brody, 'Philosophic Approaches,' in Crabtree and Miller, *Doing Qualitative Research*, p. 182.

14 Ibid., pp. 177–8.

15 Valerie Gilchrist, 'Key Informant Interviews,' in Crabtree and Miller, *Doing Qualitative Research*, pp. 86–7.

16 Congregation for the Docrtrine of the Faith, *Instruction on Respect for Human Life in Its Origin and on the Dignity of Procreation* (Vatican City, 1987).

   A practical method around the objection is to use GIFT (gamete intrafallopian transfer), in which retrieved eggs and sperm are transferred to the fallopian tube so that fertilization can occur inside the body. The Vatican's objections to masturbation and contraception can be avoided by using a fenestrated condom: the couple engage in intercourse using a condom with holes poked in it. Some sperm may escape the condom to allow natural conception, and the rest of the sperm may be taken to the laboratory for washing and later transfer to the woman's reproductive tract.

   A note about the political history of this document is reported by Dr Georgeanna Jones, one of the founders of the Jones Institute in Norfolk VA, who testified to the Vatican review committee on the use of IVF. The first ten of the twelve cardinals on the panel approved of IVF as a procedure. The eleventh member, Cardinal Caffarra, argued that separating conception from sex in IVF would require rethinking the entire body of Vatican teachings on sexuality, abortion, contraception, and homosexuality, and thus would not be acceptable. The twelfth cardinal agreed that IVF might precipitate such massive rethinking, and suggested that it might be time to conduct such a project. Cardinal Caffarra was a close associate of Pope John Paul II, however, and his minority view became the endorsed statement from the Vatican. The transcripts of the proceedings were not published, unlike the proceedings of most similar inquiries. Georgeanna Seegar Jones, personal communication, August 1988.

17 January–November 1990, supported by a grant from the ITT Corporation awarded through the Fulbright competition. Prior to this fellowship year, one month was spent

in residence at the Howard and Georgeanna Jones Institute of Reproductive Medicine, Norfolk, VA, in August 1988.

18 Aline Zoldbrod, *Men, Women and Infertility: Intervention and Treatment Strategies* (Toronto: Maxwell Macmillan, 1993) summarizes the available research in a unique scholarly book geared towards clinical counsellors and practitioners, with guidance for treatment exercises to assist patients in overcoming their psychological distress.

19 Counsellors who work with infertility patients frequently note that infertile persons go through stages of grief and recovery much like those Elisabeth Kübler-Ross described for people with terminal illnesses and those who are mourning a death. Infertility is a life crisis, and as such causes the same sorts of feelings and response patterns as other life crises do. A composite analysis of infertility coping includes stages of surprise, denial, anger, isolation, guilt, grief, and finally acceptance. Various authors present different numbers of stages, sometimes in different orders. In infertility, as with other grieving and coping processes, patients tend to shift among the stages, sometimes experience more than one at a time, and sometimes revert to previous stages believed to have been resolved or passed. Progression to acceptance thus should not be characterized as a linear process with a set timetable.

See Elisabeth Kübler-Ross, *On Death and Dying* (New York: Macmillan, 1969); Barbara Eck Menning, 'The Emotional Needs of Infertile Couples,' *Fertility and Sterility* Vol. 34, No. 4 (October 1980), pp. 313–19; Constance Hoenk Shapiro, 'The Impact of Infertility on the Marital Relationship,' *Social Casework: The Journal of Contemporary Social Work* (September 1982), pp. 387–93; Ada Armstrong, 'The Experience of Infertility: The Needs of Infertile People and the Place of a Self-Help Initiative in Western Australia,' in Patricia Harper and Jan Aitken (eds), *A Child Is Not the Cure for Infertility: National Workshop on Infertility, Report of Proceedings* September 1981 (Melbourne: Institute of Family Studies, The Citizen's Welfare Service of Victoria, 1982), pp. 15–18; Fact Sheet #9, 'Infertility and Our Feelings,' available from CONCERN, PO Box 108, Milson's Point, NSW 2061.

20 Patient interview, Sydney, April 1990.

21 Psychologist Victor Callan notes a higher-than-normal likelihood of an external locus of control among IVF patients compared with the general population. Victor J. Callan and John F. Hennessey, 'Strategies for Coping with Infertility,' *British Journal of Medical Psychology* Vol. 62 (1989), p. 350.

22 Patient interview response.

23 Sandra Lee Bartky, *Femininity and Domination* (New York: Routledge, 1990), p. 86.

24 Patient survey response.

25 Barbara Eck Menning, *Infertility: A Guide for Childless Couples* (Englewood Cliffs, NJ: Prentice Hall, 1977), pp. 118–19.

26 Patient survey response.

27 Marta Kirejczyk and Irma van der Ploeg argue, I think rightly, that reconceptualizing

infertility as a 'disease of couples' allowed IVF to be redefined as a therapy for male infertility. As long as the 'couple' gets pregnant, it does not matter who undergoes the treatments or bears the burden of risk. Marta Kirejczyk and Irma van der Ploeg, 'Pregnant Couples: Medical Technology and Social Constructions around Fertility and Reproduction,' *Issues in Reproductive and Genetic Engineering* Vol 5, No. 2 (1992), pp. 113–25.

28 See J.E. Veevers, 'Voluntary Childlessness: A Review of Issues and Evidence,' *Marriage and Family Review* 2 (1979), pp. 1–26, as cited by Victor Callan, *Choices about Children* (Melbourne: Longman Cheshire Pty Ltd, 1979), p. 15.

29 Jeremy Laurance, 'The Moral Pressure to Have Children,' *New Society* (5 August, 1982), pp. 216–18; Diane Houghton and Peter Houghton, *Coping with Childlessness* (London: Allen and Unwin, 1984), p. 45.

30 Kay Oke and Jenny Blood, social workers at Royal Women's Hospital Human Reproduction Unit, interview, 23 and 28 February 1990. See also F.A. Beach, *Hormones and Behaviour* (New York: n.p., 1948), p. 238, quoted in Germaine Greer, *Sex and Destiny* (New York: Harper and Row, 1984), pp. 38, 47. Beach lists the three separable elements of sexuality as libido, potency, and fertility.

31 Patient interview responses.

32 Houghton and Houghton, *Coping with Childlessness*, chapter 8, esp. pp. 91–7. Quotes are from two different male patients, p. 92.

33 Jan Aitken, unpublished papers and personal communication; also Harper and Aitken, *A Child Is Not the Cure for Infertility*.

34 Henry Wellsmore, 'Counselling in a Fertility Centre,' Lingard Fertility Centre, Newcastle, NSW.

35 Zoldbrod, ch. 11, *Men, Women and Infertility*, 'Medical Treatment as Rape: Sexual Problems as an Aftermath of Treatment for Infertility,' pp. 189–204. Zoldbrod argues that the perception of medical treatment as rape is not an actual rape, and thus is not a criminal form of assault by the practitioners. Rather, the woman may subjectively *experience* the painful interventions upon and repeated observations of her genitalia, especially under circumstances when she feels out of control, as a form of sexual assault. The distress of the gynecological intervention is worsened by a sense of blaming the victim, because she brought herself in for this treatment. Women who undergo repeated infertility or other gynecological interventions thus may experience emotional and sexual problems similar to those commonly experienced by rape victims.

36 Several international reviews of new reproductive technologies have criticized clinicians for inadequate testing for safety and efficacy. See, for example, World Health Organization, *Consultation on the Place of IVF in Infertility Care* (Geneva: WHO, 1990); Royal Commission on New Reproductive Technologies, *Final Report: Proceed with Care* (Ottawa, Canada: 1993); and National Health and Medical Research

Council, *Consultation Document: Long-Term Effects on Women from Assisted Conception* (Canberra, Australia, 1995).

37 Menning, *Infertility*, p. 316.

38 This story came from one of five patient support group members interviewed in an evening-long discussion in Brisbane in May 1990. She had experienced severe emotional and physical reactions to the hormone injections, as well as a punctured bladder from the trans-vaginal egg retrieval procedure. Not only was this an unsuccessful IVF cycle, but she suffered a severe peritoneal infection and lingering incontinence. Her self-descriptions focused on her 'weakness' and inability to try another treatment cycle, rather than on feelings of disgust, anger, fear, or regret that one might expect to hear under such circumstances.

Lindsey Napier, a social worker who founded the Concern NSW support group while undergoing her own infertility treatments in the 1980s, wanted to provide a safe place for patients to evaluate their options and to seek information about the emerging technologies. She left the group after several years, when it became clear to her that her original purpose had been subverted; the support group often did not support genuine choices, but instead supported renewed energies to keep trying and served as a pro-technology advocacy group. The psychological burden of choosing to end treatment seems to be too enormous even for groups to manage effectively. See also her published reflections, 'The Barren Desert Flourishes in Many Ways: From Infertility to In-Fertility,' in Renate Klein (ed.), *Infertility: Women Speak Out* (London: Pandora, 1989), pp. 188–98.

39 Patricia Harper and Jan Aitken (eds) *A Child Is Not the Cure for Infertility*. The phrase originated in the paper presented by an infertility patient at the conference. Aitken, a counsellor in private practice in Melbourne, has expounded upon the observation in several unpublished manuscripts and conference papers.

40 Patient response to written survey at Royal Women's Hospital, Melbourne, Australia; project by Belinda Leung, 1989 (unpublished). See also the post-counselling insights described by Lindsey Napier in her written account cited above.

Good Bioethics Must Be Feminist* Bioethics

LAURA M. PURDY

> Magicians know to keep the audience's attention away from the actions.
> But moral philosophers may be magicians who have tricked even them-
> selves ...
>
> Virginia L. Warren, 'Feminist Directions in Medical Ethics'[1]

Several years ago a leading bioethics journal asked me to review a paper on how physicians should deal with severely hydrocephalic fetuses. The paper carefully considered the fetus's interests, the role of the physician, the impact of the decision on society as a whole. I kept waiting for the author to notice the fetus's location inside a woman and to recognize that she has interests and perhaps even rights. He never did.[2]

If this kind of experience were an anomaly, bioethics would already be feminist. Unfortunately, it is not an anomaly and bioethics is not feminist. Quite the contrary: it is routine for women's interests to be discounted or ignored altogether. Recent feminist work documents and analyzes this phenomenon.[3] Sexism has been most apparent in reproductive matters, where, for example, plenty of work on abortion still proceeds without any reference to women's concerns; and when the new reproductive technologies were beginning to burst upon the scene some fifteen years ago, their possible impact on women seemed to be the last thing on anybody's mind.[4] Now, despite the voluminous feminist literature dealing with them, the mainstream debate seldom reflects the issues raised by this literature.

As both feminism and bioethics mature, feminists are looking beyond repro-

---

*And Allied Liberationist

duction, not only at other specific issues in bioethics, but at the field as a whole. After all, bioethics is supposed to critique the health care system, so why does it fail to see so much that is wrong? For example, where was bioethics before it became common knowledge that medical research often fails to include women? Or that it concentrates on problems that plague men?[5] How could we have been so oblivious to the gender differences in physician–patient relationships, differences that lead doctors to suppose that women need tranquilizers when the same symptoms in a man suggest a heart workup?[6] Why is it that men's views about withdrawal of care are so much more likely to be taken seriously?[7] Why, too, has it taken so long for bioethics to notice when allocation decisions leave women providing the brunt of the care?[8]

As the magnitude and pervasiveness of such gender differentials come into focus, feminist philosophers have also started to analyze the overall structure of bioethics. Many of us are coming to suspect, as Susan Sherwin argues, that 'the organization of bioethics reflects the power structures that are inherent in the health care field, which in turn reflects the power structures of the larger society' (p. 3). It hardly needs saying that despite considerable progress for women in recent years, men – mostly white, middle-class, heterosexual men – still are in charge, both in society generally and in the medical profession, and consciously or subconsciously they choose social arrangements that reflect their perceived interests. Even worse, individual practitioners may still be gripped by common sexist – even misogynist – attitudes for which medical education currently provides no antidote.[9]

The results for white women and members of other less powerful groups can be devastating. Sexist health care, for example, can rob women of physicians' respect, deprive us of safe and effective therapies, deny us the kind of birthing experiences we value, drug us into resignation at life's injustices, legitimize violence towards us, even undermine our last wishes about how to die. Consequently, we may be deprived of the kind of control over how we live that men take for granted. Although some writers question the value of such control, it is essential for the welfare of second-class citizens in societies where there is little support for positive rights.[10] An uncritical bioethics tolerates this outcome.

Bioethics is an offshoot of ethics. Academic ethics is not in the business of moral reform: it would be a waste of our beautifully trained minds for us, qua philosophers, to spend our time exhorting others to behave morally – although it may behoove us to do so, as citizens, in our spare time. It seems fully appropriate, however, for us to attend to and publicize inconsistencies in society's professed values, as well as to devote ourselves to investigating moral problems connected with equality. Yet such work has constituted only a relatively small part of the discipline of ethics, which for the most part has been preoccupied either with arcane metaethical questions or with what it regards as broader practical matters.[11]

Although this emphasis might surprise a Martian, a sociological understanding of the liberal arts generally helps explain how it might come about. It is, after all, the relatively well to do who are able to spend their lives in such delightful speculation, and few are willing to risk undermining their own psychological comfort by focusing on the moral environment that makes it possible. Indeed, the history of ethics seems to confirm this insight, since generally it either has turned a blind eye to the kinds of inequalities that now seem so apparent, or, worse still, has actively propagated them.[12] Certainly contemporary ethics usually leaves it up to feminists to bring concern for gender justice to discussions.[13]

Despite its birth in the radical 1960s, bioethics has for the most part followed its parent's example. Analyses sensitive to gender and other markers of disadvantage often have been rejected as uninteresting, bad scholarship, biased, ideological, or 'political,' thus having no place in a serious intellectual endeavor like bioethics.

This rejection has been especially pointed where gender is at issue.[14] It has been difficult for feminist voices to be heard on particular topics. The question of the relationship between feminism and established bioethics theory is still relatively uncharted territory. Feminism is, after all, but one of a number of possible perspectives from which one might approach issues in bioethics. The existence of such diverse perspectives raises the question whether there is a 'right' one (or a group of 'right' ones), or whether we are doomed to irreducible disagreement where they diverge.

My question here is whether there is anything so compelling about a feminist outlook that it must be included in bioethics. This question is meant neither to exclude concern with other socially debilitating markers, nor to imply that gender injustice is always the most urgent concern. Gender is not, *of course*, the only subordinating marker in western societies and is not necessarily the worst handicap in every situation. Furthermore, there is a hierarchy of values that hits individuals with more than one such marker particularly hard. So, despite the existence of pervasive sexism, some women are still better off than some men, and some persons of either sex are better off than other members of their sex. For this reason rectifying gender injustice need not always be our first priority, even if *awareness* of gender and the difference it makes is always crucial.

To begin, we need to know precisely what 'feminism' is, as all those to whom I have explained my project have immediately pointed out. Some still seem unsure of basic feminist theses; others, more abreast of recent controversies, wonder how one might fix upon a single feminist viewpoint.[15] In this paper I try to distinguish core theses of feminism from more debatable positions, which may be either theoretical views or positions on specific issues, such as contract pregnancy. Because they are still the subject of serious debate among feminists, it would be premature for bioethics to absorb them. However, I shall argue that what I call 'core feminism' is essential for bioethics.

Core Feminism

At the heart of all feminism – except perhaps the most aggressively deconstructionist theories – are two simple judgments. First, women are, as a group, worse off than men because their interests routinely fail to be given equal consideration. Second, that state of affairs is unjust and should be remedied. As Valerie Bryson writes, 'even in the most "advanced" nations, it remains true that positions of public power are overwhelmingly held by men; meanwhile women as a group continue to work much longer hours than men (particularly within the home) and to receive far less financial reward, while fear of sexual violence restricts their lives and they are denied full control over their own reproduction.'[16] In poorer countries, a woman's lot is often still worse in comparison with that of her male compatriots.

Some details of core feminism themselves are a matter of serious disagreement among feminists. The disagreement begins with how best to describe the ways women are worse off, and how much worse off they are. Are women discriminated against? Oppressed? Enslaved? Is the problem that they are not viewed as Kantian persons? That they are not accorded equal treatment? That their interests don't count? How bad is the problem? Are most men simply thoughtless and unaware of the issues, as some liberals assert, or are men so hostile that they would like to see women eradicated from the earth, as some radicals seem to think? Also in dispute is women's basic nature and hence the proper goals and strategies of feminism. Are women and men 'really' different? If so, then it would seem that feminism's goal ought to be validating our differences and making sure that women are as well off as men. Or are we really quite alike by nature, so the problem is to relieve women *and* men of the socialization that seems to leave us so different? Or is the truth somewhere in between?

It is understandable that even well-meaning outsiders are put off by the sometimes bitter debates about such points – sometimes I myself am. It is crucial to keep in mind, however, that they are often more academic than practical, and although their existence is sometimes taken as sufficient reason for rejecting feminism altogether, that hardly seems sensible. Disagreements about how best to liberate slaves hardly undermines the judgment that they ought to be liberated. Likewise, given the extent, pervasive nature, and consequences of unwarranted gender assumptions, it would surely be foolish to suppose that it is evident in every case how to deal with them. Widespread feminist consciousness is but a newborn in the family of ethical debate, and there is every reason to expect a fruitful maturity to be preceded by tumultuous adolescence.

How would I lay out core feminism? Many people, both men and women, still conceive of women as incomplete persons, individuals who, in Kantian terms, do not share in human dignity, since they are not capable of autonomously chosen life plans. Like Aristotle and Rousseau, they conceive of women primarily as servants whose role is to nurture others. Thus there is nothing immoral about systematically subordinating women's interests to the interests of others when they conflict. The consequences range from infanticide and starvation for little Indian girls, to more subtle forms of loss for western women. As Bryson and others point out, women, even in North America, are disproportionately absent from positions of public power and prestige, work longer hours than men for less pay, are often denied sexual and reproductive freedom, and are subject to violence from men.[17]

I suspect that the most fruitful approach to developing a more extensive notion of core feminism would proceed by emphasizing the importance of such equal consideration of interests. Equal consideration of interest would mean that women's interests would count as heavily as those of men and, where the two come into conflict, would be taken to outweigh those interests at least half the time. Such calculations would be made more complicated by the need to weight interests, with a more pressing interest sometimes trumping several less pressing ones.

This formal demand for equality constitutes the central notion of core feminism. It requires that any moral inquiry be alert to gender-related differences in treatment or outcome, that such differences be minimized or thoroughly justified, and that women's welfare be considered as important as that of men where their interests are in conflict. Fair-minded thinkers can hardly object to this approach. Nor could they reasonably object to certain attempts to flesh out the principle in particular situations. Thus, for example, how could it be moral to accept or promote social arrangements that put women, but not men, at risk of impoverishment if they choose to bear children?

What constitutes equal consideration of women's interests, however, is much less clear in many other cases. Thus, for instance, it may be as yet unknowable whether permitting paid contract pregnancy so undermines women's status that it should be prohibited, as some radicals claim. We should, in any case, be pointing out the exploitive conditions to which women are currently subjected. Fleshing out and testing such judgments will have to be an interdisciplinary enterprise. It depends, after all, on empirical judgments about the lives of women and men and on the ethical analysis of those judgments. The former fall primarily within the realm of the social sciences; the latter falls within moral philosophy.

Despite such uncertainties I would argue that there are even now many clear cases where, without justification, women's interest are accorded less weight than a man's interest in the same circumstance, to women's serious detriment.[18] We do not always need perfect understanding to clean up such cases; surely it is often possible to improve situations, even if settling them fully must await further insight.

Some theories about how society should be ordered are diametrically opposed to this approach, recommending hierarchical rather than egalitarian social and political arrangements. Aristotle, for example, thought he had reason to subject women and some men to the rule of other men. His arguments are clearly inadequate and I doubt that many contemporary thinkers would defend him on these issues. In any case, there are many different possible kinds of hierarchical theories, and presumably not all of them would justify subordinating women.

What is more interesting – and troubling – is the failure of more apparently egalitarian theorists, such as Locke, Rousseau, and Rawls, to notice the gender inequality implied by their views. In particular, in their more applied sections these writers tend to take families rather than individuals as basic, thus incorporating the public/private distinction and all the inequitable assumptions built into it. Excellent feminist work is being done on these theories, and there is no need for me to repeat it here.[19] Yet such work is often rejected in principle. This shows that core feminism and the claim of injustice inherent in it must be evaluated at a very basic level.

Objections to Core Feminism

What can be said against core feminism? Recall that core feminism says that women's interests unjustly are accorded less weight than those of men. So core feminism may be thought to go wrong in two basic ways. First, it may claim falsely that women's interests are not given equal consideration – that is, the first claim of core feminism is false. Second, although opponents may concede the point about women's interests, they may hold that this state of affairs is justifiable – a denial, that is, of the second claim of core feminism. Michael Levin takes the first path, sociobiologists often take the second.[20] I take it that the evidence for the first claim of core feminism is overwhelming,[21] and that any decent moral theory would accept the second.

Are there methological reasons for rejecting these apparently unexceptionable claims? Let us start with the judgment that women's interests are systematically discounted. What kind of claim is that? It is a mixed claim, partly moral and partly empirical. The empirical data are appropriately gathered by social science and are relatively unproblematic. If one were skeptical about the validity of social science methods, then one would have to be equally skeptical of the denial of core feminism. More controversial is the choice of what data to gather, given differing opinions about what categories are relevant. Thus Michael Levin disagrees with Bryson, contending that 'women in Western society are better off than men by every objective measure of well-being. Women live longer, enjoy better health, are less prone to insanity, alcoholism, drug abuse, and crime' (p. 7). Evaluating such contradictory positions involves a decision about what factors are most important in a good life, as well as understanding the relevant causal relationships.[22] For example, if women lack full control over their fertility, how should we rank the consequences for their welfare, and how do they compare with the factors that lead more men to become criminals?

Are there any grounds upon which this general enterprise might be rejected? The causal claims and the statistical measurements lean toward the empirical end of the spectrum. The investigations that lead to them may be relatively value free, as we have seen, although the decision about what questions to investigate is not. Doubts about specific conclusions might appropriately be raised as questions about a researcher's standards of evidence, or even her honesty. If that is really what is at issue, however, it should be discussed in those terms, not dismissed as somehow 'political.'

To judge by some comments, political contamination is so fearsome that the only acceptable motivation for research is idle curiosity. But the disinterest in human affairs suggested by that motivation is as political in its way as research motivated by concern defined as political, since it suggests either that the status quo is fine (since there is no pressing need to do the research necessary for evaluating it), or that any state of affairs would be fine (no matter how dreadful).

Such dismissal is especially unconvincing where the word 'political' is left undefined – as it usually is in these discussions. 'Political' has become a derogatory term, but its use should not lead us to reject positions without further justification. In any case, it is *issues* that are political, not positions with respect to them. Whatever 'political' is taken to mean, those who espouse one position with respect to a particular issue have no case for rejecting a different position with respect to it on the grounds that it is political. Yet this happens again and again as the unequal status quo is defined as neutral but criticisms of it are defined as 'political.'

So far we have been considering the epistemological status of the core feminist claim that women's interests are not accorded equal consideration. What now of the judgment that this state of affairs is unjust? Surely this is a paradigmatic moral judgment; discussion of the merits of hierarchy is or should be, after all, a central issue in ethics. The philosophical lever that motivates and requires it is clear for any approach that takes universalizability for granted: unequal treatment must be justified by morally relevant reasons. So what grounds might there be for asserting some philosophical impropriety here, that the debate is, after all, merely 'political'?

Perhaps questioning the assertion that women exist to nurture and serve is the sticking point – but isn't the discussion of human ends a properly moral question? Or perhaps the tender nerve is the sacred public/private distinction so closely tied to that conception of women's nature. Proponents of the traditional public/private distinction wouldn't want to have to concede that is merely a political (as opposed to a moral) arrangement, that is, one based on power rather than right. Nor can they have it both ways: either the so-called private world is a moral arrangement, in which case reasoned criticism of it must be moral talk, too, or it is a power-based arrangement, a fact that undermines their objection to allegedly political assaults on it. What feminists require here is, after all, moral consistency. Behavior that is regulated or prohibited in the public sphere among men now often may be visited upon women in the so-called private sphere with impunity. If the public/private distinction is moral, then this discrepancy requires justification. Attempting to deflect moral attention from the fact by calling criticism 'political' suggests reluctance to put at women's disposal the instruments men count on for fair adjudication of conflicts.

In short, I believe that the epithet 'political' is an attempt to preserve the domestic realm and gender matters in general from moral scrutiny. These issues are almost uniquely threatening to men's personal lives; in the worst cases, those lives are predicated on assumptions about women and justice that couldn't pass muster in a first-year course on critical thinking. Among them are the understanding that a wife will attend to children and household in order to free up the man for more socially valuable pursuits, that she will follow him wherever his career leads, and that because he provides most or all of the outside income that his wishes and desires will prevail.

A clear view of this matter would explain the emotional reactions feminist work evokes. I can't help but think back to what happened some fifteen years ago when I proposed introducing a feminism course at the small women's college where I teach. My course description was anything but inflammatory: 'An examination of the justifications proposed for different positions regarding women's role in society, including consideration of specific moral and political problems raised by such debate, such as reproductive rights, and equality in the workplace.' With nothing more to go on than this rather drab description, and apparently no interest in hearing more, my colleagues asserted, among other things, that the students would be cheated by such a course, and that it was inappropriate for a women's college. I was also asked to reassure the group that I wouldn't be indoctrinating my students. Perhaps these colleagues thought feminism means man-hating, or believed that gender issues for some reason cannot be examined with the same rigor that characterizes good treatment of other issues in moral and political philosophy. Their hostility certainly prevented any discussion of their assumptions or mine.

Such events clearly communicate that, in the words of the classic dismissal, gender is 'not a topic.' Since it clearly is a topic in the empirical sense, what is really being conveyed here is that it is an unworthy topic. Why is it unworthy? Well, of course gender, like race and so forth, is, alas, merely a particular concern, whereas philosophy is confined to the universal. However, a glance at the history of philosophy shows us that philosophers have been preoccupied with both kinds of question.[23] Why should this issue engender such emotion unless it has a deeper meaning? Moreover, it would be inconsistent for bioethics to object to an approach it so clearly utilizes.

Core feminism focuses, in any case, on very broad issues. Remember that gender is not something only women have; so noticing gender is not simply studying women.[24] Core feminism is interested in the *relationship* between women and men: what could be more universal? How is it different from studying relationships between men who fall into different categories – say, patients and physicians? Not only do these objections fail to make sense, but their obvious inadequacy once again suggests some other agenda.

If what I have said so far is right, then there is nothing epistemologically suspect about core feminism: core feminism is the expression of an ordinary moral judgment. There also is good reason for accepting it: both the statistics and the moral case for it are compelling.[25] 'Wait a minute!' some people will say; 'I'm convinced by your argument that there is in principle nothing objectionably political about core feminism, but I still see no reason to accept its premises.' Such people may hold that there is no evidence that women's interest are systematically subordinated. Or, they might believe that the disparities in question are justifiable.

As I have said, there is no space here to construct these arguments. Doubting or denying the first premise seems to me to be possible only by shutting one's eyes to the ubiquitous evidence. In any case, this level of skepticism logically implies equal doubt about the contradiction to core feminism's first premise. But when you are in such an unsettled state with respect to a belief, intellectual honesty requires that you consider evidence that could help you to make up your mind. You then must evaluate every case with any eye to possible unjust gender disparities. Even doubters must add the lens of gender to their thinking. There is not much that can be said to those who are convinced that no gender disparities exist, except what Wittgenstein exhorted in another context, 'Don't think, look!'[26]

What about those who doubt or deny core feminism's second premise? As before, doubters must be prepared to use gender analysis for testing arguments. Deniers generally hold untenable beliefs about human nature based on sociobiology or have an overly rigid conception of what it takes to keep human societies afloat.[27] They have a moral duty to reexamine their beliefs; otherwise they collude in an unfair system.

If the specific claims of core feminism are so unproblematic, why is the feminist project so often rejected in principle? Why do people claim that the issue is uninteresting, that feminist scholarship is shoddy, and/or that it is biased, ideological, or 'political'? In short, why is it thought to be intellectually disreputable, so that it need not be taken seriously by scholars? What problems and issues one finds interesting or uninteresting is surely a somewhat subjective matter, one that depends considerably on one's upbringing and situation. The question of social equality might be expected to be of substantial interest to those who have good grounds for thinking that their interests count less than those of members of other groups. Conversely, it is plausible to believe that those whose interests prevail more often will find this topic less gripping. The cynical interpretation of the claim that feminism is uninteresting is that it is the easy way to avoid challenges to one's own status. I feel some attraction to that interpretation.

One might also contend that core feminism is uninteresting because it simply aims to bring practice into line with our professed ideals, or because it raises no philosophically worthwhile questions.[28] The first version of this objection says that equal consideration for women's interests is uncontroversial: improving women's condition is merely a matter of changing behavior, not moral revolution. Unfortunately, however, many people are still obviously unconvinced of the thesis that women should be treated as equals, and the resistance to specific proposals for improvements in women's welfare by those who allege their commitment to this ideal is often so fierce as to raise doubts about their sincerity. Such resistance, of course, may be just evidence of a psychological block; but it might also signal deeper philosophical problems: persistent sexism in the work of those who intend to be egalitarian lends some support to this possibility. The second version of this objection betrays an excessively generalized and abstract conception of what constitutes worthwhile philosophy. It seems to hold that only the highest-level considerations are valuable and that lower-level work simply plays out the implications already contained in the higher. The image here is reminiscent of Thomas Kuhn's distinction between revolutionary science and normal science. But the attitude underestimates the difficulties inherent in and the value of a much lower-level work. Here, for example, taking new players into account both destabilizes old solutions and creates new quandaries.

What about the accusation of shoddy scholarship? That rejection of feminism seems no more solid. Of course there is shoddy feminist scholarship. Feminist scholarship may be shoddy because it is sloppy, ill thought out, unimaginative, poorly written, and so forth. Like all such scholarship, it should be ignored. But unless it can be shown that the core assumptions of feminism are unsound, the existence of shoddy scholarship is hardly grounds for rejecting the whole enterprise. Appalling metaphysics abounds, but nobody any longer suggests that we can do without metaphysics; the answer is to do it better.

A special problem with some feminist scholarship is that it argues for different standards of scholarship, contending that those in use are in some way biased. Such arguments not only threaten existing methods, but are especially difficult to mount, since they require people to pull themselves up by their own methodological bootstraps. Promising work is rarely perfect to start with, and the appropriate response to it is constructive criticism, not derision.[29]

Rejecting core feminism on the grounds that it is biased or ideological also is unreasonable. When accused of bias, many feminists who are not philosophers tend to retort that bias is universal.[30] This response fails to distinguish between bias and tenable points of view; it also undermines core feminism by flirting with the kind of malignant relativism that pulls the rug out from the assertions of injustice so central to feminism. In any case, unsubstantiated accusations of bias are suspect: intellectual honestly requires us to come to grips with positions and show how they go wrong.

To reject feminism on the grounds that it is ideological is equally untenable. It seems to me that the word is often used to describe philosophical systems one believes to be closed minded and unfalsifiable. Since we disagree about which we think these are, it would be preferable to describe all systems as 'philosophy' and do our evaluation of them via argumentation rather than value-laden terminology.

The last and most important objection to core feminism is that it is 'political,' and that good scholarship has no place for politics. The problem with this objection is that words like 'politics' and 'political' have come to be used in such a variety of ways that unless people stipulate how they are using them, it is not clear what they are objecting to. For example, *Webster's Ninth Collegiate Dictionary* gives the following different meanings for 'political': '1. Of or relating to government, a government, or the conduct of government; 2. Of, relating to, or involving politics, and especially party politics.' The *Oxford English Diction-*

ary also suggests: '3. Of, belonging, or pertaining to the state or body of citizens, its government and policy, especially in civil or secular affairs; public, civil, of or pertaining to science or art of politics. 4. Belonging to or taking a side in politics or in connexion with the party system of government; in a bad sense, partisan, factious.' Furthermore, *Webster's* adds under 'politics,' 'the total complex of relations between people in society.'

'Politics' and its cognates thus have radically different descriptive meanings. Worse yet, sometimes these terms are used in purely descriptive ways, but at others they are used in derogatory ways. We see something of these senses in (4) above. 'Political' can mean partisan. To be partisan is not necessarily to be biased, although the word can be used to imply bias. Bias can take several forms: leaping to conclusions on the basis of too little evidence or evidence of the wrong kind; ignoring evidence that undermines one's conclusion, and so forth. It also may imply the kind of bad faith that leads people to be less alert to or even knowingly to commit these errors. Another common assumption is that whereas moral argument involves reasoned discourse, political discourse is instead rhetoric that aims at making the weaker argument appear to be the stronger; or it is a mere epiphenomenon of power. Political discourse may also be rejected because it is motivated by anger, but of course even angry people may have good arguments.

Naturally, like 'politics,' many words have widely differing meanings, but the problem is that the context often leaves us in doubt about the subtleties of a given use. For example, consider Sherwin's comment that 'subordination of one group of persons by another is morally wrong as well as politically unjust.'[31] Precisely what distinction is she making here?

General rejections of the political in scholarship are still more puzzling.[32] Of course we should be avoiding biased, partisan work, but that scholarship should not be messing with government, party politics, civil affairs, or political philosophy are vastly different theses. Surely it is reasonable to demand that discussions about these matters be, first and foremost, clear, with well-defined terms. This is such a fundamental point, and the solution so obvious, that one can hardly avoid the suspicion that the obfuscation is intentional. One interim solution is to refuse wherever possible to use 'political.'

Ethics or Politics?

One way to limit the use of 'political' is to recognize how much it overlaps with the 'ethical' or 'moral.'[33] Some thinkers – including some pioneers in bioethics – seem to think that the scope of ethics is narrow and should be limited to immediate personal relationship, say, between doctor and patient or between nurse and doctor. But conceiving of ethics in this way cuts it off from broader structural issues. The model is some versions of act-utilitarianism that ignore universalizability as well as the subtler aspects of particular situations. Working in such a shrunken framework can be an interesting exercise and is often necessary for making decisions in an imperfect society. It is important to return always to the big picture, however, because only thus is it possible to see why some problems recur repeatedly.

Sticking to narrow contexts tends to support the status quo at the expense of human welfare. It fails to question why people find themselves in unfavorable circumstances, and it mindlessly applies what appear to be the relevant moral rules. Suppose, for example, that an individual physician, Sue, is trying to decide whether to do an abortion for Mary. If Sue accepts a narrow definition of health and believes that her job is to help Mary achieve health, she might conclude that it is inappropriate for her to do the abortion. Sue might also believe that social justice for women requires that women have access to abortion, however, and she knows that no other agency provides that service. Therefore she does the abortion for Mary. Sue's decision is, I would argue, a moral one, not exclusively a social or political one, even though it may be seen as transcending the traditional boundaries of medical ethics. Bioethical decision-making thus conceived ranges over all human activity, drawing upon both values embedded in the context of health care and those exemplified by broader moral principles.

My perspective closely reflects Ezekiel Emanuel's conception of the logical structure of bioethics. As he argues in *The Ends of Human Life*, the apparently 'endless irresolution' of specific problems in bioethics arises because the values intrinsic to health care cannot resolve the conflicts that arise within it. Instead, they demand recourse to broader principles of political philosophy, defined as that which 'is primarily concerned with the proper ends of human activities and what people should and should not do to realize those ends' (p. 13). He goes on to say: 'How we confront and resolve them will both reflect and affect our understanding of ourselves as human beings, of the good life, of social justice, of the proper way to care for the disabled, debilitated, and dying. Medical ethics is a measure of our own moral vision; these questions force us to articulate our ideals and values, our ethical understanding, and to assess their worthiness' (p. 4). According to him, the liberal political philosophy widely accepted in the United States discourages law and public policy from advancing particular notions of the good (p. 7). Hence, health care ethics reflects the splintered values of the political conceptions underlying it.[34]

Emanuel's general diagnosis makes sense; it is not clear, however, why these higher principles are principles of political philosophy rather than principles of plain old ethics. What is ethics, if not a discipline 'concerned with the proper ends of human activities and what people should and should not do to realize those ends'? Perhaps Emanuel sees judgments in political philosophy as those about which reasonable people may disagree, whereas moral judgments are those we are compelled by reason to accept. In my opinion, however, that approach would overestimate both the compelling nature of ethical judgments and the freedom from constraint inherent in political philosophy. So, although I believe that Emanuel has the general picture right, I think that we are unable to reach a consensus about many issues in bioethics because of the pluralism of our *moral* beliefs.

Achieving clarity about the boundaries and areas of overlap between the moral and the political realms seems in any case long overdue. It would makes sense to label as 'political' the theory that deals directly with government, but much of political theory does not. Most of the material in the political theory courses I took, for instance, could just as well have been labelled 'moral theory.' The lines seem even more blurred today when leading political theorists, such as Susan Moller Okin, Michael Walzer, and Emanuel himself, are so active in what it seems reasonable to call 'ethical' theory.

Clear thinking necessitates this kind of conceptual housekeeping. In its absence, dust and cobwebs infiltrate the scene, and we find it hard to see what is wrong with rejections of work as 'political.' Once the metaphysical Pledge has been applied, however, the primarily moral nature of the enterprise emerges. Positions seen by some as threatening can no longer be deprived of standing on allegedly epistemological grounds. That in turn forces the would-be moral gate-keepers to recognize and come to terms with radical challenges.

Thus we see clearly that ethics that turns a blind eye to particular forms of unfairness is broken and in need of repair. The tendency to discount women's interests is, as I have suggested, pervasive in bioethics: it requires constant vigilance to penetrate the apparently seamless discussions that leave no moral space for women, as did the paper on hydrocephalic fetuses. What is distinctive about bioethics is that women are especially at risk in the medical establishment: erroneous or self-interested assumptions about our bodies and minds are close to the surface, and the delivery of care is so value laden that it cannot help but reflect them. Bioethics that fails to be alert to women's vanishing interests is, whether intentionally or not, biased: it condones the promotion of all other interests at the expense of those of women. In short, there is no 'safe' neutral territory between biased bioethics and feminist bioethics.

Rethinking gender assumptions from scratch is a major undertaking. But because the issues are so much clearer in bioethics, it may be possible for those who think there is no gender injustice to confine their inquiries to that field. What, after all, do women want from the health care system? Like men, we want help in staying healthy. We want safe, effective, respectful therapies when we are ill or injured. In addition, because reproduction happens in our bodies, we also want help in carrying out our goals with respect to it. Other legitimate life goals also may require medical support. We generally want to keep on living as long as we are content with the quality of our lives. In dying, we want our wishes about that process respected, and we want no unnecessary pain or suffering. Practices that repeatedly leave women worse off with respect to these aims should be evidence enough of my contentions and should be targets for change.

Whither Feminist Bioethics?

I have been arguing that what distinguishes feminist from biased ethics is the premise that a woman's welfare is as important as anybody else's. Biased ethics turns a blind eye to women's needs even as it attends to the needs of others. Biased ethics fails to scrutinize denials of core feminism (and the equivalent cores for other disadvantaged groups) and is all too ready to accept attempts to justify discrimination and discrepancies in welfare.

Feminist ethics documents how existing practices harm women unfairly and unjustifiably, and it focuses on how to avoid such outcomes. Feminists, writes Alison Jaggar, 'seek to identify and challenge all those ways, overt but more often and more perniciously covert, in which western ethics has excluded women or rationalized their subordination. Its goal is to offer both practical guides to action and theoretical understandings of the nature of morality that do not, overtly or covertly, subordinate the interests of any woman or group of women to the interests of any other individual or group.'[35] I have argued that the moral minimum for those who wish to escape biased ethics is to recognize that because women and men are now so dissimilarly situated, even apparently gender-neutral principles may well affect them very differently.

Contrary to popular belief, this approach does not imply the determination to see gender bias everywhere. It does imply the resolve to root it out where it exists. Considering how oblivious people – including feminists – have been to even blatant instances of bias, our alertness to its more subtle manifestations is necessary, even if it strikes unsympathetic souls as a paranoid conviction that bias is everywhere.[36]

How to proceed? Enough good feminist bioethics exists to light the way for those of good will who are unsure of how to begin. The path is rocky, given the disputes among feminists alluded to earlier, but openness to the idea that traditional approaches are inadequate is a good start. Awareness of possible gender inequity is compatible with a variety of positions on the kinds of disparities that exist between women and men. Of course it will matter whether we are liberals who emphasize equality of opportunity or radicals more interested in welfare; whether we are reasonably optimistic about the potential for harmonious relations among humans or members of FINRRAGE. Those who start with such different assumptions will often reach different conclusions about particular issues, but active awareness of possible gender inequity will help set the framework for fruitful dialogue. The basic point is that checking for gender problems should become as integral to bioethics as is checking for spelling errors: just as we no longer let work 'go public' before passing it through a spell check program, it shouldn't appear without a gender check. If we attend to this, then, to the extent that the health care establishment takes bioethics seriously, the most obvious discrepancies in care will diminish.[37]

As I have suggested, we need to keep a weather eye out for possible gender injustice. But is that all there is to it? I'm not sure; it certainly is a start. What about the more sophisticated and demanding recommendations coming from new feminist work in bioethics? Both Sherwin and Warren emphasize how sexist ostensibly neutral theories can be. From there they go off in different directions, although their suggestions intersect at some points. Warren distinguishes between substance and process, arguing that in both we need to become more sensitive to male perspectives that we now take as the whole story.[38] For example, she believes that such a perspective concentrates on situations where competition is a central element, or it focuses on their competitive aspects; inquiries are often transformed into a power struggle. Sherwin argues that feminist bioethics requires of us a new attention to context, reconsiders the nature and importance of basic moral concepts, such as relationships and character, and always keeps the political dimension in mind.

Eradicating unjust gender discrepancies in bioethics will certainly entail some fundamental rethinking. We shall have to pay close attention both to what problems we address and to the ways we deal with them; we shall certainly have to reanalyze basic concepts and principles, even if some will not emerge intact. Fortunately, the more general work in feminist ethics is a fruitful source of inspiration. Where it will lead is anybody's guess, although it seems safe to say that bioethics will look very different when we are done. Pleasurable as it is to indulge in such speculation, it is time to roll up our sleeves and set to work.

Notes

Thanks to Hilde Nelson for casting a critical eye over this manuscript and for several useful comments. This paper was originally published as part of the Introduction to *Reproducing Persons* (Ithaca: Cornell University Press).

1 Virginia L. Warren, 'Feminist Directions in Medical Ethics,' in *Feminist Perspectives in Medical Ethics*, ed. Helen B. Holmes and Laura M. Purdy (Bloomington: Indiana University Press, 1992), p. 33.

2 The happy ending here is that the author radically revised his paper and it was ultimately published.

3 See Susan Sherwin, *No Longer Patient* (Philadelphia: Temple University Press, 1992), and Holmes and Purdy, *Feminist Perspectives in Medical Ethics*. There are also quite a few articles on specific topics written from a feminist point of view.

4 See Laura M. Purdy, 'The Morality of New Reproductive Technologies,' *Journal of Social Philosophy*, 18 (Winter 1987): 38–48. Written in the late 1970s and therefore somewhat dated, the article discusses this question.

5 See Sue V. Rosser, 'Re-visioning Clinical Research: Gender and the Ethics of Experimental Design,' in Holmes and Purdy, *Feminist Perspectives in Medical Ethics*.

6 For a recent eye-opening look at the medical establishment, especially gynecology and obstetrics, see John M. Smith, *Women and Doctors* (New York: Dell, 1992). He cites a 1990 AMA report, 'Gender Disparities in Clinical Decision-Making,' which notes significant gender differences in critical matters such as kidney transplants, cardiac catheterization, and diagnosis of lung cancer (p. 18).

7 See Steven M. Miles and Allison August, 'Courts, Gender and the Right to Die,' *Law, Medicine and Health Care*, 18(1,2): 85–95.

8 See Warren, 'Feminist Directions in Medical Ethics.'

9 This is a point repeatedly emphasized by Smith, *Women and Doctors*.

10 Doubts about the value of control are to be found in the literature on ecofeminism and in Daniel Callahan's recent book, *The Troubled Dream of Life* (New York: Simon & Schuster, 1993).

11 In particular, it has tended to define problems faced by men as more important than those faced by women. Thus, for example, there is a long history of just war theory, but relatively little on childrearing.

12 The dismal record of ethics with respect to women is by now well known. See, for example, the writings of Aristotle, Kant and others in Rosemary Agonito, *A History of Ideas on Women: A Source Book* (New York: G.P. Putnam's Sons, 1977). It also seems to me that traditional ethics has been remarkably oblivious to class inequality and matters of race. Of course, it may turn out that earlier writers in ethics were more sensitive to these issues than is now apparent from what we take to be the history of ethics.

13 I suspect that Michael Levin's contempt for the issue is widely shared. In an unusually frank preface to his book, *Feminism and Freedom* (New Brunswick, NJ: Transaction Books, 1987), he writes: 'The reader may be puzzled, as I myself have sometimes been, that a philosopher should devote several years of his finite existence to feminism, when he could be thinking about the problem of induction or a hundred

other intrinsically more interesting topics ... I could mention that what made me a philosopher in the first place was impatience with ignorance and irrationality, salient traits of feminist writing' (p. x). No doubt he feels the same way about discussions of other kinds of inequality. For an excellent treatment of recent moral and political theory, see Susan Moller Okin, *Justice, Gender, and the Family* (New York: Basic Books, 1989).

14 In some circles, 'feminism' has become such a dirty word that using it immediately ends serious discussion, even where framing the issue without using it hardly raises eyebrows. My suspicion is that feminism is more fundamentally threatening to the establishment than claims, say, of racial injustice. I do not know whether that is because threats to the gender status quo are more basic, or whether they are simply more immediate, given the relative numbers of white women and members of other racial groups in academe. In any case, a number of articles written from a feminist point of view have slipped past the gatekeepers in the last fifteen years, although it was not until 1992 that the first book-length works were published. See Sherwin, *No Longer Patient*, and Holmes and Purdy, *Feminist Perspectives in Medical Ethics*.

15 For example, a fundamental divide among feminists is between what Catharine Stimpson has called the 'minimizers,' and the 'maximizers.' The former want to minimize the meaning of sex differences, the latter want to valorize what they see as basic differences between the sexes. See Catharine R. Stimpson, 'The New Scholarship about Women: The State of the Art,' *Ann. Scholarship*, 1 (2) (1980): 2–14; cited in Ann Snitow, 'A Gender Diary,' *Conflicts in Feminism*, ed. Marianne Hirsch and Evelyn Fox Keller (New York: Routledge, 1990), p. 14. The consequences of these kinds of fundamental divisions are painfully evident in the more specific debates on issues like pornography and reproductive technologies.

16 Valerie Bryson, *Feminist Political Theory* (New York: Paragon House Publishers, 1992), pp. 261–2.

17 As Robin Morgan points out, even Kurt Waldheim, former UN Secretary General, wrote that 'while women represent half the global population and one-third of the labor force, they receive only one-tenth of the world income and own less than one percent of world property. They are also responsible for two-thirds of all working hours' (cited on p. 1 of Waldheim's 'Report to the UN Commission on the Status of Women,' in *Sisterhood Is Global*, ed. Robin Morgan (New York: Anchor Books, 1984).

18 Again, for an excellent bibliography, see Sherwin, *No Longer Patient*; see also individual articles in Holmes and Purdy, *Feminist Perspectives in Medical Ethics*.

19 See, for example, works such as Susan Moller Okin, *Women in Western Political Thought* (Princeton: Princeton University Press, 1979) and her *Justice, Gender, and the Family*; see also *The Sexism of Social and Political Theory*, ed. Lorenne M.G. Clark and Lynda Lange (Toronto: University of Toronto Press, 1979); Nancy J. Hir-

schmann, *Rethinking Obligation: A Feminist Method for Political Theory* (Ithaca: Cornell University Press, 1992); and Virginia Held, *Feminist Morality: Transforming Culture, Society, and Politics* (Chicago: University of Chicago Press, 1993).

20 See Levin, *Feminism and Freedom*, and sociobiologists such as E.O. Wilson, *On Human Nature* (Cambridge, MA: Harvard University Press, 1978); and R. Dawkins, *The Selfish Gene* (Oxford: Oxford University Press, 1976.)

21 For a brief overview of the claim that women are worse off, see Sherwin, *No Longer Patient*, ch. 1, especially 13–19.

22 For instance, we need to know why women live longer and why more men go insane, if those claims are true. These facts, per se, do not necessarily tell us that women or men are more unjustly treated. Thus women may live longer because of their stronger biological constitution, even though men get more effective medical care; men may have a higher incidence of insanity for genetic reasons or because their overblown expectations of their just deserts fail to be met, rather than because of unfair treatment.

23 See also the work of Stephen Toulmin, 'The Recovery of Practical Philosophy,' *Arts & Sciences*, Northwestern University, Spring 1988; and Albert R. Jonsen and Stephen Toulmin, *The Abuse of Casuistry: A History of Moral Reasoning* (Berkeley: University of California Press, 1988).

24 Just as race is not something predicated only of people of color, class is not what only the poor have, and sexual orientation not what only homosexuals have. See Elizabeth V. Spelman, *Inessential Woman* (Boston: Beacon Press, 1988).

25 For an excellent summary of facts and issues, see Sherwin, *No Longer Patient*, ch. 1.

26 See Ludwig Wittgenstein *Philosophical Investigations*, section 66.

27 For an excellent discussion of the pitfalls of sociobiology as applied to human behavior, see Philip Kitcher, *Vaulting Ambition* (Cambridge, MA: MIT Press, 1985). For more socially oriented discussions, see Pauline Bart's response to Melford E. Spiro's *Gender and Culture*: 'Biological Determinism and Sexism: Is It All in the Ovaries?' in *Biology as a Social Weapon*, ed. Ann Arbor Science for the People Editorial Collective (Minneapolis: Burgess Publishing Company, 1977). There are many other discussions of possible social arrangements; for example, see John Stuart Mill, *The Subjection of Women*, and *Feminist Scholarship: Kindling in the Groves of Academe*, ed. Ellen Carol DuBois, Gail Paradise Kelly, Elizabeth Lapovsky Kennedy, Carolyn W. Korsmeyer, and Lillian Robinson (Urbana: University of Illinois Press, 1985).

28 Thanks to Daniel Callahan for reminding me of this argument.

29 See, for example, some of the pieces in Claudia Card's recent anthology, *Feminist Ethics* (Lawrence: University Press of Kansas, 1991).

30 For example, see a recent sympathetic review of *Issues in Reproductive Technology I: An Anthology* (New York: Garland Press, 1992), a feminist collection edited by Helen B. Holmes. The reviewer, Lois B. Moreland, writes: 'of what value is a femi-

nist anthology? By definition, its perspective is biased. It is gender-centered. Its vision is limited' *Politics and the Life Sciences*, 12(2) (August 1993): 301.

31 Sherwin, *No Longer Patient*, p. 56.

32 See, for example, Karen Lehrman's recent attack on women's studies, 'Off Course,' *Mother Jones* (September/October 1993): 45–51, 64, 66, 68. She accuses some women's studies classes of being political and praises what she takes to be non-political mainstream treatments of the same issues, yet she never defines the word or asks what is central about the feminism that informs women's studies curricula.

33 I use the two terms interchangeably.

34 Emanuel distinguishes three other possible positions on this issue of the source of values used in health care ethics, and he argues, convincingly I believe, that his own political conception is superior. First, there is the teleological view, which holds that all the relevant values are intrinsic to the health care enterprise. Second, there is the applied ethics view, which derives the values in health care ethics from more general moral principles. Third, there is a view that recognizes two moral worlds competing for center stage in health care ethics: a professional role morality and what he calls 'common' morality (pp. 26–9). He comments: 'Each of these approaches should be rejected. Professional ethics is not separated from, derived from, or to be balanced against political philosophy. Instead, it is best to see that the intrinsic ends of a profession are incomplete; they need specification and balancing through political philosophy. A complete account of the purposes of the profession – a specification of its ends, a balancing of its internal ends, a balancing of its internal ends with nonprofessional ends – requires political philosophy. Professional ethics can be fully articulated only by references to political values. Professional ethics and political philosophy are not in conflict or at cross-purposes, but professional ethics is insufficient without the values articulated in political philosophy' (p. 29). Ezekiel J. Emanuel, *The Ends of Human Life: Medical Ethics in a Liberal Polity* (Cambridge, MA: Harvard University Press, 1991).

35 Alison Jaggar, 'Feminist Ethics: Some Issues for the Nineties,' *Journal of Social Philosophy*, 20(1–2) (Spring/Fall 1989): 91–107, 91.

36 The problem here is that developing a feminist consciousness seems to be akin to having not one scale but a series of scales drop from one's eyes. The quantum nature of the experience is reminiscent of Plato's view of how we are to come to know the forms. Fortunately, the recipe is somewhat clearer!

37 I take it for granted that women should be treated at least as well as men; men should not, of course, drop to women's current level. We shall then have something like equal consideration in care.

38 See Warren, 'Feminist Directions in Medical Ethics.'

Reflections of a Sceptical Bioethicist

CHRISTINE OVERALL

Introduction

In the course of much of my scholarly work over the last decade I have been perceived as a bioethicist. I have served as a so-called expert witness in ethics at an inquest into the death of a baby born at home; I have worked as a bioethics consultant for the Royal Commission on New Reproductive Technologies; and I have spoken on television, radio, and in print as an academic who specializes in bioethics. Although I have sometimes described my work as including bioethics, or more specifically, reproductive ethics, I none the less *think* of what I do as feminist philosophy, both theoretical and applied. Within my work, then, bioethics is not a distinct field, but rather a branch of feminist philosophy, and interesting for precisely that reason. It was not because reproductive issues fall under bioethics that I became interested in them; rather, it was because of the centrality of reproduction to many women's lives, its connections with the status of children, and the role of reproductive practices in perpetuating sexism.[1] Similarly, my interest in sexuality issues and in AIDS arose not out of a preoccupation with health care, per se, or with what is conventionally defined as bioethics; it originated from a concern for the connection of these issues with problems of oppression, definitions of sexuality, and questions about inequities allotted to marginalized peoples.

Another reason that I think of my work as being feminist philosophy rather than bioethics is that while feminist philosophy gives me moral, political, and intellectual inspiration, contemporary bioethics by contrast makes me somewhat uneasy. This paper represents my attempt to articulate and evaluate some of the characteristics of bioethics that cause me discomfort.

Margaret Urban Walker says, 'it flies in the face of the professional self-image of supposedly disinterested searchers after timeless moral truth to recognize that a moral philosophy is a particular rhetoric too, situated in certain places, sustained and deployed by certain groups of people.'[2] But philosophers need to think carefully about what bioethicists are doing – and how, for whose benefit, and for what reasons. The case of bioethics should make us self-conscious about the content and social value of our work as philosophers and about the cultural construction of subfields of philosophy.

Although I welcome the opportunity to voice my scepticism, I am also diffident about the legitimacy of generalizing, as I will, about the entire field. After all, the field of bioethics encompasses both clinical practice and academic research; bioethicists embrace a wide variety of moral perspectives, from utilitarianism to Kantianism to situation ethics to ethics of care, and they investigate a diverse field of issues, ranging from familiar questions about honesty and truth-telling to problems about the latest technologies of genetic manipulation.

Some of my observations, therefore, will have the air of caricature; they are to some extent stereotypes of the field of bioethics and its participants. I hasten to acknowledge that I do not regard all bioethicists as exemplars of the problems to which I am pointing, and I do include myself among those who must answer to the criticisms I am making.

My usual approach to philosophical issues is by means of what might be termed philosophical piecework: pessimistic of the possibility of developing an overarching theory, I have typically chosen to work at relatively detailed and specific problems, in the hope that a more general illumination might thereby indirectly be achieved. It is possible that this approach itself has contributed to – or at least failed to challenge – some of the very problems in bioethics that I cite later in this paper.[3] Now, however, I want to confront the givens that I have heretofore not discussed, using a politically motivated analysis and critique derived from feminist philosophy. My aim is not simply to bring a feminist and radical perspective *to* bioethics, as already constituted, but rather to interrogate the field itself and how its constitution is able to co-opt radical dissent, including some dissent from a feminist perspective.

I have in mind bioethics primarily as it is ordinarily represented and practised in university courses, at conferences, and in textbooks and journals – what might be called academic 'bioethics-as-usual.' My understanding of and approach to bioethics are those of an academic, not a clinical practitioner. I do not have clinical experience of and background in the day-to-day practice of bioethics in hospitals and other health care settings. Indeed, my lack of experience in clinical bioethics has angered at least some of those who have read my work; they think I lack the authority to speak about bioethics at all. I shall say more below about bioethical credentials and the general questions of epistemic and moral expertise that this charge raises. For now I merely point out that I have not been provided with evidence, even by my critics, that the clinical practice of bioethics differs significantly from its typical academic representations.

I shall lay out my scepticism using a classical bioethical approach: the case study. My aim in so doing is not to find a moral resolution to the case, but rather to use it to illustrate some conditions and characteristics of bioethics that are deserving of scepticism. I shall argue that there is a need for scepticism about (1) the existence of bioethics as a distinct field and the generation of bioethical problems; (2) the success and acceptance of bioethics within academia, medicine, and the culture generally; and (3) the political and moral conservatism of bioethical theory.

The case study, which I shall refer to as the Glover case, is taken from Robert Veatch's 1977 book, *Case Studies in Medical Ethics*, and is entitled 'This Won't Hurt a Bit.'

Clara Glover brought Tommy and Michael, her two sons ages four and two, to Dr. Stephen Huntington, the family pediatrician, for routine examinations. Michael, the older boy, was getting ready to enter kindergarten, so he needed a medical form filled out for school. Dr. Huntington had a reputation for being kind and gentle with children, always willing to take a worried mother's call. He had been practicing pediatrics for twenty-seven years and had learned many tricks of the trade.

He began Michael's examination by looking at his throat, ears, and eyes. When he got to the examination of the fundus of the eye, he made use of a clever idea he had learned from a tip in *Medical Economics*, a widely read magazine distributed to physicians free of charge for the advertising. He showed Michael his ophthalmoscope and asked, 'Would you rather see a doggie, a kitten, or a butterfly?' Michael replied, 'A doggie.' Lawrence Garner, who sent in the tip to *Medical Economics*, remarked that the child will usually pick the first. Dr. Huntington, following the advice from the magazine, told Michael he was going to shine the light into his eye. Michael should look into it to see if he could see the doggie. Michael did not seem to see anything and began to get restless, so Dr. Huntington said, 'The doggie is a little afraid, but I'll get him to come out for you. I see him, do you? He has one black eye and one white eye.' Michael did not appear convinced but looked into the ophthalmoscope a bit longer. Dr. Huntington, having completed his examination of the right eye, now told Michael he thought the doggie had jumped into the other eye. The examination of the fundus was completed.

Examination of the heart and lungs and a blood pressure reading followed, building up to what they all knew was the climax. Michael was required by state law to have a rubella immunization. The nurse had been preparing the syringe carefully outside the vision of Michael and his mother. Dr. Huntington opened a drawer and took out a wrapped piece of hard candy. He handed it to Michael's left hand while simultaneously reaching for the vaccine-filled syringe. He took hold of Michael's right arm, inviting

Michael to unwrap the candy with his left hand and teeth. As Michael glanced over to the syringe, Dr. Huntington said, 'This won't hurt a bit.' Michael winced slightly as the needle went in. His mother left the office marveling at what a wonderful doctor Dr. Huntington was.[4]

It has been suggested to me that this case is not, or is no longer, typical of medical practice today. I am not sure that this is correct. But in any case, I employ the Glover case not because I think it is necessarily a typical situation, but rather because it is useful for raising two main questions about bioethics-as-usual. First, how is bioethics constituted? Second, why is bioethics both successful and conservative? I also want to use the case as a point of departure for some remarks on the so-called ethic of care, and for observations about the deployment, in oppressive systems in general and in medicine in particular, of the concept of the child.

How Is Bioethics Constituted?

To being with the obvious: the Glover case is a problem or set of problems in bioethics. It is, presumably, classified as such by reference to the sorts of people and the types of activity involved. In this case there is a physician, a mother, and a child; the activities described include communicating with and ministering to a child. What is important to note is that there is nothing particulary unusual about the situation. It does not depict a medical crisis. Indeed, many readers of the Glover case may find it trivial or even unproblematic, especially in contrast with the other problems – ranging from 'Black Lung Disease and National Health Insurance' to 'Reporting the Epileptic Motorist' to 'Sickle Cell and Black Genocide' – presented in the Veatch text. It is the presence of a doctor, the health care context, and specifically medical activities that constitute the case as a bioethical problem or set of problems.

Walker asks, '[W]ho or what decides what *is* a "case" – a moral problem – in the first place, as well as what sort of case – subject to what principle or principles – it is?'[5] Abortion is virtually always regarded as a central and persistent bioethical problem (arguably forcing women, especially feminists, to devote extensive effort to arguing for women's control over their own bodies[6]). Yet by contrast, in the United States the absence of universal state-supported health care and in Canada the deplorable living conditions of many native people often are not recognized as central bioethical problems (and if they were, their recognition might impel governments to defend themselves – or to change their own policies). What Ivan Illich calls the 'ethical status of medicalization'[7] – that is, the gradual incursion of medicine into, for example, sexuality,[8] reproduction,[9] disability,[10] the emotions, nutrition,[11] childhood, old age, and dying – is seldom recognized as an issue within bioethics. Nor are the marketing of infant formula and bottle feeding, the effects of environmental degradation on health, the drugging of athletes, or physicians' widespread participation in the certification of deviance, incompetence, and insanity recognized as such.[12]

As Susan Sherwin points out, 'work in bioethics is largely defined in terms of what may be characterized as the narrower field of medical ethics; attention is focused on the moral dilemmas that confront physicians, and the doctor's point of view is generally adopted.' Moral problems faced by nurses, occupational therapists, pharmacists, social workers, technicians, orderlies, and nursing assistants usually are omitted.[13] Bioethicists commonly demonstrate great interest in issues of power within the patient-provider relationship, focusing on autonomy and paternalism, informed consent, and control of information; there is relatively little discussion of power inequities – and I would include here male/female and adult/child inequities – within the larger social sphere.[14] As a result, the Glover case normally would not be considered an instantiation of generally unequal gender and/or age relationships, of the oppression of children, or of that of mothers. Instead, in bioethics-as-usual, patients are considered both equally vulnerable and equally used to expressing their autonomy; there is little discussion of connections between social status and health care practices.[15]

It is important to ask not just why only certain problems and not others get recognized *within* bioethics, but also why bioethics is a distinct and well-developed field, and ethical issues arising from other significant areas of human interest and activity are not. The ethics of medicine is sharply distinguished from and highly developed compared with the bodies of issues arising in connection with nutrition, work, leisure, and sport. Since there is a subsection of applied ethics devoted to health care, why is there not a subsection devoted to the ethics of nutrition and eating? Or the ethics of purchasing and consuming? Or the ethics of what Virginia L. Warren calls 'housekeeping issues'[16] – the ongoing, often domestic, everyday moral issues that all of us face, within a variety of roles and institutions?

Most surprising of all (to me), why is the ethics of child care and childrearing not a distinct field within applied ethics? Why shouldn't the Glover case be interpreted as a case in child care ethics at least as much as bioethics? Admittedly, there has been some philosophical attention to ethical issues of child care (Sara Ruddick's work[17] is one example), but not enough to constitute it as a distinct field – with courses, consultants, conferences, journals, grants, etc. – in the way that health care ethics is constituted. Consider the following moral problems one might encounter in the experience of childrearing: what kind of education to provide for a child; how much to give a child within an acquisitive, materialistic culture; how to help a child to understand and deal with the harms of racism and sexism; whether a child should be engaged in paid work; how seriously to take appeals to peer group activities and standards; how to balance the division of responsibilities between parents' paid work and time with a child in a fulfilling and fair way; and how much independence a child needs and deserves to have. Most of these issues are, of course, fairly specific to middle-class families, and there are other, often more serious, issues for persons from working class and poor backgrounds. They are, in any case, *moral* issues, not merely practical ones; they are questions about what children and their care-givers must do, what kinds of people they should be, and what adult/child relationships ought to be like.

Why isn't the ethics of childrearing a large and important area within applied ethics? Probably, in terms of numbers, these issues are far more frequently encountered by both non-philosophers and philosophers than are the typical health care problems within bioethics. Arguably, they may be even more important than health care questions, and have a greater and wider effect.

The point I am making is *not* that mothers, or parents in general, have special moral insights (though that may sometimes be true[18]). Nor am I making claims about mothering or maternal/child relationships as models for other forms of ethical reasoning.[19] Nor am I making a point about the worthiness of special cases and issues involving children to be considered morally interesting and problematic; for in fact I think they are sometimes recognized as such. Instead, I am making a point about the definition of subfields in ethics, about where boundaries are drawn, and about what sets of problems are thought both to hang together and to be especially worthy of focus and examination.

I am not opposed to carving up the field of philosophy, per se, but we need to ask the political questions: To what end is it carved up? What gets left out? What does the carving up reinforce? Whom does it benefit? Whom does it fail to help, or even harm? Part of the reason there is no developed 'child care ethics' field may be that it is mostly women who are involved as child carers, and it is children to whom they minister. On the other hand, there is a field called 'bioethics' because this culture respects physicians, who are usually male, far more than it respects children or mothers.

Moreover, the constitution and apparent uniqueness of bioethics is parasitical upon the constitution and apparent uniqueness of health care. Health care seems special and singular because of characteristics such as the often extreme state of the patients – disabled, diseased, or dying; the existence of defined locations for health care; the scarcity of health care resources; the tendency to situate health problems primarily in the individual patient rather than in her social and physical environment and her relationships to it; medicine's commitment to the technological fix; and the social location of special expertise within health care providers. These characteristics provide a certain unity to medicine and hence to bioethics. Yet almost all of these characteristics could have been otherwise – that is, health care could be otherwise provided – and they obscure the social and ethical continuities of health care, as currently constituted, with the rest of the culture.

Why Is Bioethics Both Successful and Conservative?

The definition and boundaries of bioethics and its use of certain cases promote conservatism in approach: the moral question in bioethics is almost always taken to be: what should be done *within this given set of circumstances*?[20] As Sherwin pointedly observes, 'Conferences, textbooks, and journals of medical ethics are chiefly occupied with establishing an ethical rationale for existing practices within the field of health care.'[21]

In the ordinary, bioethics-as-usual construal of the Glover case, the moral questions seem to concern how the doctor can, within moral limits, coax or compel the child's acquiescence and cooperation in necessary medical treatments. To that question there are several different but standard bioethical answers. First, Veatch, the author of the text in which the case appears, includes discussion questions for the case that direct the reader's attention to such consequentialist factors as pleasing Michael's mother, comparing short- and long-range consequences, and contrasting the impact of one instance of patient deception with the impact of a pattern of patient deceptions. While he alerts the reader to the potential dangers of public 'mistrust of the medical profession,' he also implies that 'good, on balance' was produced through Huntington's deception of Michael.[22]

Second, one could interpret the Glover case as raising questions about traditional, key bioethical concepts such as autonomy, respect for persons, competence, paternalism, and the allocation of scarce resources such as time and money. From this ethical perspective, bioethics-as-usual would likely conclude that Michael lacks the competence to be treated as a fully autonomous patient; that Dr Huntington is justified in exercising some form of paternalistic behaviour towards him; but that, given Huntington's willingness to devote time to careful examination of his patient, questions should be raised about the moral appropriateness of his strategy for handling children.

A third and more recent approach to the case would involve the invocation of the so-called ethic of care, which calls for the establishment and maintenance of caring, responsible relationships with patients.[23] 'Caring for involves responding to the particular, concrete, physical, spiritual, intellectual, psychic, and emotional needs of others,'[24] with a focus not on moral principles, but on the immediate activity of nurturing.[25] 'The central directive of an ethic of care,' says Eve Browning Cole, 'is that I should act always in such ways as to promote the well-being of both the others to whom I am in relation and the self which is relationally constituted.' This requires 'a caring and attentive conscientious *presence* within one's moral situation, a sensitivity to the needs and desires of others, and a basic dispositional willingness to do what I can to create situations in which those needs can be met.'[26] From this perspective it could be argued that Huntington's examination strategy establishes a short-term connection with Michael and his mother, but that it does not augur well for his long-term relationship with the boy because it may foster distrust in Huntington's reliability.

While all of the standard bioethical approaches just described appear to rely on important moral values, all three, either alone or even somehow in tandem,[27] are regrettably conservative in moral and social terms. For not one is likely to challenge the framework or the social conventions of the problem. All three interpret the Glover case in terms of the expertise of the physician and the moral decisions he must make. In this encounter the physician is the holder of knowledge, authority, and power; the ethical questions appear to concern the justification of his use of information and his exercise of authority and power. By virtue of its place in a bioethics textbook and standard bioethical approaches to it, the Glover case is not about, or not primarily about, accepted practices of disease prevention, the child care role of mothers, the relationships between women and men, the education of children, or the connections between adults and pre-schoolers. Instead, as Warren points out, 'The main relationship questions in medical ethics now involve competitions for power, status or authority. Who should have the moral authority to make the final decision: the patient or the physician (in the autonomy/paternalism debate), the physician or the nurse (in nursing ethics)?'[28] Thus Veatch himself, for example, argues that a central problem for clinical ethics is 'identifying the primary decision maker.'[29]

The problem with this focus on identifying the moral and medical decision maker is partly a matter of emphasis – it distracts attention from other important questions – and partly a matter of misconstruction of the issue. It presupposes that moral and medical problems are to be resolved by giving to one or two persons – usually physicians – the power to trump the views of others, and it assumes that no other approach to conflict or ambiguity is possible.

In this way, the fetishization and essentializing of medical expertise is reproduced and endorsed by bioethicists. For many bioethicists, it is uncontroversial that physicians should be centre stage. Eike-Henner Kluge, for example, says that medical ethics 'assumes that there are ethical principles that ought to guide the conduct of *physicians* and that these apply to all doctors regardless of personal and cultural differences ... [T]he principles themselves are the same because they are anchored in the *nature of the profession itself.*[30] Moreover, professionalization and hierarchy within medicine are accepted by and reduplicated within recognized bioethical problems, approaches, and practices. Bioethicists – and I include myself here – often acquiesce in and benefit from the power of medical professionalization, of science, and of the health care industry. The bioethicist is a professional advice giver; an often full-time paid purveyor of practical wisdom. Just as the medical expert cures the disease, the ethical expert resolves the moral problem and arrogates to him/herself the moral authority for so doing. As Cheryl Noble points out, bioethicists are fitting experts for an 'era accustomed to solving its problems by delivering them to the correct set of problem solvers. Why shouldn't there be philosophical experts to deal with moral problems just as there are experts to deal with environmental and engineering problems?'[31]

Even the most recent apparent changes in the role of the bioethicist have not altered the bioethicist's status as expert. Thus, for example, although Walker chronicles and lauds a 'shift in emphasis [in bioethics] from issues of content to those of *process* – from what the ethicist knows, to what the ethicist does or enables,'[32] she does not question the bioethicist's situation as an expert who '"facilitates" a social process of moral negotiation and mutual accountability.'[33] So on this account of the bioethicist's role, the bioethicist becomes a sort of moral therapist – and is potentially manipulative in that capacity. For it is difficult for ethics to be a conversation, a dialogue, or a mediation, where the participants are socially located at distinct points, with very different amounts of knowledge, control, access to resources, and decision-making abilities. As Giles R. Scofield points out, 'What [bioethicists] know and believe, their biases and prejudices, all these subjective variables will influence how they frame issues and how they go about deciding whose voice needs to be heard more. Even such factors as who pays their salary may influence their perceptions about voice.'[34]

Just as medicine constructs a hierarchy of experts, so also does philosophy. Within academic philosophy the professional hierarchy seems partly based on the degree of abstraction and distance from so-called 'real life' issues: the closer a philosophical field comes to the messy details of human existence, the lower it is in the philosophical chain of being. (The position of a subfield is perhaps also partly related to who engages in it; my guess is that women are inclined to do applied philosophy, and the relatively lower reputation of the area may not be coincidental.)

Although applied ethics tends to be at or near the bottom of the philosophical heap, it is interesting that within applied ethics bioethics gets special billing, perhaps partly because it primarily involves, or revolves around, the expertise of men. Not all bioethicists are trained philosophers (some are physicians or lawyers, for example), but, whatever their background, bioethicists get respect. Bioethics is, relatively, a prosperous form of applied philosophy, a form that has been successfully institutionalized in less than three decades, not only inside academia, but within the health care professions. Barry Hoffmaster quotes a former dean of an Ontario medical school who described bioethics as 'the biggest growth area in medicine.'[35] According to K. Danner Clouser, 'bioethics brought fame and fortune to philosophy, a public notice and acclaim it had never had: it brought burgeoning classes and massive opportunities for funding. It brought to philosophy a new air of excitement ... Philosophers were needed – even wanted!'[36] Indeed, I suggest that bioethics is so successful as to constitute a philosophical industry: consider the journals, books, courses, committees, research boards, guidelines, codes, conferences, funding opportunities, granting bodies, foundations, consultants, hospital staff, and university positions now devoted solely to bioethics.[37]

I do not think that the signal success of bioethics is, in itself, a problem; I am sceptical about it largely because its success contrasts so interestingly with the reputation and development of other actual and possible areas of applied ethics, and because the allotment of resources to bioethics may also affect its content. In Veatch's words, with respect to clinical ethicists, 'The fact that the ethicist is on the clinician's turf, is paid by the health professional system, and gradually develops identification with clinical professionals, all cast doubt on the legitimacy of the clinical ethicist's role.'[38] Veatch points out that a clinical ethicist passes an initial screening in order to be hired, or even tolerated, by the clinic; this screening makes it more likely that the ethicist will have originally been trained as a health professional, will have a world view like those of health care providers, will be case oriented, and will be committed to a form of ethical situationalism.[39]

Thus, there is mutual reinforcement between bioethics and medicine. While the professionalization and hierarchism of medicine influence bioethics, the construction of bioethics as a field of exclusive and specialized professional expertise in turn reinforces the apparent uniqueness of health care and, by extension, of what medical professionals, especially physicians, do. While I do not deny that bioethicists, as Peter Singer argues, often have produced unconventional 'solutions' to bioethical problems,[40] bioethicists rarely, if ever, challenge the physician's rather exclusive authority, expertise, and power, or give attention to the moral issues faced by other health care providers, or more generally question the normal assignment of health preservation and enhancement to specialized experts. Bioethical issues are seen as problems *within* professional ethics;[41] the formation, deployment, and effects of bioethics as a whole are seldom examined and evaluated. (It is therefore hardly surprising that views of 'outsiders' of the fields should be both resented and regarded as illegitimate, or that attempts should be made to distinguish who is a 'real' bioethicist and who is not.) Thus, bioethicists' imitation of medical expertise contributes to both the conservatism and the success of bioethics.

Of the three standard bioethical approaches I earlier described, the ethic of care might be thought to have more radical potential than the others. Derived from attention to women's practices, especially as nurturers, caring has been thought by some feminists to provide an iconoclastic alternative to orthodox ethical theories. So it is important to ask why the ethic of care is both easily interpreted in conservative terms, and embraced fairly happily within bioethics as a professional field.[42] Whatever the potential of the ethic of care, its effects have been hijacked by contemporary bioethics.[43] In the words of Rosemarie Tong, 'what worries me is the Tradition's willingness, even eagerness, to accommodate feminine and maternal approaches to ethics ... Pessimistically interpreted ... the Tradition's "welcome party" may be motivated by the realization that feminine and maternal ethics are unlikely to end its moral monopoly.'[44] The current emphasis on the ethic of care represents the co-optation of women's varied practices of nurturance, which is transmogrified into 'care' – genderized, often biologized, essentialized, stereotyped, and individualized.

It is not hard to see why. An ethical focus on caring tends to construe the objects of care as rather passive; it can therefore be used to encourage and validate the acquiescence of patients, along with the omnipotence of some care-givers (physicians) and the altruism and self-sacrifice of others (nurses). The recent and growing emphasis on a certain sort of contextualization in bioethics[45] also makes assimilation of the value of caring easy. The fact that an ethic of care seems either to preclude generalization (because of attention to specific context and the particularities of *this* relationship) or only to permit generalizations so sweeping as to be useless[46] shows why it is easily co-opted for traditional ends within bioethics. While the ethic of care bids us be attentive to the needs of particular others, it seems indifferent to where those needs came from. The ethic of care focuses on specific social relationships as moral givens; it can thus be applied conservatively, without challenging the framework within which bioethical issues are posited.

The extraordinary success of bioethics and its pervasive conservatism throughout many theoretical incarnations are related. These characteristics are a function of its parasitism on health care as it is currently practised. Bioethics tends to reiterate the hierarchism, individualism, professionalism, and separatism of medicine, and to co-opt the radical potential of progressive analyses of the medical profession. Consequently, in the words of Warren, 'It may be time for moral philosophers to question not only the power relationship between physicians and patients, but that between themselves and those they would instruct.'[47]

An Alternative to Bioethics-as-Usual

Moral evaluation of a bioethical case requires that we first understand the terms of its construction and description. In the words of Arthur L. Caplan, 'Often, in the confused world of practical affairs, it is not clear exactly what the moral problems that require resolution are. Moral expertise is sought, not for problem resolution, but for problem individuation and identification ... Occasionally, those involved in practical affairs are not even aware that a moral problem exists. The task of those with moral expertise may be to create moral perplexity where none existed.'[48] This task is partly a matter of perception, that is, what we *notice* and thereby deem important in a situation. Howard Brody calls it a 'pattern recognition skill.'[49] As Jean Grimshaw remarks, 'the process of attention is itself part of the moral struggle, not merely the final choice or the behavioural outcome.'[50]

Of course, it makes a difference what sort of moral perplexity is generated and where we place our attention. The placing of attention has a political dimension.[51] Here I take issue with Hoffmaster, who claims, 'Philosophical ethics cannot account for the "deeper" or "hidden" values that function at a cultural level and figure prominently but inconspicuously in decisions.'[52] I am suggesting instead that bioethicists have a responsibility to attempt to unearth the deep and hidden cultural values that both help to determine patterns of social interaction and also often to deflect critical attention from systemic inequity.

What is necessary, then, is attention to the wider context of bioethical problems. But by 'context,' I do not mean only the specific details of a moral situation, or the personal identities of the protagonists,[53] or merely local values.[54] Admittedly, awareness of context in all of these senses may be both relevant and important; for the more traditional approach, what Walker refers to as 'shear[ing] off complicating, possibly "irrelevant" details to magnify "repeatable," even "universalizable" features general enough to map cases onto available theoretical categories,'[55] often jettisons what is most significant in and crucial to a moral dilemma. Yet awareness of context in these senses is not sufficient, because once identities, relationships, and local values are recognized within a moral problem, there remain questions about what patterns and themes they reveal and the perspective from which the patterns and themes should be evaluated.

I advocate that we follow Walker's advice 'to pierce through the rhetoric of ethics to the *politics of ethics*.'[56] The alternative to bioethics-as-usual is the development of the theory and practice of what I shall call *bio(medical)politics*, which requires a political critique of health care boundaries, cases, moralities, practices, and policies, bearing in mind both medicine's continuities with other oppressive institutions and its unique instantiations of power differentials. Attention must be placed, not only on individual persons, considered as particular units, but on the social values and practices that help both to constitute and to set limits on what individuals can do and be.

The pervasive medicalization of many aspects of human life often disguises their political construction: 'Political analyses of the unequal power of women and men, of white people and people of color, of First World and Third World people, of the rich and the poor, of the healthy and the disabled ... [have] been almost entirely absent from the literature of mainstream medical ethics, although the institutions in which health care is provided are deeply implicated in the maintenance of structures of oppression.'[57] Bioethics cases are characterized immediately and extensively by the vulnerability of some of their participants and by the power imbalance between participants. A significant part of what bioethicists should therefore call attention to in case studies are the oppressive cultural patterns they often embody. Contextualization in the sense of attention to the political and social context of moral problems is essential; that is, we must examine the 'connections between specific practices and the patterns of dominance in society.'[58]

An Example: (Systematic) Infantilization in Health Care and in Bioethics

The Glover case can be used to illustrate how the perspective of bio(medical)politics may enlarge standard interpretations of problems in bioethics. The Glover case is not simply a situation with undesirable long-term consequences, or a puzzle about truth-telling to children, or a failure to develop an adequately caring relationship, although it is all of these. It also has something to tell us about accepted practices of disease prevention, the child care role of mothers, the relationships between women and men, the education of children, and the connections between adults and preschoolers.

The situation can be seen as a representation of two disadvantaged groups of people – women, especially women as mothers, and children – within a culture that systematically devalues members of both. Michael Glover is not permitted to participate in the proceedings as a developing person. Nor is his mother's personhood recognized: her views on and hopes for her children are not mentioned or even solicited, but she has, in any case, apparently been co-opted by the physician's pseudo-expertise with children.

Despite Huntington's reputation for kindness, his story about the 'doggie' in the ophthalmoscope, and his failure to warn Michael about the injection and explain its importance in terms the child could understand, amount to both a profound inability to communicate on a respectful basis with children and a culturally approved attempt to deceive in the interests of securing the cooperation of a type of being commonly assumed to be less than human and therefore not deserving of information. For in North America, children are not persons; indeed, they are not even second-class citizens. Oppression begins and is learned in childhood, and power over children is more readily acquired than almost any other kind of power.[59] Not even children deserve to be treated like children. Grimshaw remarks: 'The cult or mystique of medical authority and expertise, as it permeates much of medical practice, tends to objectify or *infantilise* people, to deny them the status of participants in discussion or decisions about their condition or welfare and to render them powerless or fearful to ask questions or insist on information or participation.'[60] In Michael Glover's case we see the literal, the unnecessary, and the unwarranted infantilization of a patient. But infantilization within the health care system is not confined to children. From the perspective of bio(medical)politics, the concept of infantilization can be applied more broadly to illuminate important and problematic features of a variety of health care contexts.

It is no coincidence that in a culture where there is little or no concerted attention to moral issues arising from child care, where children themselves are often virtually invisible, there is none the less an implicit commitment to the perpetuation of inappropriate adult/child distinctions within many other human interactions, in a way comparable to the pervasive genderization of society. By 'adult/ child division' I mean a systematic cultural pattern of classifying human beings, regardless of actual age, maturity, or level of development, into either the powerful and privileged category of adult, or the powerless and disadvantaged category of child. While I do not deny that some adult/child distinction should be made, I do deny that we make it fairly and appropriately, and that it is relevant elsewhere in human relationships.

There is no word for this pattern. 'Ageism,' discrimination on grounds of age, is not the right term, since this form of oppression is a matter not only of age differences, but rather of distinctions based on lack of experience, lack of education, and apparent ignorance, weakness, smallness, or vulnerability. 'Adultism,' the privileging of the interests, needs, and experiences of adults, refers to but one application of the adult/child division. For the adult/child division is not confined to relationships between older people and young people. Merely getting older does not necessarily protect one from being oppressively placed in the child position; in fact, it is a not-infrequent experience of very elderly people, who may be regarded by younger adults as inept, incapable, ignorant, and incompetent[61] – in other words, they are infantilized. Infantilization can also be manifested among adults of about the same age who have different educations and world experience. When a person is or is thought to be childlike – that is, lacks or is thought to lack experience, education, knowledge, or physical skills – s/he is often inappropriately classified and treated by others as, in social and political terms, a child.[62] A number of different social roles, statuses, and conditions may serve as stimuli for infantilization, including looking young, being a health care patient, being female, being a student, being a member of a so-called 'visible minority,' and coming from a poor or working class background.[63]

What I am suggesting is that our cultural views about and evaluations of children, inappropriate as they are, none the less serve as an archetype and model for treatments of other human beings who are not literally children, in terms of age or development. What is needed, then, is a term to refer to the social construction and invidious deployment of the category 'child.' The most accurate term I can offer is 'systematic infantilization.'[64]

In a culture committed to systematic infantilization, it is not surprising that medical patients are infantilized, not only by physicians,[65] but also by other health care workers such as nurses. Infantilization of patients is not a social anomaly but an enactment of one of our deepest held values: those who are weak, vulnerable, frail, or helpless deserve to be treated like (the cultural stereotype of) children. The knowledge, experience, emotional stability, and capacity to decide of patients of any age – but especially those who are female and/or very young or very old – are consistently underestimated. In medical institutions, the standard hospital gown is reminiscent of the bib of infancy; patients are routinely referred to by their first name or by diminutives such as 'dear'; they are often condescended to or discussed as if they were not present. They are believed to need non-demanding amusements, or to require regular naps; they must be protected from overstimulation and from interference by other child-patients or visitors from the adult world.

Bioethics-as-usual fails to recognize the infantilization of patients and to situate it within the broader social context of systematic infantilization. Instead, it positions bioethicists themselves as adults in relation to other participants in the health care system. Thus, Veatch suggests that clinical ethicists should see both patients *and* clinicians as their 'patients.'[66] Caroline Whitbeck suggests that the obsession of bioethics with issues of paternalism is derived from a preoccupation with infants' needs for human 'interference' in order to survive. 'These interferences on the parent's (or at least the father's) part are recognized as morally justifiable, and serve as a model ... for other possibly justifiable acts that limit or hinder the self-determination of another for that person's own good. Such acts are labelled "paternalistic."'[67]

The institutionalization of systematic infantilization within medicine also helps to explain why the ethic of care has been so readily acceptable within bio-ethics, since it was originally modelled on maternal/child relationships.[68] Conventions of systematic infantilization cross gender boundaries, so the fact that the ethic of care is derived primarily from the practices of women does not protect it from potentially oppressive applications and implications. Maternal/child relationships are easily corrupted within a culture that does not respect children and others with a comparable lack of experience, education, or power.

Conclusion

Sensitivity to the instantiation of inequalities within health care will not, of itself, resolve bioethical problems. What it will do is provide a much fuller appreciation of the structure, ideology, and causal mechanisms of these problems and make it less likely that we, as philosophers, buy into and reinforce inequity within health care.

Using the perspective of bio(medical)politics generates differences from bioethics-as-usual at both a micro and a macro level of analysis. Within the existing health care system, at the micro level, the perspective of bio(medical)politics calls attention to unfair treatment and the operation of oppression. It advocates non-maleficence, the promotion of self-determination, mutual realization,[69] integrity,[70] and respect.[71] Practitioners of bio(medical)politics are committed to problematizing the role of the bioethicist and to the development and dispersion of ethical 'expertise' among all community participants.

Just as important, however, the perspective of bio(medical)politics also requires, at the macro level, attention to the structure and nature of the health care system itself and its relationship to the rest of culture. With respect to what is provided, why, by whom, and to whom, practitioners of bio(medical)politics should be committed to a radical re-evaluation of health care. Such a re-evaluation requires a challenge to the invidious partitioning of health concerns from those of nutrition, education, disease prevention, exercise and sport, and childrearing. Gilbert Meilaender worries that 'expanded definitions of health will extend medical authority into too much of life while at the same time expanding the notion of "health needs" through an analysis focusing on gender, race, and class.'[72] But the rejection of the compartmentalization of health care need not result in the inevitable expansion of medical authority. The point is to redefine health preservation and enhancement, not to reduplicate existing processes devoted to them. Rather than simply claiming that 'all of life and life's activities are therapeutic,' we need to grasp, in Janice Raymond's words, that 'a good life is conducive to good health.'[73] We need a commitment, as practitioners of bio(medical)politics, to bringing about the conditions that promote good lives.

The absence of some things – attention, respect, love, physical affection, validation, adequate nutrition, exercise, fun, relaxation, and meaningful work – along with the presence of others – stressful jobs, poor housing, bad food, inadequate education, dangerous and unhealthy environments, violent relationships, oppressive social structures, and the emphasis on acquisition of material possessions – contribute to health problems. Bio(medical)politics should be committed to asking whether existing cultural values, practices, and institutions are inevitable. This perspective rejects the patterns of genderization and systematic infantilization within health care and is sensitive to the contribution of forms of oppression – sexism, heterosexism, racism, classism, and so on – to health problems. It challenges the cultural commitment to beauty, youth, and technological perfectionism and is cognizant of issues of disability[74] and the social construction of illness, deviance, and 'craziness.'[75] The commitment of bio(medical)politics to non-maleficence as a micro-principle implies, on the macro level, ending sexism, systematic infantilization, and other oppressive systems that cause widespread harm and a dedication to the empowerment and liberation of women,[76] people of colour, children, persons with disabilities, and others – without privileging an incessant self-focus that encourages preoccupation with one's own or one's group's own injuries to the exclusion of those of others or to the exclusion of general strategies for liberation. Practitioners of bio(medical)politics should be committed to the deconstruction of the feminine,[77] or more generally the deconstruction of gender, and, ultimately, to the demise of gender and all other invidious uses of social categories.

Bioethics-as-usual is both a highly successful and a conservative academic field. It reflects the hierarchism, individualism, professionalism, and separatism of medicine and is able to co-opt the radical potential of some progressive analyses of health care and the medical profession – including those, such as the ethic of care, that are derived from women's experience. The alternative, I suggest, is the self-reflective and self-critical theory and practice of bio(medical)politics, which can highlight the political constitution of health care boundaries, cases, moralities, practices, and policies, with special attention to the ways in which systematic infantilization has pervaded the practice of both traditional medicine and traditional bioethics.

Notes

I wish to thank Wayne Sumner of the University of Toronto Department of Philosophy, whose provocative questions about the nature of bioethics inspired the writing of this paper. I also thank Jerry Bickenbach, of the Queen's University Department of

Philosophy, as well as the participants in the Queen's University Department of Philosophy Summer Colloquium, especially Sandra Taylor, Michael Fox, Sue Hendler, and Stephen Leighton, for their helpful comments.

1 So-called reproductive ethics encompasses far more than specifically medical activities; for example, it includes a concern for the effects of the workplace and of environmental contaminants on reproductive health.

2 Margaret Urban Walker, 'Moral Understandings: Alternative "Epistemology" for a Feminist Ethics,' *Hypatia* 4, 2 (Summer 1989): 24.

3 Indeed, I recently withdrew from a project on medical genetics precisely because my role, as conceived by the project's main investigators, was to have been that of an ethical tinkerer, fiddling with the details of medical practices of genetic testing, without in any way challenging their social context, their value, or their general ethical implications.

4 Robert M. Veatch, *Case Studies in Medical Ethics* (Cambridge, MA: Harvard University Press, 1977), pp. 149–50.

5 Margaret Urban Walker, 'Keeping Moral Space Open: New Images of Ethics Consulting,' *Hastings Center Report* 23, 2 (March–April 1993): 34, her emphasis.

6 See also Virginia L. Warren's discussion of standard problem definition and choice within applied ethics, which, she argues, often keep women 'on the defensive'; Warren, 'Feminist Directions in Medical Ethics,' *Hypatia* 4, 2 (Summer 1989): 75.

7 Ivan Illich, *Limits to Medicine: Medical Nemesis, The Expropriation of Health* (London: Marion Boyars, 1976), p. 103, fn. 211.

8 Susan Sherwin, *No Longer Patient: Feminist Ethics and Health Care* (Philadelphia: Temple University, 1992).

9 Christine Overall, *Ethics and Human Reproduction: A Feminist Analysis* (Boston: Allen & Unwin, 1987); idem, *Human Reproduction: Principles, Practices, Policies* (Toronto: Oxford University Press, 1993).

10 Jerome E. Bickenbach, *Physical Disability and Social Policy* (Toronto: University of Toronto Press, 1993).

11 Janice G. Raymond, 'Medicine as Patriarchal Religion,' *The Journal of Medicine and Philosophy* 7 (1982): 200.

12 See Illich, *Limits to Medicine*.

13 Sherwin, *No Longer Patient*, pp. 3–4.

14 Ibid., p. 4.

15 Ibid.

16 Warren, 'Feminist Directions in Medical Ethics,' p. 78.

17 Sara Ruddick, 'Maternal Thinking,' in Joyce Trebilcot (ed.), *Mothering: Essays in Feminist Theory* (Totowa, NJ: Rowman and Allanheld, 1984), pp. 213–30.

18 Not by virtue of the role identity itself, but by virtue of the experience usually associated with it. Mary Briody Mahowald has developed the interesting notion of 'paren-

talism' as an alternative to the one-sidedness of both paternalism (acting on the basis of the patient's assumed welfare, independent of his/her wishes) and maternalism (the fostering of autonomy and independence) in health care. Parentalism involves mutual caring, protection from harms, and the fostering of autonomy; Mahowald, *Women and Children and Health Care: An Unequal Majority* (New York: Oxford, 1993), pp. 32, 262.

19 As do Ruddick, 'Maternal Thinking'; and Virginia Held, 'Non-Contractual Society: A Feminist View,' in Marsha Hanen and Kai Nielsen (eds), *Science, Morality and Feminist Theory* (Calgary: University of Calgary Press, 1987), pp. 111–37.

20 The conservatism of bioethics, in both Canada and the United States, is likely to be exacerbated by the economic conservatism and financial retrenchment of 1990s-style health care.

21 Sherwin, *No Longer Patient*, p. 87.

22 Veatch, *Case Studies*, pp. 150–1.

23 Nel Noddings, *Caring: A Feminine Approach to Ethics and Moral Education* (Berkeley: University of California Press, 1984).

24 Joan C. Tronto, 'Women and Caring: What Can Feminists Learn about Morality from Caring?' in Alison M. Jaggar and Susan R. Bordo (eds), *Gender/Body/Knowledge: Feminist Reconstructions of Being and Knowing* (New Brunswick, NJ: Rutgers University Press, 1989), p. 174.

25 Joan C. Tronto, 'Beyond Gender Difference to a Theory of Care,' *Signs: Journal of Women in Culture and Society* 12, 4 (Summer 1987): 648.

26 Eve Browning Cole, *Philosophy and Feminist Criticism: An Introduction* (New York: Paragon House, 1993), p. 107, her emphasis.

27 Carol Gilligan claims that the two main moral perspectives she identifies, justice and care, are related, like background and foreground in figure-ground pictures; Gilligan, 'Moral Orientation and Moral Development,' in Eva Feder Kittay and Diana T. Meyers (eds), *Women and Moral Theory* (Totowa, NJ: Rowman and Littlefield, 1987).

28 Warren, 'Feminist Directions in Medical Ethics,' p. 80.

29 Robert M. Veatch, 'Clinical Ethics, Applied Ethics, and Theory,' in Barry Hoffmaster, Benjamin Freedman, and Gwen Fraser (eds), *Clinical Ethics: Theory and Practice* (Clifton, NJ: Humana Press, 1989), p. 16. Autonomy is a characteristic that the physician (and bioethicist) grants to or recognizes or accepts (or not) in the patient. Helen J. John suggests that a focus on autonomy has the effect of 'bypass[ing] criticism of social arrangements and institutions by centering attention on personal choice'; John, 'Reflections on Autonomy and Abortion,' in David H. Smith (ed.), *Respect and Care in Medical Ethics* (Lanham, MD: University Press of America, 1984), p. 277.

30 Eike-Henner Kluge, 'Medical Ethics and Women,' *Canadian Medical Association Journal* 142, 8 (1990): 878, emphasis added.

31 Cheryl Nobel, 'Ethics and Experts,' *Hastings Center Report* 12, 3 (June 1982): 7.
32 Walker, 'Keeping Moral Space Open,' p. 33, her emphasis.
33 Ibid., p. 38.
34 Giles R. Scofield, Letter, *Hastings Center Report* 23, 5 (September–October 1993): 45.
35 Barry Hoffmaster, 'Philosophical Ethics and Practical Ethics: Never the Twain Shall Meet,' in Hoffmaster, Freedman, and Fraser (eds), *Clinical Ethics*, p. 201.
36 K. Danner Clouser, 'Bioethics and Philosophy,' *Hastings Center Report Special Supplement* 23, 6 (November–December 1993): S10.
37 Significantly, many of them have an overtly conservative history. For example, Betty A. Sichel suggests that institutional ethics committees originated in the United States at least in part to avoid federal interventions into difficult health care cases and to 'protect health care institutions and personnel against malpractice claims'; Sichel, 'Ethics of Caring and the Institutional Ethics Committee,' *Hypatia* 4, 2 (Summer 1989): 46–7, 48.
38 Veatch, 'Clinical Ethics, Applied Ethics, and Theory,' p. 20.
39 Ibid., pp. 22–3.
40 Peter Singer, 'How Do We Decide?' *Hastings Center Report* 12, 3 (June 1982): 10.
41 I owe this point to Jerry Bickenbach.
42 For example, Sichel argues that the ethic of care is already well in use within institutional ethics committees ('Ethics of Caring and the Institutional Ethics Committee'). Sara T. Fry says that it has been adopted by the nursing profession in the United States; Fry, 'The Role of Caring in a Theory of Nursing Ethics,' *Hypatia* 4, 2 (Summer 1989) 88–103.

    Proceed with Care, the final report of the Canadian Royal Commission on New Reproductive Technologies, outlines the moral theory the commission purportedly used to arrive at its recommendations. Its 'Ethical Framework,' based on a research paper by liberal philosopher Will Kymlicka, is described as an 'ethic of care,' which 'gives priority to ... mutual care and connectedness and tries to foster it ... rather than being concerned only with resolving conflicts that have already occurred.' Significantly, the framework is also said to encompass 'eight guiding principles,' which 'serve as a prism for moral deliberations'; Royal Commission on New Reproductive Technologies, *Proceed with Care: Final Report of the Royal Commission on New Reproductive Technologies* (Ottawa: Minister of Government Services Canada, 1993), p. 50. Two of the eight – 'individual autonomy' and 'equality' – are standard bioethics textbook fare. Others – such as 'appropriate use of resources' and 'accountability' – are so general as to be almost empty. And most of the rest – 'respect for human life and dignity' is the most egregious example – can easily be enlisted in the service of a right-wing procreative agenda. The Royal Commission's 'Ethical Framework' is a good example of the potentially conservative results of an attempt to combine traditional bioethical notions with an ethic of care.

43 For extensive criticisms of the ethic of care see the Review Symposium on Nel Nod-dings, '*Caring: A Feminine Approach to Ethics and Moral Education*,' *Hypatia*, 5, 1 (Spring 1990). A central criticism of caring is that its history and its contemporary interpretations are gendered. See Tronto, 'Beyond Gender Difference to a Theory of Care,' and Jean Grimshaw, *Philosophy and Feminist Thinking* (Minneapolis: University of Minnesota Press, 1986), pp. 215ff.

44 Rosemarie Tong, *Feminine and Feminist Ethics* (Belmont, CA: Wadsworth, 1993), p. 226. The extent of the welcome given by the Tradition to the concept of caring is indicated, at least in part, by the fact that in the Queen's University Library computer system, the key word 'caring' calls up 206 items, the phrase 'ethics and care' calls up 171, and 'care and health' no fewer than 2,809 – although of course not all of the latter can be assumed to be about ethics of care.

45 See, for example, Sherwin, *No Longer Patient*.

46 Tronto, 'Women and Caring,' p. 181.

47 Warren, 'Feminist Directions in Medical Ethics,' p. 85.

48 Arthur L. Caplan, 'Moral Experts and Moral Expertise: Do Either Exist?' in Hoffmaster, Freedman, and Fraser (eds), *Clinical Ethics*, p. 82.

49 Howard Brody, 'Applied Ethics: Don't Change the Subject,' in Hoffmaster, Freedman, and Fraser, *Clinical Ethics*, p. 197.

50 Grimshaw, *Philosophy and Feminist Thinking*, p. 234.

51 Ibid., p. 239.

52 Hoffmaster, 'Philosophical Ethics,' p. 209.

53 More and more attention is being paid to them. See, for example, Walker, 'Moral Understandings.'

54 See Tronto, 'Beyond Gender Difference to a Theory of Care.' Neither am I referring merely to what is perhaps the newest interpretation of problem context, as 'a *narrative* understanding of moral problems and moral deliberation,' according to which 'we need to know how the parties are, how they understand themselves and each other, what terms of relationship have brought them to this morally problematic point' (Walker, 'Keeping Moral Space Open,' p. 35, her emphasis).

55 Walker, 'Keeping Moral Space Open,' p. 35.

56 Walker, 'Moral Understandings,' p. 24, her emphasis.

57 Sherwin, *No Longer Patient*, p. 84.

58 Ibid., pp. 55, 57.

59 As a society we are not committed to meeting children's special needs, and this is evident in how the social environment is structured. One obvious example is public washrooms: the sinks and toilets are too high for young ones to use comfortably, the paper towels are out of reach, the water in the tap is burningly hot, and there is seldom any facility to enable parents to change diapers or breast feed in comfort. While access to public buildings is becoming more widely recognized as an important issue

for disabled persons, it is never considered in connection with children, who have trouble negotiating steep stairs, cannot reach elevator buttons, and fall easily on slippery, hard waxed floors. Public institutions like banks, post offices, and government buildings are forbidding places to little children, and public events that are not suitable for children, such as conferences, workshops, films, lectures, and exhibits seldom, if ever, offer adequate child care.

The social environment is not accommodated to children, and on that basis alone North American society must be charged with indifference to our offspring. This lack of concern for children's needs is also a symptom of a wider social pattern of segregation of children – segregation that, if applied to any other group of human beings, would be considered immoral and illegal. There are apartment buildings, hotels, and restaurants that not only do not welcome children but sometimes actually forbid their presence. Children are banished from workplaces and confined to age-stratified institutions called 'schools.' Daycare is inadequate, expensive, and often non-existent. Instead of welcoming children into everyday adult activities, we encourage them to take part in substitute behaviours: games and toys that are imitations of real human work, entertainment that distorts and confines their understanding of the world, and lessons that make them hate what they are learning.

Children have virtually no voice in the society in which they live. Denied many of the most basic ways of expressing their views, for example, by voting or changing their place of residence, children are very seldom listened to and are unable to affect social policy. Even on the level of personal interactions it is a common observation in grocery stores or on buses that children will ask questions and make comments to adults and be utterly ignored or, at best, laughed at. Many children routinely find that they must make requests, three, four, or five times before finally the urgency in their voices gets noticed. Children are thought to be nuisances. How many adults are even willing to assume that children have ideas and opinions worth hearing? As Shulamith Firestone remarks, the segregation of children from adults indicates 'disrespect for, [and] a systematic underestimation of, the abilities of the child'; Firestone, *The Dialectic of Sex* (New York: William Morrow 1979), p. 83.

So North American children are not welcomed in adult society, are segregated from it, and are ignored. But the treatment of children is even worse than this. Children are deliberately used; indeed, the exploitation of children is so widespread and common as to be taken for granted. Children's tastes and interests are often powerfully manipulated in order to sell consumer goods, goods that may fail to benefit them and may even harm them. A huge toy industry, a burgeoning market for snack and fast foods, and an entertainment industry that cultivates passivity and non-thinking all testify to the money to be made from selling to children.

Perhaps not surprisingly in a society where children can be so effectively exploited as consumers, they are not only urged to buy commodities; they actually *become* commodities. Children are regarded as a type of consumer good to be acquired only if we can afford them and they fit our 'lifestyle.' Parents are encouraged to want only the highest-quality children: prenatal diagnosis and other reproductive technologies are supposed to ensure that less than perfect offspring are eliminated, and later on, music, art, sports, and other forms of training and child-betterment schemes are devoted to producing top-notch child products.

What all of these aspects of our behaviour towards children suggest is that children are viewed as possessions (Janet Farrell Smith, 'Parenting and Property,' in Trebil-cot, *Mothering*), as items that can be purchased, improved upon, and even (with the advent of contract motherhood) sold. If they are adults' possessions, then it follows – does it not? – that adults can do what they like with them. That attitude is all too obvious in the behaviour of the horrifying numbers of adults who subject children, both their 'own' and those that 'belong' to other people, to cruel physical, sexual, and psychological abuse, sometimes in the name of 'discipline.' Hundreds of thousands of children are routinely exposed to severe and almost unremitting torment as part of the experience of 'growing up.' Others are not actively hurt, but they suffer from neglect, deprivation, and serious malnutrition.

60 Grimshaw, *Philosophy and Feminist Thinking*, p. 222, emphasis added.

61 Donald S. Klinefelter, 'Aging, Autonomy, and the Value of Life,' in Smith, *Respect and Care in Medical Ethics*.

62 This classification is founded upon certain implicit metaphysical assumptions about what a child is: a non-person, less than fully human, uncivilized, incomprehensible by ordinary human standards. When older human beings are infantilized, these assumptions have been inadvertently transferred to them.

63 In this context, infantilization partly intersects with classism (see Firestone, *The Dialectic of Sex*).

64 Infantilization is not to be confused with infantilism, which is immature ('childish') behaviour manifested by an adult. While infantilism is not particularly commendable, those who manifest it do not necessarily deserve to be infantilized.

65 In *The Silent World of Doctor and Patient* (New York: Free Press, 1984), Jay Katz repeatedly mentions, without much elaboration, the tendency of physicians to regard their patients as children. He suggests that 'the childlikeness so often displayed by patients is triggered not only by pain, fears, illness, and memories but also by how physicians view and respond to patients,' 101.

66 Veatch, 'Clinical Ethics, Applied Ethics, and Theory,' pp. 14, 20.

67 Caroline Whitbeck, 'Why the Attention to Paternalism in Medical Ethics? Review Essay of James F. Childress's *Who Should Decide? Paternalism in Health Care*', *Journal of Health Politics, Policy and Law* 10, 1 (Spring 1985): 183.

68 See Noddings, *Caring*.

69 Caroline Whitbeck, 'A Different Reality: Feminist Ontology,' in Carol C. Gould

(ed.), *Beyond Domination: New Perspectives on Women and Philosophy* (Totowa, NJ: Rowman & Allanheld, 1983), p. 65.

70 Janice G. Raymond, *The Transsexual Empire* (London: Women's Press, 1979), p. 150.

71 See also Sherwin's very thorough discussion of the ways in which a feminist approach transforms bioethics (*No Longer Patient*, pp. 92–5).

72 Gilbert Meilaender, 'A Feminist Medical Ethics?' *Hastings Center Report* 23, 3 (May–June 1993): 44.

73 Raymond, 'Medicine as Patriarchal Religion,' p. 213.

74 See Susan Wendell, 'Toward a Feminist Theory of Disability,' *Hypatia* 4, 2 (Summer 1989): 104–24.

75 These are connected to gendering in certain ways (as evidence, for example, if one deviates from gender expectations).

76 We can see health care and bioethics as gendered, and can criticize their politics, without (1) supposing that women are ultimately better than men or biologically very different; (2) adopting conspiracy theories about medicine's attack on women – for example, the catastrophizing in much of feminist reproductive ethics (see most of the articles in the journal *Issues in Reproductive and Genetic Engineering*) is probably a mistake; or (3) presupposing a uniquely female moral point of view as the only legitimate response to bioethical issues.

77 Barbara Houston, 'Rescuing Womanly Virtues: Some Dangers of Moral Reclamation,' in Hanen and Nielsen, *Science, Morality and Feminist Theory*, p. 241.

Theory versus Practice in Ethics: A Feminist Perspective on Justice in Health Care

A Methodological Proposal

My main concern in this essay is to dismantle the widely accepted distinction between conceptual and practical questions in ethics and bioethics. In the usual organization of ethical activity, conceptual and practical activities are treated as distinct and separate tasks. The conceptual category includes matters such as the pursuit of questions aimed at developing systems for investigating moral claims and also efforts to clarify the nature of the terms, principles, and arguments that are used in moral discussions. The practical category is thought to encompass the explorations of questions that arise out of the human experience of trying to live as a moral agent, including efforts to propose, critique, and defend solutions to identified moral problems. While most theorists assume that there are connections between these two tasks, the precise nature and strength of those connections tend to be unexamined.

Within this familiar model for organizing ethical thought, it is generally agreed that, of the two broad types of concerns, the conceptual questions are the more truly philosophical. Indeed, conceptual questions are usually addressed as paradigmatically philosophical, best approached as purely abstract, theoretical problems that demand a relatively high level of philosophic inclination and experience. In contrast, practical problems are thought to represent questions that confront all moral agents when they discover contradictions or ambiguities among their personal beliefs about moral behaviour. Since identifying and exploring practical questions is an activity demanded of all moral agents, and since philosophers do not seem to be especially good at actually living morally, it is not at all clear that practical ethics even requires any special philosophical acumen. Indeed, there are debates in the philosophical literature about whether the study of actual moral problems is appropriately addressed within philosophy at all.

The field of bioethics is defined largely in terms of its focus on concerns that are principally on the practical side of this divide; so philosophers, while prominent within bioethics, tend to have a somewhat uneasy relationship to the field. Because the problems studied in bioethics seem virtually to announce themselves to conscientious agents, it seems that recognizing them does not require any special philosophical expertise; moreover, responding to them often seems to require more practical wisdom than analytic skill. While philosophers are inclined to stress the conceptual issues underlying particular problems (e.g., definitions of life, death, and personhood), most acknowledge that discussion usually originates and concludes in the practical domain. Many quite modestly assign themselves the limited tasks of clarifying what is 'really' at issue in ethically problematic cases and fitting particular ethical questions into a larger moral structure. Some philosophers engaged in bioethics describe their work as simply helping to analyse a problem into its component features in order to make clear which factor should dominate when those who are ultimately responsible for implementing decisions seek a solution to a moral problem.

This vision of a bifurcated ethics landscape is not limited to philosophers, but is widely assumed within the interdisciplinary field of bioethics. Many who approach bioethics from different disciplines have learned to expect philosophers to contribute to moral deliberations primarily at the level of conceptual analysis. Some even appear to assume that this dichotomy within ethics represents an efficient division of moral labour and that all necessary philosophical input can easily be summarized in the initial stages of bioethical investigation simply by adopting some variation of the 'Georgetown mantra' – an appeal to the principles of autonomy, beneficence, non-maleficence, and justice as the strategic theoretical tool necessary for resolving most sorts of moral dilemmas.[1] It is not uncommon to find practitioners treating these four principles as an adequate summary of all necessary conceptual effort when they engage in practical ethical problem-solving. They proceed to address specific moral dilemmas without any felt need to attend any further to the conceptual dimensions of moral deliberation, leaving those niceties to philosophers. Trusting that this efficient division of moral labour has generated reliable interpretations of the values represented by the central principles, some bioethicists seem to believe that all that remains is empirical study to determine how the central moral principles work out in the actual world of health care.

Confronted with such a stark interpretation of the tasks of applied ethics, many philosophers are highly critical of the sort of mechanistic model of bioethics in which moral principles are accepted as given and the real work of ethical deliberation involves primarily empirical investigation into the specifics of application. Yet it is philosophers themselves who have invited this model of bioethical activity by their commitment to distinguishing the philosophical or conceptual aspects of moral deliberation from the practical dimensions of moral life. They have deeply entrenched the idea that a distinction exists between the abstract theoretical dimensions of ethical thought and the practical work of analysing dilemmas – this distinction is so deeply entrenched in philosophic thought, in fact, that its existence is generally accepted as a truism in need of no real argument.[2] In so far as debate exists around this matter, it is chiefly confined to the question of which realm is the legitimate sphere for ethical thought. The majority of philosophers has long favoured the view that the philosopher's role is exclusively in the abstract conceptual realm, though a vocal and rebellious group argues for the prominence of practical reasoning free of the restrictive constraints of theory.[3] Some philosophers active in the field of bioethics have gone farther yet and come to despair of the usefulness of abstract ethics altogether.[4] Despite these ongoing disagreements about which element is primary, few philosophers have challenged the general view that they are separate and distinct activities.

I want to dispute this common assumption, however, and I shall argue that the two sorts of ethics tasks are inextricably linked. In support of this thesis, I shall explore the concept of justice and show how important it is to attend to the intimate interrelationship of conceptual and practical concerns when we invoke this central concept in health care discussions. I shall argue that the connections between theoretical and practical concerns run both ways; that is, both that the conceptual discussions of the terms of the debates about justice in health care cannot be adequately addressed in abstraction from the practical questions at issue and also that the practical proposals we might make about justice in health care must involve important theoretical decisions. Neither task should be pursued in isolation of the other. We should reject all models of ethics that envision practitioners engaged in a deductive exercise of developing and then applying settled concepts to practical dilemmas. We ought also to reject models of bioethical reasoning that suppose we can resolve specific questions merely by gathering particular sorts of data without reflecting on the concepts and principles that guide our deliberations.

This proposal may seem mundane, since no one argues explicitly that we can pursue either agenda in the absence of the other. When phrased in the stark terms of mutually exclusive practices, the idea of rigidly dividing ethical activities is easily rejected. It is widely appreciated that we need to know something about conceptual matters in order to attend to practical concerns, and it is also commonly recognized (though with more ambivalence) that we cannot adequately pursue theoretical questions without considering their implications in the practical domain. Despite this surface agreement, however, it seems very common in practice to find theorists and practitioners doing exactly that. Philosophers who engage chiefly in ethical theory often restrict their discussion to purely abstract considerations, and, in so far as they attend to the practical repercussions of their proposals, they confine themselves to hypothetical, and often fanciful, examples. At the same time, much of the research conducted in bioethics focuses only on the details of application of widely accepted (though vague) principles, and no efforts are made to examine or question the values that are invoked. Further, even those who do explicitly acknowledge that there must be some connection between theory and practice tend to be quite vague about the precise nature of that connection; they generally leave unexpressed both the details as to the specific sorts of data that are relevant to theory-making and also the type of conceptual work that is essential to good practical analysis. Yet failure to specify the details of that conception can undermine both projects, for it often results in neglect of elements that are ultimately important to each of these areas of concern.

I am convinced that we need a more explicit expression of the importance of doing theory and practice together, and, in the course of arguing for a more self-conscious connection between these two domains, I shall spell out some of the particular ways in which those links are to be made. I shall look at the central question of justice in health care as a specific example of how these issues must be investigated in tandem. By spelling out the outlines of a particular interpretation of the concept of justice in the context of health care discussions and contrasting it with other approaches that are less committed to doing both levels of analysis together, I hope to demonstrate why theoretical and practical concerns must be explored in concert with one another.

In addition, I shall use this area of moral debate to raise a further objection to the familiar picture of moral analysis reviewed above in which practical moral issues are taken as given and are readily apparent. This picture is problematic because it ignores the moral dimensions that are involved in the actual framing of practical moral questions – the step that is commonly assumed to be self-evident and non-controversial. The identification and characterization of practical moral problems themselves must be recognized as morally complex activities in need of study so that we can see that they too require moral reflection. Moreover, the same point applies to the questions pursued primarily at the conceptual level: the concepts we choose to invoke in organizing our moral thoughts and the ways we choose to interpret those abstract ideas have important moral consequences when they are applied to actual moral life; therefore, they also must be made subject to moral review. This means that even the methodology we rely on should be evaluated not only in terms of its internal coherence and intuitive plausibility, but also in moral terms that take into account the effects that its use is likely to produce on the world.

Part of the task of bioethics, then, is to become sensitive to and critically engaged with the ethical issues involved in the decisions of which questions are studied, how they are formulated, and what conceptual tools are brought to bear on them. Since all these features are likely to influence the answers we entertain, we need to reflect on the choices we make regarding each. As I contrast a distinctly feminist concept of justice in health care with more traditional views, I shall identify some of the overlooked moral dimensions of these matters and point out how this feminist conception radically changes the focus of concern and, hence, the outcomes recommended.

Feminist Reflective Equilibrium

Because this proposal is, in many respects, similar to the idea of reflective equilibrium proposed by John Rawls,[5] it is useful to spell out both the similarities and the differences between our approaches. Like Rawls, I am recommending a dialectical type of process for ethics in which we are to explore theoretical questions by simultaneously examining the practical effect of the theoretical proposals we entertain and by searching for theoretical expressions of our initial moral values. In his conception, ethical theory is to be developed by engaging in an ongoing practice of shifting our focus back and forth between the level of abstract, theoretical concepts and principles and that of our considered moral judgments. Each level is envisioned as correcting and informing the other until our intuitions at both levels can be brought into line with one another. Since neither is sufficient in itself or logically prior to the other, both levels of reflection are necessary to the construction of adequate moral views. In order to ensure an adequate scope to these reflections, Rawls recommends that we look at a wide range of moral alternatives and weigh competing moral ideals before settling on any particular one; this can best be achieved by taking into account the considered moral views of others as well as our own.

While there is much wisdom in the methodology that Rawls proposes, I find this conception of reflective equilibrium to be in need of refinement. For one thing, he describes this practice in entirely abstract terms and ideals. The comparison of views he proposes is done entirely at the level of generalizations and rules, so there is no requirement for us to attend to the specific details of particular human lives. As Rawls envisions it, our conceptual and theoretical commitments are to be developed and tested against considered moral judgments, which themselves are merely abstract generalizations about moral behaviour. (In his later work, Rawls makes clear that what he has in mind is general views such as 'slavery is wrong' and 'religious differences should be tolerated.'[6]) He does not demand that we reflect on the actual details of any particular moral dilemmas in this exercise, and, when he practices reflective equilibrium himself, his reflection is confined to hypothetical and fundamentally abstract circumstances (especially the conditions of the original position).[7]

In contrast, I propose that we go beyond the general and the hypothetical and include practical concerns and observations of real life in this process. In my view, we should strive to ensure that any ethical proposals we come up with address the specific concerns that are generated by attention to our actual world. We ought to evaluate the adequacy of any theoretical proposals by considering very carefully what effect they have on actual moral problems within existing circumstances and arrangements. We can still speak in terms of the metaphor of reflective equilibrium, but we should demand that the equilibrium we pursue involve a third element, namely, attention to the practical world of moral life, in addition to the two levels of abstraction that Rawls proposed.

Further, I think that it is important to make certain, when we entertain the considered moral views of others, that we do not follow Rawls in restricting the scope of that injunction to examination of developed moral theories, but that we explore the moral views of a wide range of people. In so far as the differences in experience of this diverse group inform their various moral judgments, we should investigate the moral relevance of those differences. In this task, it is especially important that we take steps to secure access to the experiences and judgments of those whose voices are least likely to be heard in traditional ethics debates by virtue of their relatively disadvantaged positions in society.

I am concerned, then, that Rawls is silent about the sorts of social and political considerations that are associated with existing patterns of oppression.[8] I have argued elsewhere that moral reasoning ought to take account of the social and political dimensions of the actions and policies it reviews; I consider these factors to be essential aspects of moral evaluation that must be reflected in our moral commitments.[9] More specifically, in a world in which powerful systems of oppression and domination have a significant and unjustifiable impact on the relative privilege or disadvantage of members of different social groups, such systemic forces must be seen to be morally objectionable. Because systemic oppression, such as sexism and racism, has devastating consequences on many human lives, and because it is manifestly unjust, it is a matter of moral urgency that we identify, condemn, and find ways to eliminate these sorts of forces from our society. Listening to the voices of those who are harmed by these oppressive forces will help us to recognize and address the moral injustice of oppression.

In the light of the centrality that concerns about oppression play in feminist moral thought, I use the term 'feminist ethics' to identify those approaches to ethics that direct us to include attention to these sorts of features of social and political life in our moral deliberations. My methodological proposal, then, is that ethics and bioethics proceed by a practice that might be called 'feminist reflective equilibrium,' in which we make a conscious effort to consider questions of domination and power as morally relevant concerns when we explore the conceptual and practical dimensions of issues in bioethics.

This form of reflective equilibrium differs from the one proposed by Rawls in several important respects. Most obviously, it ensures that we pay attention to the systemic forms of power differentials that are represented by patterns of oppression and privilege. In addition, it is self-consciously situated within the specific social and political contexts in which it is conducted. That is, this notion of feminist reflective equilibrium is occupied with the real-life concerns of particular social and political arrangements, in awareness of the fact that oppression can take many different forms and have many different effects and that it is likely to look very different from different social perspectives. Feminist reflective equilibrium requires us to examine the salient details of the actual social relations that it is meant to address. Rather than striving to identify a set of eternal moral truths, this methodology is aimed at identifying moral ideals that are explicitly relative to a specific time and place.

I cannot share Rawls's faith that the perspective of a single rational moral agent can be reliably generalized to offer a universal perspective. Attention to political difference makes it clear that we must insist on the active engagement of persons from diverse social positions in the pursuit of moral insight. In the light of the established difficulty those in privileged groups have in even perceiving oppression, it is especially important that we secure the active participation of those for whom part of their oppression consists in their exclusion from discussions of ethics. Rather than disqualifying victims of oppression from moral discussions of oppression by virtue of their 'special interest' – as many moral theorists do – my proposal of feminist reflective equilibrium works from the assumption that everyone has a stake of some sort or other in existing patterns of oppression and that adequate moral analysis requires that we acknowledge this social fact and find ways of ensuring that moral concerns are not obscured by the self-interested ignorance of any particular group. Thus, whereas Rawls envisioned a process of reflective equilibrium that seems to be aimed at producing timeless, static, universal rules for ethics,[10] the feminist version I am proposing promotes a process that is collaborative, situated in time and place, dynamic, and sensitive to the ways in which one's own experience may limit one's moral vision.

In order to make my methodological point clear, I shall now engage in some of the conceptual and practical work that I am recommending. To illustrate my position, I shall sketch out some proposals about how feminist ethics suggests that we understand the concept of justice in health care contexts, and I shall contrast my interpretation with some familiar, non-feminist alternatives. I shall pay particular attention to the fact that the alternative (non-feminist) conceptions in the literature purport to be apolitical and disinterested with respect to questions of oppression and domination. As such, they represent themselves as evolving within a philosophical framework in which the theoretical work of concept formation is done in isolation from the particular circumstances in which that concept will be invoked. I shall argue that these alternative conceptions are not as apolitical and abstract as they claim to be, but, because of their proponents' unwillingness to acknowledge their practical and political roots explicitly, these conceptions are insensitive to important moral dimensions of the very contexts they are meant to address. I shall also use this particular area of ethical reflection to point out why I think it is important to recognize the moral dimensions of choosing and framing ethical problems for analysis at both the theoretical and the practical levels.

The Traditional Approaches to Justice in Health Care

Let us begin, then, with the most familiar bioethical formulations of the ethical issues associated with questions of justice in health care. Typically, arguments about justice in health care are defined as being about accessibility to health care services and about the associated question of who should pay for those services. There is a vast literature addressing this topic and most of it focuses on two basic questions: (1) What should be the basis for access to health services? (2) How are particular resources to be allocated when the demand exceeds the supply? (These are commonly categorized as questions of macroallocation and microallocation, respectively.) I shall limit my remarks to the first question, since it is the more fundamental of the two.

The issue of access to health services is often formulated in terms of the question: Who is to pay for these services? In either version, the discussion is typically cast in the language of rights. In most cases, those who argue in favour of socialized medical services choose the first formulation and argue that universal access to needed health care must be assured in response to a universal positive right to health care – a right that is ultimately grounded in a particular theory of justice. In contrast, those who place greatest value on individual liberty rights usually opt for the second formulation. They define coercive taxation for the purpose of paying for the health care of others as a violation of individual liberty, and so they oppose the conditions required to fund any form of socialized medicine program. Hence, the traditional debate tends to be about the nature of rights and the primacy to be placed on positive and negative rights.

Of course, other positions between these two poles are found in the literature. Some authors try to steer a middle course in which they argue for partial socialization of medical services, suggesting, for example, that the state fund only 'essential' medical services at a 'basic' level. Others demand that we factor in questions of personal responsibility for health and illness by subsidizing the forms of health care that are associated with unavoidable illness but not by guaranteeing provision of health services for conditions brought about by unhealthy practices, such as drug or alcohol abuse. Despite the intuitive appeal of the various intermediary proposals, it has proved extraordinarily difficult to translate them into practice; and for practical purposes, we still are left with the central question of whether or not any significant amount of health care should be socialized, and so we are back with the original problem.

Note that this debate, although ultimately of enormous practical and political significance, is carried out as if it were an abstract contest about the concepts of justice and rights, where each side constructs the issue and the central concepts differently. Both sides approach the issue as one of determining the proper meaning of these general moral terms; both assume that those meanings can then be invoked in a purely deductive argument in favour of their own preferred social policies, although that is not how their own reasoning usually proceeds. Rather, proponents on both sides of this issue tend to be well aware of the policy implications of their conceptual commitments before they make them. Hence, there is, at best, something disingenuous about the implied suggestion that the conceptual work is being done in abstraction from any political concerns.

This same phenomenon can be widely observed in other areas of health care ethics. For instance, it seems clear that within the abortion debate, although conceptual commitments are usually argued for in a priori fashion, such decisions are, in fact, seldom made before their practical implications are identified and accepted. Competing definitions of personhood, rights, and the ontological and moral status of the fetus all are claimed to be, ideally, purely theoretical concerns. In practice, however, I believe that conceptual choices generally are shaped by political values – at least to the degree that the practical outcomes that advocates prefer are built into the concepts they promote. I find that few people are willing to make these sorts of conceptual choices without ensuring that their choices do not require them to support a policy on abortion that they consider unacceptable. In other words, despite the misleading structure of many arguments on abortion, the definition of central concepts does not generally precede the practical policy proposals they suggest. Neither do they simply follow slavishly from those policy preferences. In so far as theorists are engaged in

moral debate about abortion, they recognize the importance of careful conceptual analysis of the theoretical commitments they are willing to entertain; such
analysis may well lead to modification – though seldom outright rejection – of
their initial practical intuitions.

The traditional deductive model of ethical deliberations would judge this sort
of interactive theorizing objectionable. Even Rawls, who proposes reflective
equilibrium as a dialectical rather than a purely deductive methodology for
arriving at our theoretical commitments, urges us to approach practical policy
issues by distancing ourselves from the actual effect of those theoretical commitments; in his scheme, we are first to agree on the general moral principles
that will generate the morally justifiable policy before we look to see what
effects they will have in practice. In contrast, I consider this common interplay
to be a clear example of the inevitability of proceeding on both practical and
theoretical levels at the same time. Not only are moral deliberations actually
carried out in this way, but it is how they should be conducted. It is at least as
great a mistake to try to decide on the personhood status of the fetus without
considering the implications of that conceptual decision in the real world as it is
to assume that one can come to a firm view about the moral or political legitimacy of abortion without considering the sort of beings that fetuses are. Both
levels of thought are essential to adequate moral reflection in the context of
abortion; similarly, both levels are essential when questions of justice in health
care are reflected on.

What is generally wrong with the debates about abortion and justice in the
provision of health services is not that political implications are usually operating in the background of each position, but that denying their legitimacy rele-
gates them to the background and keeps us from evaluating those political
concerns appropriately. Specifically, these moves prevent us from evaluating
the role of various theoretical proposals in support of competing abortion policies that maintain or challenge existing patterns of oppression. But if we consciously accept the fact that political values are relevant to ethics, we can make
these suppressed concerns visible and, hence, we can evaluate competing theoretical proposals more adequately.

Feminist ethics has been quite explicit about acknowledging the relevance of
the political consequences of moral decisions in its ethical deliberations.
Although that explicitness exposes feminist ethicists to criticism from tradition-
alists who believe ethics can and should be done in the absence of political calculations, their self-conscious focus on questions of power and privilege
actually ensures that they are more aware of and hence better able to address the
kinds of considerations that I believe most theorists actually engage in when
evaluating issues in bioethics. Feminist reflective equilibrium makes visible the

kinds of political values that I believe do – and should – enter into all discussions of justice in health care, and that fact makes it easier to weigh the hidden assumptions that may be biasing thought at both the conceptual and the practical level of analysis.

Consider now how feminist ethics sheds light on the other methodological concern that I have raised, namely, the question of how moral issues are formulated. As in other areas of health care ethics, a feminist perspective on the matter of justice in health care will find it necessary to address the traditional arguments on the subject, even as it extends and redefines them substantially. Because feminist reflective equilibrium asks us to consider the impact of particular principles and policies on existing patterns of oppression in society, it is able to observe difficulties inherent in various arguments about socialized medicine that often remain invisible in bioethics debates. For example, most libertarians oppose publicly funded health care by appealing to individual rights to freedom from taxation; they stress the importance of leaving individuals the choice to decide for themselves how much of their income should be invested in health insurance. But if we investigate the impact of these principles on different groups in society, we can see that such freedoms are inevitably restricted to the privileged, whose incomes they help preserve. Efforts to respect libertarian principles universally will have the effect of abandoning the worst-off members of society to a non-exercisable, and hence empty, formal freedom. Feminist focus on the workings of oppression in our society make clear the problems inherent in rhetoric that presents all health care as an optimal consumer good, described in the language of personal choice, no matter what the urgency of a patient's need.

Expanding the Agenda

Feminist approaches to justice in health care have other benefits as well.[11] For instance, they generally extend the range of concern far beyond the established boundaries of the traditional debate, where discussion is often limited to deciding who is to pay for health services. They recognize the necessity of identifying and addressing many other complex issues that fall under the rubric of justice in the context of health care. By virtue of their explicit concern about matters of oppression and privilege, feminist approaches make clear that even though our highly valued, universal (though increasingly precarious), socialized health care system in Canada would seem to resolve the questions of the traditional debate – that is, who is to pay and who is to have access to health services – many problems of justice remain. For instance, though its coverage is far more extensive than that of the United States, it still leaves many gaps: health care costs tend to be narrowly defined in terms of doctors' and hospital fees, and this arrangement excludes provision for many other important health needs (e.g., prescription drugs, special diets, home nursing). Also, poor women often have to contend with potentially insurmountable problems in pursuit of health services, such as arranging for transportation to the clinic and finding child care while they are being treated.

In addition, because feminism is highly sensitive to the disproportionate number of women and children living in poverty and to the continuing economic disparity between women and men, it directs our attention to the moral significance of the strong correlation that exists between economic status and health. Despite several decades of widespread feminist activism and now nearly universal rhetoric in support of equality of opportunity and pay equity, it is still the case that women in North America face significant economic disadvantages relative to men of the same race, class, and ethnic background: on average, women earn only two-thirds of what men do and they are much more likely than men to be living in poverty. The fact that people with low incomes are much less likely than others to have access to adequate nutrition, proper exercise, home and work environments free of toxins, and needed stress management programs surely falls into the category of justice in health care, but if is often overlooked in discussions of this topic.

We also ought to reflect on the fact that women are likely to find themselves responsible for seeking health care services far more often than men do, even though they usually have fewer resources with which to work. Their reproductive needs are more frequent and more complex than are those of men and their dependence on health professionals for reproductive health care is exacerbated by the fact that all aspects of their relatively complex reproductive lives (menstruation, contraception, pregnancy, childbirth, lactation, menopause) have been subject to medical surveillance and control. As well, the existing sexual division of labour means that women are generally the primary caregivers at home, so they are the ones usually assigned the role of monitoring and maintaining the health of other family members. They are expected to recognize illness in children, elderly or disabled relatives, and sometimes in husbands, and it is usually women's responsibility to obtain medical care when a problem is identified. In health care, as in other spheres, questions of justice regarding the sexual division of labour in society have repercussions in the uneven demands put on women to negotiate their way through an expensive, complex, and often intimidating health care system. Here, as elsewhere, injustice in the public sphere is inseparable from injustice in the private sphere: each is replicated and reinforced in the other domain.[12] Bioethical discussions should reflect the fact that ongoing injustice in the domestic and economic spheres produces unjust restrictions on many different levels with respect to access to and responsiveness of health care services.[13]

Moreover, many other questions beyond the matter of funding must be raised about how health care services are distributed. There seems to be a marked discrepancy in the effectiveness of medical treatments made available to women and men. In a 1990 report to the American Medical Association, Richard McMurray documented a series of areas in which women are significantly less likely than men to receive the diagnostic and therapeutic interventions considered to be medically appropriate for their conditions (e.g., women are only 10 per cent as likely to be referred for cardiac catheterization as are men with the same symptoms). In cases where the proposed therapy is especially controversial, however, women may receive more than their share (e.g., psychosurgery is performed twice as often on women as on men).[14]

There are significant and disproportionate gaps in medical knowledge about treatments for women. The overwhelming majority of medical research to date has been done on men; often the data simply are not collected to determine how best to treat women for the same diseases.[15] Studies of heart disease, for example, are almost universally conducted on men, even though heart disease is as big a killer of older women as it is of men. The record is even worse on certain diseases that particulary affect women. For example, although it is now estimated that breast cancer will affect one in nine women in North America, until very recently breast cancer research received only a very small proportion of cancer research funding.[16]

If we look at particular groups of women and consider questions of multiple oppression, the picture becomes even more grim. Black women in the United States are four times as likely to die in childbirth and three times more likely to have their newborns die than are white women.[17] They have three times the rate of high blood pressure and are twelve times more likely to contract HIV.[18] Lupus affects black women at three times the rate of white women and the disease is barely researched or understood.[19] In Canada, native women contract cervical cancer at many times the rate of white women,[20] and aboriginal adults report some level of disability at more than twice the level of the population at large (31 per cent compared with 15 per cent, according to Statistics Canada[21]). The injustice represented by such examples extends beyond questions about provision and mode of payment for medical services; it is a matter of differential societal responses to the conditions that afflict different groups in society.

It is a mistake, then, for the traditional debate to presume or suggest that payment for actual medical services provided and the allocation of scarce medical resources are the only major issues of justice that arise in health care contexts. There are many different ways in which women in general, and some groups of women in particular, get less than their fair share of needed health care services. While the many types of failure to provide for the health needs of oppressed groups have been widely documented, to date only feminists and other political reformers have been inclined to investigate these non-monetary dimensions of the justice in health care question.

Most bioethicists who are concerned with the practical question of identifying the criteria for a just health care policy have accepted the standard formulation of the question of justice in health care as one of access to or payment for medical services. In so doing they have settled for an unjustifiably narrow focus of concern; and theorists, occupied as they are by abstract concerns and hypothetical original positions, have failed to observe the limitations of a model of justice that concentrates solely on distributions of defined services. Both have overlooked, and to some extent obscured, important issues that are visible in other formulations of the question of justice in health care. However, this is not merely a matter of academic omission; it translates into serious failures in resulting policy. To the extent that those in the practically oriented group have been insufficiently critical of the conceptual tools they work with and the theorists have been insufficiently sensitive to the practical limits of the concepts they promote, both groups have been instrumental in maintaining biased policies of health care distribution.

Feminist Approaches to 'Justice' and 'Health Care'

Yet even if we expand the scope of our investigation of differential benefits and burdens associated with the health care system to deal with these sorts of concerns, it will still not be sufficient to capture all the forms of injustice that feminist critics have revealed as inherent in our health care system. To capture these further dimensions, we need to rethink the central concepts of the discussion and extend the meanings of the terms of this debate beyond the traditional measures of justice as fairness in the distribution of defined health services. The terms of the debate – both 'justice' and 'health care' – must be made subject to feminist re-visioning. In revising these concepts we change the scope of the questions to be explored under the rubric of justice in health care. By making these changes we shall be able to see more clearly how conceptual decisions have significant practical import in this sphere of bioethical study and to understand why the social realities we inhabit need to be reflected in the concepts we use in our ethical deliberations about the world.

Beginning with 'health care,' then, we should first observe that this term usually is reserved for the services that happen to be offered within existing health care systems. As I noted above, the services that are at issue in most discussions of justice in health care are largely those that health care professionals, especially the most powerful among them (doctors), perform. In fact, however, while this conception may seem to fit the health care needs of a certain advantaged portion of the population, it is inadequate for capturing the actual health needs of many members of society. A more effective, and arguably more efficient and fair, health care system would allow patients access to forms of treatment outside the domain of allopathic medicine if they have been proved effective in some types of cases, for example, herbal remedies, special diets, acupuncture, and massage therapy, even if most physicians lack expertise in their practice.

Moreover, as is well known but often forgotten, most of the dramatic improvements in the morbidity and mortality rates of western nations are attributable not to expensive, technological medical services, but rather to progressive improvements in such ordinary human requirements as basic hygiene and nutrition. Conversely, many of the continuing health care problems in western societies can be explained by the fact that large segments of the population still suffer from inadequate access to the necessities of life and health: proper nutrition, clean water, adequate housing, prenatal care, safety from physical violence, protection against toxic chemicals in the environment, and a strong sense of self-esteem.

Thus, rather than simply arguing for more universal provision of health care services as they are now defined, we should rethink the foundation of the arguments put forward in defence of a positive right to health care. Arguments for universal health care typically are based on a recognition of the importance of good health to individuals' sense of well-being and to their opportunity to participate fully in their communities.[22] These arguments should be reformulated to include not only medical services but all of the controllable conditions that contribute to good health. We ought not to restrict our attention to the artificial boundary that is implicit when we limit our focus to the concerns and activities of physicians. A more foundational analysis of the standard of justice in the domain of health would begin with a much broader conception of health care that includes all measures that contribute to opportunities for improved health, for example, protection against avoidable threats such as environmental poisons, physical assault, and psychological abuse.

Provision of basic necessities such as safely and adequate nutrition is likely to go further towards ensuring a greater distribution of health in the population than the purchase of the latest magnetic imaging machines. It is also more likely to ameliorate some of the unjust burden of illness that is now borne by those whose very oppression is a significant contributing factor to their illness. In other words, a more inclusive health care system of this sort would not only be more effective at fostering health more equitably across the population, it would

also be better able to help reduce injustice in society. In contrast, current definitions of health care tend to exacerbate existing injustices by addressing only
specific forms of treatment once illness sets in. By dividing the public purse into
rigid categories that distinguish health care services from social services and
then promising to provide citizens only with equal levels of the former, we create a social environment in which we condemn some people to preventable illness and then argue about whether we can afford to treat them.

By revising our initial conception of health care we shall be able to place a
higher priority on preventative and protective health measures and to empower
individuals to assert a right to health that is more fundamental than their derivative right to medical care. While political and economic realities may make it
impractical at this time to provide everyone with everything that is required to
ensure the good health of each, there is a meaningful sense of a right to health in
which the ideal we should be striving for is to assure everyone an equal chance
at good health at least in so far as this is a condition amenable to social, economic, or political adjustments. Such a right would include, at least, efforts to
provide a safe environment, an adequate diet, clean water, health education, and
an opportunity to develop self-esteem. Obviously such an ideal would organize
political and social priorities quite differently than the current system does.

Moreover, all of these factors should be seen as public responsibilities, since
they are inaccessible to most individuals acting independently. This fact is
clearest in the case of ensuring access to clean water and a non-toxic environment; for these conditions of health are beyond the scope of most individuals'
power and initiative and can be achieved only through public efforts.[23] More
sustained political argument will be necessary to achieve agreement on the
importance of insisting on public responsibility for ensuring the other goods
identified as requirements for individual health. In support of that argument, we
shall need to show that women, children, blacks, native people, gays, and lesbians (among others) all are at risk of being subjected to systemic (and systematic) violence in their daily lives and that, as individuals, they often are unable
to protect themselves from such violence. In the face of existing levels of sexism, racism, homophobia, anti-Semitism, and classist prejudice in our communities and the documented evidence of well-organized campaigns of hatred and
anger directed against certain groups, it is probable that only the state has the
institutional power and authority to protect most victims of discrimination from
assault. Further, in the absence of collective action and public education, it is
often difficult for individuals within oppressed groups to develop the self-
esteem that is essential to their psychological health. Such facts imply that the
state is obligated to do more than simply pay the bills for treatment after the
health damage is done; it should assume responsibility for protecting these

dimensions of the health of all its citizens, especially those who are most vulnerable to the health hazards of oppression. Within bioethics, then, health care should be understood to involve all measures that positively contribute to health, including measures aimed at preventing, not merely treating, illness.

These broader concerns for health lead us into the case for re-evaluating the other concept that is central to this discussion. Feminists have reason also to challenge traditional understandings of the term 'justice.' Discussions of justice are usually taken to be concerned with establishing a fair distribution of benefits and burdens among members of a society. When the issue is health care, the presumption is generally that we need to determine a fair mechanism for providing and allocating a certain level of health care services (however they may be defined). But as Iris Marion Young has argued, the distributive paradigm that is assumed by most justice theorists is inadequate; it does not capture all the relevant considerations that should be addressed under the concept of justice.[24] Young argues that justice cannot be reduced simply to questions of distribution of some limited set of resources, because such reductions avoid important questions of social structure and organization. Moreover, the distributive paradigm focuses attention on a particulary atomistic conception of persons in society that fails to recognize that persons are socially interconnected, not independent, beings. In particular, it avoids examination of the social relations that control the application of distributive policies.

Most seriously, from the perspective of feminist ethics, the distributive paradigm actually obscures rather than challenges the moral offence of oppression and domination. In an effort to avoid explicit sexism or racism, those who adopt the distributive paradigm of justice typically commit themselves to gender, race, and class neutrality in their deliberations. They consider individuals only as generalized abstractions, and they assume a certain measure of interchangeability among them. In maintaining the focus of their attention at the level of abstract rather than particular individuals, however, they are unable to address or account for the specific differences that work to the disadvantage of certain groups. Traditional justice theorists deliberately remain ignorant of the ways in which their own assumptions include and perpetuate biases in the application of their principles, relying on the false hypothesis that all persons will be affected similarly by abstract policies. In failing to look specifically at the differential impact of their conceptions and principles of justice on oppressed groups, they inevitably ignore, and, in fact, render invisible important questions about justice.

Another way of clarifying the gaps in solely distributive notions of justice is to ask that any account of justice also include attention to questions of *injustice*. As Judith Shklar observes, it is important to consider injustice as a distinct entity that exists beyond the absence or failure of the conditions demanded by traditional measures of justice.[25] She defines injustice as a social category that is largely shaped by political understandings and commitments, and she argues that injustice often reflects the social decision to create misfortune out of certain sorts of difference (e.g., skin colour). Attitudes of sexism, racism, classism, heterosexualism, ageism, and ablism are oppressive, both singly and collectively, to those on the unfavoured side of the divisions they construct and represent. These attitudes and the practices they support constitute forms of injustice that are usually ignored by the traditional focus on justice as distribution, because distributive theories are designed with the deliberate intent of masking or ignoring precisely these sorts of differences. Therefore, the subtlety and complexity of the harms of oppression cannot be fully represented by the measures of a distributive model. Like Young, Shklar perceives that the usual models of justice are inadequate to capture the experience of injustice because they choose to attend to different things.

Of course, distributive questions are still important within feminist ethics. The demand is not to abandon such investigations but to recognize that they are only part of the much broader moral question of justice. Young's concept of social justice recognizes that the elimination of institutionalized oppression and domination is an important aspect of justice. In contrast to the more familiar distributive paradigm where persons are regarded simply as possessors or consumers of goods, this feminist theory of social justice allows us to see people as responsible moral agents who create the social institutions that determine social, political, and economic privileges and constraints; it encourages us to evaluate those institutions in terms of a wider range of criteria. Moreover, by directing attention to the social context in which goods or opportunities are distributed, her conception of justice has the further advantage of providing a better basis for considering even the familiar questions of distribution. Most distributive accounts focus on questions of comparison of narrowly construed outcomes. Young's account expands this focus and provides us with a larger set of relevant information for evaluating patterns of distribution. Thus, it actually offers greater promise of ultimately achieving truly just distribution patterns in matters of health and other goods. Developed in recognition of the social inequities that are associated with domination and oppression, this feminist conception of justice is, therefore, more adequate than the traditional alternatives for investigating questions about justice within health care contexts.

Conclusion

This sketch of a feminist perspective on justice in health care does not, of course, constitute an exhaustive theory of justice. If I am right about what such a theory involves, it will turn out that a comprehensive and empirically adequate theory of justice in health care cannot be produced by a single theorist working in the abstract. A full theory of justice in health care will require a much more detailed investigation of the workings of oppression and the role of health care within those forces. It will also require a much wider conversation, where the views of other members of society, especially those who are differently oppressed, are sought and considered. The demands of feminist reflective equilibrium cannot be satisfied by a single researcher but require a collaborative process of dialogue and reflection. This paper is meant to provide support for the project of engaging in such conversations and to offer some methodological direction to questions that will need to be addressed.

I have sought to show that traditional (non-feminist) formulations of the question of justice in health care ethics tend to restrict inappropriately the focus of our ethical attention and discussion. To the degree that theorists have attempted to settle on the formulations of the key concepts of justice and health care in advance of exploring their role in setting health care policies, they have produced concepts that do not capture all relevant dimensions of the concerns they represent. Similarly, so long as those involved in the formation of health care policies accept existing theoretical formulations uncritically, they fail to include relevant aspects of existing injustice in their proposals. Both approaches have the effect of narrowing our conceptions of what constitutes the important ethical questions to be raised and also our sense of what sorts of answers we should pursue in response. I draw on feminist work to spell out a richer set of concepts that reflect the ways in which bioethical work needs to engage with both theoretical and practical issues simultaneously if it is to develop a reliable understanding of justice in health care.

This exploration is not meant to be unique but to be illustrative of the sort of work that needs to be done in other areas of health care ethics; for example, similar kinds of examination should also be brought to bear on discussions of the widely used concepts of autonomy, beneficence, and non-maleficence in health care ethics. Similarly, problems that are usually assigned to the practical end of the theoretical-practical divide of bioethics also would benefit from recognition of the importance of considering other possible formulations and approaches to the issues they represent. (Consider, for example, how investigations differ depending on whether we define a question as one of discontinuing life-sustaining treatment or of doctor-assisted suicide.) When engaging in bioethical discussions at either the conceptual or the practical level, we should not merely accept the formulation of problems as they arise but must continually question the constructions of the problems we study. It is as important to explore the questions that remain beneath the surface of the presenting structures as it is to try to respond to established areas of moral concern. We need to be prepared to restructure and to expand the existing agenda of health care ethics.

Moreover, we should be wary of any philosophic or practical policing that proposes that abstract conceptual work can and should be done in the absence of exploration of its practical political and ethical consequences (and vice versa). The concepts we are offered to work with inevitably structure our thinking. Some concepts encourage narrow conservative thought that works to preserve the oppression-laden status quo, while others encourage expansive liberatory alternatives. One of the measures of adequacy for ethical concepts should be the implications that arise from application of that concept to practical problem-solving. All moral agents have reason to take an active role in critically examining the concepts with which they work and the ways in which existing and proposed social institutions affect patterns of oppression. All of us should learn to be selective about our choices of proffered ethical concepts and proposed strategies. Ethics cannot be done adequately if we concentrate on either the practical or the theoretical level of reasoning alone. These two dimensions of ethical thought are ultimately inseparable, and to the extent that we try to pursue one in the absence of the other, we are bound to wind up with distorted and unreliable results.

My own view is stronger yet. I do not think it sufficient simply to agree that theory and practice are connected. We need to clarify exactly how they are connected so we can understand and evaluate the nature of particular interactions. Feminist reflective equilibrium proposes some specific criteria and strategies to appeal to when we engage in this dual-layer process of moral deliberation. It draws on the sensitivity of feminists, and others who are committed to eliminating oppression, to the ways in which political values are related to moral ones. Unlike their traditional counterparts, most feminists do not find this interaction to be morally or theoretically problematic; rather, they urge others to become more attentive to the ways in which their own moral values reflect political ones (though the latter may be unconscious).

Once we recognize the extent of these sorts of connections, we can appreciate how important it is for feminists and other ethicists to take particular care to make certain that the conceptual tools we rely on do not perpetuate the very injustice we seek to dismantle. Often, the best way of ending oppression requires new, or at least modified, conceptual tools as much as it does reformed or rebuilt social institutions. We shall need to experiment with competing options to find the ones most compatible with our ethical ideals, and we are more likely to engage in such examinations when the true structure of our moral values is clear to us. Feminist reflective equilibrium is aimed at clarifying that structure and adding some moral constraints to the process.

Notes

Earlier versions of this paper were presented to the philosophy departments at University of Toronto and Dalhousie University. I am grateful for the helpful comments offered by both those audiences. I am especially indebted to the thoughtful responses of Richmond Campbell, Sue Campbell, and Duncan MacIntosh.

1 This irreverent caricature of the work of Tom L. Beauchamp and James F. Childress, *Principles of Biomedical Ethics*, 4th edition (New York: Oxford University Press, 1994), is clearly oversimplified, but unfortunately, so too is the way in which many practitioners tend to interpret the role of these principles. Beauchamp and Childress themselves do not propose that interpreting these principles is ever straightforward, nor do they claim that the four principles will suffice for addressing all ethical dilemmas encountered in health care contexts.

2 For example, the 'History of Ethics' article in the *The Encyclopedia of Philosophy* begins by 'separating purely philosophical thought from the practical advice, moral preaching, and social engineering which it illuminates and from which it receives its sustenance,' Raziel Abelson and Kai Nielson, 'History of Ethics,' *The Encyclopedia of Philosophy*, vol. 3., ed. Paul Edwards (New York: Collier-Macmillan, 1967), p. 82. The 'Problems of Ethics' entry continues with the assumption of this distinction and, while acknowledging that historically, philosophical ethics attended to practical as well as conceptual questions, it reports that contemporary analytic philosophers are concerned with 'knowledge of the distinctive uses or roles of moral language or, to use another idiom, knowledge of the meanings of moral concepts'; Kai Nielson, 'Problems of Ethics,' ibid., p. 118.

3 See, for instance, the arguments offered in *Anti-Theory in Ethics and Moral Conservatism*, ed. Stanley G. Clarke and Evan Simpson (Albany: State University of New York Press, 1989).

4 See, for example, Barry Hoffmaster, 'The Theory and Practice of Applied Ethics,' *Dialogue* 30 (3): 213–34 (Summer 1991); Annette Baier, *Postures of the Mind: Essays on Mind and Morals* (Minneapolis: University of Minnesota Press, 1985).

5 John Rawls, *A Theory of Justice* (Cambridge, MA: Harvard University Press, 1971). Rawls himself picks up on the idea of reflective equilibrium introduced by Nelson Goodman in *Fact, Fiction, and Forecast* (Cambridge, MA: Harvard University Press, 1955).

6 John Rawls, *Political Liberalism* (New York: Columbia University Press, 1993).

7 Norman Daniels has amended Rawls's initial proposal, suggesting we be sure to engage in what he calls 'wide reflective equilibrium,' to ensure that attention is paid to relevant background theories in this exercise. But Daniels, too, seems to confine his set of concerns to abstract, general, theoretical considerations. He does not explicitly engage with concrete and particular moral contexts in his description and

employment of wide reflective equilibrium. Norman Daniels, 'Two Approaches to Theory Acceptance in Ethics,' in *Morality, Reason and Truth: New Essays in the Foundations of Ethics*, ed. David Copp and David Zimmerman (Totowa, NJ: Rowman and Allanheld, 1984).

8 For a detailed definition and discussion of oppression, see Iris Marion Young, *Justice and the Politics of Difference* (Princeton: Princeton University Press, 1991).

9 These arguments and explanations of feminist ethics are spelled out in Susan Sherwin, *No Longer Patient: Feminist Ethics and Health Care* (Philadelphia: Temple University Press, 1992).

10 This seems to be the goal of Rawls in *A Theory of Justice* (1971). In his later work (*Political Liberalism*, 1993), he is more explicit in that he proposes that we use this methodology to obtain political consensus in the actual world. Yet even this degree of situatedness is not adequate from the perspective of feminism, because the tendency of oppression to be internalized makes it possible to achieve consensus on oppressive arrangements. Feminist reflective equilibrium is designed to resist consensus that may be achieved through the forces of oppression. See Sherwin, *No Longer Patient*, chapter 3.

11 Note that I speak of feminist approaches in the plural, because feminist ethics, like feminism itself, admits of many distinct perspectives. I shall focus on certain elements that I believe are common to many of these distinct approaches, but that is not to say that they would be endorsed by every feminist, nor that they exhaust the list of concerns that can be raised under the label of feminism.

12 Susan Moller Okin, *Justice, Gender, and the Family* (New York: Basic Books, 1989).

13 Mary Briody Mahowald, *Women and Children in Health Care: An Unequal Majority* (New York: Oxford University Press, 1993).

14 Richard J. McMurray, 'Gender Disparities in Clinical Decision-Making,' Report to the American Medical Association Council on Ethical and Judicial Affairs, 1990.

15 Rebecca Dresser, 'Wanted: Single, White Male for Medical Research,' *Hastings Center Report* 22(1): 24–9, Jan 1992.

16 A newsletter of the Breast Cancer Action group reports that $4 million Canadian went to breast cancer research in 1991 when 5,000 Canadian women died of breast cancer, while $33 million went to AIDS research, a disease that killed seventy-two Canadians that year – Montreal *Gazette*, 27 April 1992, B2. In their second report on breast cancer, the Parliamentary Sub-Committee on the Status of Women on Breast Cancer (*sic*) was able to identify approximately $3.1 million as targeted specifically to breast cancer research (Barbara Green, Chair of Sub-Committee on the Status of Women, *Breast Cancer: Unanswered Questions* (Ottawa: Supply and Services Canada, 1992), 23. Some improvement is now in sight: since release of that report, the federal government promised to spend $20 million on breast cancer research over the next five years (*Globe and Mail*, 16 Dec. 1992, A9).

17 Ruth H. Gordon-Bradshaw, 'A Social Essay on Special Issues Facing Poor Women of Color,' in *Too Little Too Late: Dealing with the Health Needs of Women in Poverty*, ed. Cesar A. Perales and Lauren S. Young (New York: Harrington Park Press, 1986).

18 Angela Y. Davis, 'Sick and Tired of Being Sick and Tired: The Politics of Black Women's Health,' in *Black Women's Health Book: Speaking for Ourselves*, ed. Evelyn C. White (Seattle: Seal Press, 1990).

19 Ibid.

20 L.A. Gaudette, E.M. Illing, and G.B. Hill, 'Canadian Cancer Statistics 1991,' *Health Reports* 3(2): 107–35, 1991; L.A. Gaudette, R.-N. Gao, S. Freitag, and M. Wideman, 'Cancer Incidence by Ethnic Group in the Northwest Territories (NWT) 1969–1988,' *Health Reports* 5(1): 23–32, 1993.

21 Statistics Canada, *1991 Aboriginal Peoples Survey* (Ottawa: Minister of Industry, Science, and Technology, 1994).

22 For example, Norman Daniels, *Just Health Care* (Cambridge: Cambridge University Press, 1985).

23 In fact, there has been substantial public agreement about the value of public funding for these purposes (though arguably insufficient public financing).

24 Young, *Justice and the Politics of Difference*.

25 Judith N. Shklar, *The Faces of Injustice* (New Haven, CT: Yale University Press, 1990).

Gender Rites and Rights:
The Biopolitics of Beauty and Fertility

KATHRYN PAULY MORGAN

Taught from infancy that beauty is woman's scepter, the mind shapes itself
to the body and roaming round its gilt cage only seeks to adorn its prison.

Mary Wollstonecraft, Vindication of the Rights of Women (1792)

An Instructive Parable of Privilege

Once upon a time, not long ago, I was asked to give a workshop to a group of
women on the subject of 'Older Women's Sexuality.' When I inquired about
what was meant by 'older' and about the ages of the women at the workshop I
was told that the women would be in their sixties to late seventies but would not
be classified as 'extremely elderly.' The workshop was to be held at the home
of one of the members. I agreed to give the workshop, although I felt a little
strange, since I was not yet a member of the age group in question.

The appointed day arrived, a dreary, gray, cold February day, and I arrived at
the address I had been given. I entered the elevator, pressed the button for one
of the upper floors, then stepped out with the realization that her floor was *her
floor* and that the elevator opened out into her polished mahogany foyer. I was
surrounded by mirrored walls, elegant antiques, and large vases overflowing
with fresh lilies, irises, roses, freesias, and birds of paradise. In the dining room
the table was laid with fine crystal, cutlery, china, linen napkins, and serving
plates bountifully filled with crêpes, aged veined cheeses, nuts, and dressed sal-
ads. Around me glided the 'older women' – elegant, white, tanned, blonde, pen-
cil-thin, with unwrinkled faces, youthful in appearance.

Dear reader, I must confess that I went into a kind of ontological free fall! I
wondered whether I had arrived on another planet. I wondered whether the

apparent food on the table was, in fact, real food. I reasoned that it couldn't be, because the pencil-slim women were actually putting the food-like objects into their mouths and swallowing them. I wondered whether the young-looking women were the older women I was coming to speak to or whether there was some other group – perhaps hidden? – who would come out later when it was time to begin the workshop. Not so. Pretending that nothing was untoward with my philosophical sensibility, I chatted, shared the (maybe) food, listened to historical narratives, looked at photographs that persuaded me that these women were the older women, gave my workshop, and fled – fled down to what I regarded as 'my world,' 'my planet,' a place where such ontological free fall and alienation of embodiment could not occur.

I was wrong. This is what I returned to in 'my world':

1. A seminar is held in my advanced Women and Health class in which five of the young women described how their boyfriends were putting pressure on them to have breast augmentation. When one young woman in the class confessed that her father performed cosmetic surgery, another woman turned to her saying, 'That's GREAT! He could do your whole body!'
2. A copy of *HomeMaker* magazine drops through my front door mail chute (free of charge, since I live in one of the designated 'right' neighbourhoods in Toronto) with an article on elective cosmetic surgery for women, which announces in bold type: **'For many women, it's no longer a question of *whether* to undergo cosmetic surgery – but what, when, by whom and how much.'** [1]
3. A clipping from *US Air Magazine* arrives in my philosophy department mailbox, advertising the Pittsburgh Institute of Plastic Surgery (which it itself refers to as PIPS) advocating breast augmentation by saying, 'If enlarging your breasts will help you achieve your personal goals call us at 1-800-321-7477' [2] (at which point my fingers wandered to my touch-tone phone to see if that spelled 1-800-BREASTS and speculated about whether breast augmentation could really help me with my writer's block).
4. A fax arrives at my home with a column from the *New York Times* about the surgical/aesthetic experiences of the avant-garde female artist Orlan, who arranges cosmetic surgical interventions in her body as carnal feminist political sculpturing. [3] In the course of the interview, Orlan remarks, 'I am a feminist, and I want to use plastic surgery to perpetuate my ideas. It's a critique of beauty and a critique of cosmetic surgery ... I have given my body to art.' Orlan undergoes her surgeries under local anaesthetic, arranges for the media to be present, has galleries where the viewing audience can fax the operating room during the surgery, and arranges for artwork resulting from

the surgery, including videos and 'reliquaries' of petri dishes of fat removed from her body. The columnist remarks, 'Orlan's [work] has explored the role of identity in an era in which technology has made the body malleable.'

5. At the supermarket, my eye is caught by the September 1994 cover of *Mirabella* because, in addition to the expected heroic-size beautiful face, there is an unmistakable computer chip floating prominently next to the face. When asked about the identity of the cover model, the photographer, Hiro, answers coyly that 'she's something of a split personality ... that it wasn't easy getting her together. Maybe her identity has something to do with the microchip floating through space.'[4]

Clearly, I was wrong. The site of my ontological free fall was no alien planet. It is my world; it is our world. How are we to participate in it? How are we to understand it? How are we to evaluate it from a moral and political point of view? Since I believe that as a feminist philosopher it is important to reflect 'from the ground up,' my next move involved listening to the consumers and the practitioners of elective cosmetic surgery who form one of the most dramatic subcultures in which the radical malleability of the human body is being explored. Listen to their voices.

Voices of the Advertisements

Voice 1:   '[I]f your features don't quite seem to fit and are causing you lots of heartache, fear not: Plastic surgery can fix your flaws.'[5]

Voice 2:   'The next morning the limo will chauffeur your loved one back home again, with a gift of beauty that will last a lifetime.'[6]

Voice 3:   'Plastic surgery ... will gradually become as common as eyeglasses, braces and hearing aids and be just as useful.' (brochure, Washington, DC, cosmetic surgery clinic)[7]

Voices of the Consumers

Voice 4:   'I'm a teacher and kids let school teachers know how we look and they aren't nice about it. A teacher who looks like an old bat or has a big nose will get a nickname.'[8]

Voice 5:   'We hadn't seen or heard from each other for 28 years. Then he suggested it would be nice if we could meet. I was very nervous about it. How much had I changed? I wanted a facelift, tummy tuck and liposuction, all in one week.' (a woman, age forty-nine, being interviewed for an article on 'older couples' falling in love)[9]

Voice 6: 'It's just not about what *he* thinks. He says that he's satisfied with my breasts ... and, well, it's probably true, too. But *I'm* not. *I'm* the one who wants it done and what does it matter what he says? I'm doing it for myself and not for someone else.'[10]

Voice 7: 'I'll admit to a boob job.' Susan Akin, 1986 Miss America[11]

Voice 8: 'This is different from buying luxury items ... It deals with self-esteem. I admit we're looking Anglicized, but we're social animals, and we have to adapt to society.' (music teacher, 27, South Korea)[12]

Voice 9: 'I came to see Dr X for the holiday season. I have important business parties, and the man I'm trying to get to marry me is coming in from Paris ... I do it to fight holiday depression.'[13]

Voices of the Surgeons

Voice 1: 'Women need it for their holiday ball gowns.'[14]

Voice 2: 'The skin you were meant to have is buried underneath the surface and unfortunately people cannot see the skin you were meant to have.' (comment made to a woman inquiring about cosmetic surgery for her nose)[15]

Voice 3: 'It's the ultimate in re-cycling.' (spoken triumphantly by a plastic surgeon who has just sucked and centrifuged the fat cells from the upper thighs of a young woman and forcibly shoved them through a circular series of punctures around her breasts, on the TV show '20-20')[16]

Voice 4: 'The way I look at it is, kids have been getting braces for years, and that's quite accepted ... This is just taking it one step further to noses, chins, cheekbones, and ears.'[17]

Voice 5: 'You know, don't you buy clothes ... don't you get your hair done, don't you wear makeup, so you'll look good? ... putting on makeup, you're just a step away from cosmetic surgery.'[18]

Voice 6: 'It's hard to say why one person will have cosmetic surgery done and another won't consider it, but generally I think people who go for surgery are more aggressive, they are the doers of the world. It's like makeup. You see some women who might be greatly improved by wearing makeup but they're, I don't know, granola-heads or something, and they just refuse.' (Dr Ronald Levine, director of Plastic Surgery Education, University of Toronto, vice-chairman of the Plastic Surgery section of the Ontario Medical Association)[19]

Voice 7: '[P]atients sometimes misunderstand the nature of cosmetic surgery. It's not a short cut for diet or exercise. It's a way to override the genetic code.'[20]

Voice 8: 'If you have your implants removed, you will be suicidal.'[21]

Look at the surgical instruments in figure 1.[22] Think about the Abdominal Scissors cutting into your belly. Think about the Nasal Hump Cutting Forceps cutting into your nose. Think about the Scalpel making incisions around your hairline, your jawline, circling your breasts. Look at the Eye Needles coming closer and closer. Think about Orlan experiencing her body as clay to be sculpted by these needles and knives, these scalpels and sutures. Think about your loved one 'coming home with a gift of beauty that will last a lifetime.'

The voices are momentarily silent and the instruments are at rest. What are these voices saying to us? How are we to understand these complex and varied descriptions, intentions, goals, scenarios and judgments? My questions reflect a genuine epistemic and political bewilderment when I, as an ageing (like most mortals) feminist philosopher/woman, try to reflect critically on contemporary practices and individual choices in the area of elective cosmetic surgery. Do these decisions and practices signal a new domain of liberation – or oppression – or both? How are we to think, to feel, and to evaluate practices and choices at the limits of human carnal malleability?[23]

I search for theories and frameworks that might lead to insights, to a consistent set of moral feelings and values, and to policies and norms. I reject those that turn out to be unilluminating or that further intensify my bewilderment. I pay particular scrutiny to those theories that might prove treacherous, serving as ideological camouflage, that function to intensify the oppression of human beings through the differential institutional structures of gender, race, and class. What if the same theory generates both positive and negative outcomes?

My search for an adequate theory and set of practices is guided by three sets of interrelated moral questions:

1. The question of agency
   Do I have the right to choose elective cosmetic surgery?
   If I have the right, should I choose it?
2. The question of moral emotions
   How should I morally feel about others' choices to have elective cosmetic surgery?
   What factors are morally and politically relevant with respect to the justifications of these feelings?
   Is it possible, with any sense of moral integrity, to respect individual choices as indicators of active self-determination while, simultaneously, rejecting the ideological and material systemic norms and practices constituted out of and sustained by those very choices?

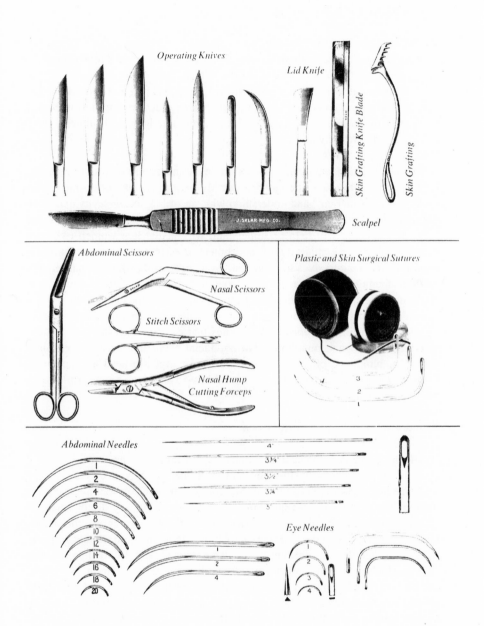

Figure 1 The Instruments

3. The question of universalizability
   Can I apply different stands of appraisal to my own choices regarding elective cosmetic surgery than to others' choices?
   Should the same or different standards of moral and political appraisal apply to individual choices and to the systems of practices and norms constituted out of individual choices? Is one a moral judgment, the other a political one? Why / why not?

We need an adequate theory that will help us understand why, until recently, breast augmentation was the most frequently performed kind of cosmetic surgery in North America[24] and understand why, according to *Longevity* magazine one in every 225 adult Americans had *elective* cosmetic surgery in 1989. We need a theory that will help us understand why actual live women (who are overwhelmingly the majority of consumers for elective cosmetic surgery) choose to reduce ourselves to 'potential women,' participating in anatomizing and fetishizing our bodies as we buy 'contoured bodies,' 'restored youth,' and 'permanent beauty.' In the absence of any demonstrable medical advantage, we need a bioethical political theory to help us understand the burgeoning market and demand for interventions in our bodies that can and do result in infection, bleeding, embolisms, pulmonary edema, facial-nerve injury, scar formation, skin loss, blindness, crippling, and death.[25] We urgently need a framework. Until now, mainstream bioethics has not addressed either the issues or the question of frameworks.[26]

Framework I. A Rights Framework

Rights discourse is at the centre of much bioethical reasoning. It is also at the heart of many liberation struggles and continues to play a pivotal role in women's health movements. One of the central critical moves that makes rights discourse so powerful is the question of access itself. For any disenfranchised individual or group, coming to see oneself as a legitimate bearer of rights and as having valid access to the protections of those rights in a culture that respects rights is critical to individual and collective empowerment. Being able to cite a right to bodily privacy and a right to bodily self-determination as central domains of human entitlement has been crucial in gendered and racialized struggles for individual and collective erotic and reproductive rights.[27] Perhaps a rights framework will provide us with the theory we are searching for.
   In my analysis of a rights framework, I am using a model developed by Veatch as indicative of the kinds of priorities built into much orthodox bioethical reasoning when it begins from a liberal, rights-based starting point.[28]

Veatch's model focuses on five important moral maxims:

(1) Produce Good and Not Harm
(2) Protect Individual Freedom
(3) Preserve Individual Dignity
(4) Tell the Truth and Keep Promises
(5) Maintain and Restore Justice

In this model, the assumed moral and political dynamic between patient/client/ consumer and health care provider involves trust and confidence. All relevant participants are seen as the bearers of rights whose autonomy needs to be preserved (albeit in asymmetrical ways). Although there are clear differences with respect to knowledge and access to relevant health care goods and services, all relevant participants are seen as sharing ethical authority and responsibility in the exchange. These practices and moral and political assumptions clearly distinguish rights-based liberal health care models from a variety of paternalistic health care models.[29]

It must be acknowledged that there are sleazy, exploitative, manipulative cosmetic surgeons who perceive elective cosmetic surgery performed on women simply as a self-aggrandizing, masculinity-enhancing, extremely profitable profession. On a recent television talk show one cosmetic surgeon described himself as 'perfecting God's handiwork'![30] While this physician was unusually blatant about assessing the cosmic significance of his labours, there is a recurrent Pygmalion theme in the surgeons' narrative literature. Nevertheless, I wish to set this set of surgeons on the moral sidelines, since their objectifying gaze and surgical practices disqualify them for consideration within the boundaries of the rights framework under consideration here.

With respect to the first rights maxim, 'Produce Good and Not Harm,' both cosmetic surgeons and the recipients of their surgical services generally concur that good, not harm, is produced – even when there is considerable risk, postoperative pain, and complications.[31] With respect to the second rights maxim, 'Protect Individual Freedom,' cosmetic surgeons offer their services at public rates, thereby preserving the freedom of individual consumers. I know of no documented cases where a surgeon coerced a client to undergo (more) surgery against her will, although admittedly the line between persuasion and psychological coercion can get blurred at times.[32] At the level at which a rights-based model operates, the conditions for free choices are satisfied for the women and men in question. Indeed, the surgery so clearly appears to satisfy the conditions of freedom that it is called 'elective,' and there are usually no prior medical conditions whatever that would weaken the client's capacity for choice.[33]

With respect to the third rights maxim, 'Preserve Individual Dignity,' no significant issues are raised. Although cosmetic surgeons sound defensive at times, there is no reason to think that practising their profession intrinsically threatens their individual dignity. Nor, if we are to accept the narratives of clients, do clients feel that their dignity has been threatened. If anything, they feel it has been enhanced by undergoing the various surgical procedures and transforming themselves.[34] Ironically, this sense of dignity may be further protected by the establishment of free-standing cosmetic surgery clinics and salons, a move that guarantees that clients will not have to undergo the disabling and infantilizing effects of most hospital rules, procedures, and settings. (Although this move takes the practice of most elective cosmetic surgery out of the eye of any kind of hospital and professional monitoring, I regard this as a pragmatic concern rather than a difficulty intrinsic to the practice of cosmetic surgery in its present cultural context. Market considerations alone would suffice to maintain standards among practitioners, with negligence and malpractice not only being highly publicized but being visible on the surface of bodies of clients in a way in which few other surgical procedures are.)

The fourth rights maxim says 'Tell the Truth and Keep Promises.' The impression that most cosmetic surgeons give is that they go to great lengths to tell the truth about what they are capable – and incapable – of doing and to keep their limited promises. The more conscientious say that they rule out various motivations among the consumers, saying that they cannot cure a dying marriage or produce a new life for a woman or man in question. Similarly, the consumers have the most to gain by being explicit about what they want cosmetically from their surgeon, although, in dealing with highly selective surgeons, they may choose to be less than fully explicit about all their motives.

The situation with respect to the fifth rights-maxim, 'Maintain and Restore Justice,' is somewhat more complex. With respect to considerations of equality of opportunity, in some ways the practice of cosmetic surgery is simpler than many other fields of health care (e.g., expensive organ transplants, access to expensive reproduction technologies). Cosmetic surgeons do not appear to behave in any kind of exclusionary ways. Routinely cited grounds for discriminatory practice, such as sex, age, sexual orientation, race, ethnicity, disability status, marital status, and income, do not appear to play any major role, although there may be differential pressures deriving from the culture at large. Radical cosmetic surgeons could claim that by participating in, for example, the creation of transsexualled and transgendered embodied subjects, they are participating in an important critique of oppressive gender constraints ascribed on the basis of allegedly 'given' sexual properties. Where access to a particular procedure is limited – for example, women defined as 'generally fat' are not seen as 'suitable candidates' for liposuction –justifiable medical reasons are advanced by surgeons for this exclusion. The services are increasingly available to those who can afford them in terms of money and time, and surgeons are targeting their advertising to increasingly large groups diversified by race, class, and sexual self-definition.

Apparently such advertising is effective, since adolescents across a variety of cultures and ethnic backgrounds are seeking cosmetic surgery. More and more women who work in low-waged sectors of the economy are also encouraged to save up their money for their surgery. Access is becoming increasingly broad as cosmetic surgery is becoming normalized as an aspect of 'looking after oneself.' Although the price of various procedures is high, there is no difficulty in principle with cosmetic surgeons operating with sliding scales to accommodate economically disadvantaged women and men. Some surgical procedures could be performed as a form of pro bono professional activity. In general, the results of the surgical procedures performed appear to be satisfactory (although some gruesome failures sometimes make headlines in tabloid newspapers), and technologies that women and men consume and recommend to others continue to be created.

If we raise questions about the allocations of scarce medical resources, there are at least two sides to the issue. As one cosmetic surgeon remarks, 'Perhaps it's difficult for someone who is waiting for cancer surgery to understand, but my patients pay taxes and have a right to use the public hospitals too ... *Doing a breast augmentation is just as important for me as a plastic surgeon as taking someone else's breast off may be for another surgeon* ... There is also the question in this time of rationed revenues, of additional revenue for the hospital' (emphasis added).[35] Most physicians who have been the target of complaints that valuable operating room time should not be used for non-essential surgery like facelifts and breast augmentations have opened their own clinics and salons.

With respect to considerations of justice, cosmetic surgeons can make two responses to the criticism that elective cosmetic surgery violates norms of equitable allocation. First, they can argue that though the surgery may be elective, it is as significant *for themselves* (as in the above quotation) as are other forms of surgery whose importance is not questioned. If we accept this kind of argument-by-parity, then we have to be able to give an ethical and political reading of those situations in which not having a breast augmentation is as potentially devastating in its consequences as postponing or not having a mastectomy or lumpectomy in the case of a malignant breast tumor. Although this argument has an initial implausibility, there are possible readings of elective (not reconstructive) breast augmentation narratives that might render it more persuasive as a response (although I personally do admit to a continued sense of moral horror at the above quotation).[36]

A second response might involve reversing prima facie negative moral perceptions by arguing that performing elective cosmetic surgery in hospitals where there is no obvious shortage of operating rooms is, in fact, advantageous for the hospital and for the health care system at large. Rather than producing an unjust allocation of resources, the additional revenue generated through elective cosmetic surgery could be reallocated to areas in which the hospital and health care system may need such revenue. It might be used, for example, to raise the salaries of intensive-care nurses so that more urgent surgery could be performed. Thus, the cosmetic surgeon might conclude, elective cosmetic surgery could be seen not only as maintaining and restoring justice but as, in fact, justice maximizing, since it could lead to a more equitable distribution of health care resources than would be possible without it.

What have we learned, then, from this critical application of rights-maxims in the area of cosmetic surgery? Very little, I am afraid. On the side of the purchaser of services, the central liberal maxim that operates on a presumption of freedom is 'It's my body and I'll cut it if I want to!'[37] On the side of the providers of cosmetic surgery, there is no obvious violation of any of the rights-maxims cited above. Perhaps the parallel maxim might be 'It's your body and I'm qualified to cut it if you want me to!' (This may be one reason why discussions of elective cosmetic surgery do not make their way into any of the canon-defining literature in the field of bioethics.) Yet there are, I would argue, further insights to be gained, deeper levels of philosophical illumination, and more complicated moral and political issues that need to be examined with respect to the choices and practices around elective cosmetic surgery. While I acknowledge that the autonomy/rights/justice-based paradigm of bioethics has brought into focus some important moral dimensions that we would not want to discard at the level of practice and ideology, I believe that other salient features can come into sharp focus only through a significant paradigm shift.[38]

Framework II. A Paradigm Shift to Bioethical Politics

In his article 'Toward a Philosophy of Technology,' Hans Jonas distinguishes between pre-modern and modern technology.[39] Characterizing modern technology, Jonas remarks that the relationship of means and ends is no longer unilinear but circular, so that 'new technologies may suggest, create, even impose new ends, never before conceived, simply by offering their feasibility ... Technology thus adds to the very objectives of human desires, including objectives for technology itself.'[40] In 1979 Jonas was making predictions; we are living the reality of those predictions. In advanced capitalist societies we have become increasingly accustomed to regarding ourselves as both technological subject and technological object, transformable and literally creatable through biological engineering. Biotechnology is pervading more and more aspects of our daily lives and is assuming increasing control in the most private and formerly sequestered domains of fertility, the erotic, birthing, and dying.

I want to shift the focus of our understanding of elective cosmetic surgery away from the lived embodied choices of individual human beings engaged in a process of carnal self-definition with the rights-preserving assistance of their surgeons. I believe that we need to consider the structural material and ideological context in which these choices are taking place and to situate these choices in this larger framework. I call this larger framework the Domain of Bioethical Politics,[41] and my visualization of it is shown in figure 2. In contemporary capitalist cultures, this domain is marked by several distinguishing features. Four of these are as follows:

1. Technological Mediation of the Natural
2. The Production of Living Beings as Natural Artefacts
3. Epistemic and Political Dominance of Experts
4. (Latent) Phenomenological Frame of Coercive Voluntarism

One of the most striking features of modern technology is the extent to which it now mediates many human life experiences that were, until recently, thought to be aligned with the 'animal' or 'prehuman' natural side of human nature, carrying with it an emphasis on the 'givenness' of certain aspects of human existence. Birth, fertility, dying and death; bodily appearance; the so-called 'natural appetites' such as hunger and thirst; sexual identity and erotic desire; feelings, affects, personality, and temperament – all have been cited by philosophers, psychologists, and other students of human existence as constituting the domain of the given and natural in human existence. Now we are witnessing and participating in technologies that mediate our lived experiences in these domains. New reproductive technologies, new death technologies, new psychopharmaceutical technologies, new forms of prenatal genetic and endocrinological intervention, and new technologies in cosmetic surgery are producing metamorphoses of individual and species human existence. These metamorphoses lead to the production of what I call 'natural artefacts,' artefacts created and influenced by human design and intervention out of living matter, out of living human matter.[42]

Since human choices in the domains of the natural are increasingly technologically mediated, we have become increasingly dependent on the technolo-

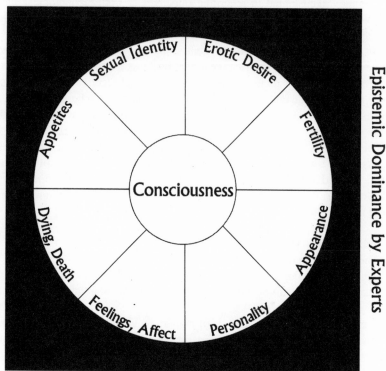

Dimensions of Human Natural Artefacts

Biotechnology-mediated Domains

Epistemic Dominance by Experts

Sexual Identity

Erotic Desire

Appetites

Fertility

Consciousness

Dying, Death

Appearance

Feelings, Affect

Personality

Phenomenological Frame: Coerced Voluntarism

Figure 2 The Domain of Bioethical Politics

gies, on access to the technologies, and on those experts whose knowledge and power create and control the technologies. Consequently, there is both greater epistemic and political dependence on experts, who rise to a position of dominance in defining and creating what is regarded as 'natural,' 'normal,' and 'healthy' alongside the correlative definitions of the 'unnatural,' the 'abnormal,' and the 'pathological.' I argue that various descriptions that emphasize individual choice and maintain that various expert mediations are done solely for reasons of benevolence, altruism, and therapeutic outcome camouflage the extent to which the lived experience of voluntary choice, at the micro level, is really occurring in a context of powerful but diffuse ideological pressures and constraining material structures. I call this the latent Phenomenological Frame of Coerced Voluntarism.

The Zoom-Lens at Work: Focusing the New Paradigm on Beauty and Fertility

Virtually all the parables and examples that have informed my reflections about cosmetic surgery have involved women. Women are also the focal point of most of the advertising, the surgical practices, the commodification of the results, and the public celebration of the practices. Although women are mentioned briefly in the context of Framework I, the Rights Framework, gender is not easily thematized as problematic in the context of a rights-based, liberal theoretical model.[43] As a feminist philosopher, I am interested in examining the role of gender in relation to the actual practices and the cultural construction of elective cosmetic surgery. Is the prevalence of women in this set of practices simply a demographic fact without consequence, or does gender function here as a central systemic structure with attendant moral and political consequences?[44] In what follows I shall argue for the second of these alternatives. I want to understand what the contemporary technologizing of the Natural means in the lives of women, particulary in the areas of appearance and fertility. In order to do this, I shall use concepts such as disciplinary bio-power, the political technology of the body, and the notion of women's bodies as natural artefacts, concepts that have no obvious role to play in Framework I.

Virtually every culture has a set of categories, symbols, and ritualized practices associated with Nature. Often they carry with them gendered and racialized associations. Some cultures regard the domain of the Natural as a limit to be preserved with respect, kinship, affiliation. Other cultures operate with a view of the domain of the Natural as primitive, open for exploration and domination, something to be tamed and exploited. In western cultures women's oppression has been 'justified' by assimilating Woman to Nature, to the domain of the Natural, where the 'natural' is set up in binary opposition to 'culture,' to the 'fully human.' To give credibility to theories of the naturalized inferiority of women, western European and North American scientific traditions have often sought to demonstrate empirically how women, and women's bodies in particular, are essentially pathological approximations to men and the bodies of men.[45] As a result, the assimilation of Woman to the Natural coupled with empirical demonstrations of natural pathology have led to oppressive misogynous structures of material, social, and political control by men. Male physicians have played a prominent role in this oppression.[46]

In the latter cultures what is designated the 'natural' functions primarily as a 'frontier' rather than as a 'limit' or 'barrier.' While genetic identity, human sexuality, fertility, reproductive outcome, and longevity previously were regarded as open to variation primarily in evolutionary terms, biotechnological cultures see them as domains for creation and control. Often the role assigned to technology is that of transcendence, transformation, control, exploitation, or destruction; correlatively, the technologized object or process is conceptualized as inferior or primitive, in need of perfecting transformation in the name of some 'higher' purpose or end, or as deserving of eradication because it is seen as harmful or evil. Cosmetic surgeons, for example, see human bodies as a carnal site of challenge. As one plastic surgeon remarks, 'patients sometimes misunderstand the nature of cosmetic surgery. It's not a short cut for diet or exercise. *It's a way to override the genetic code*' (emphasis added).[47]

Given the oppressive consequences of associating women with the Natural in capitalist, racist, patriarchal cultures, it is not surprising that women themselves should envision access to technological control as a way of severing this connection.[48] Modifying the original quotation from Mary Wollstonecraft, we now need to ask whether still being taught from infancy that youth, beauty, fertility, and heterosexual affiliation are women's sceptre, women's bodies are coming to shape themselves to women's minds. We also need to ask whether, with this inversion, women's artefactual bodies serve as new kinds of cages, new kinds of prisons – or both. As more and more experts and technicians administer to and transform women's bodies in terms of appearance and child-bearing, we need to ask whether RoboBeauty and RoboFertility do represent a genuine advance for women or whether new forms of oppression are entering our lives.

How do these remarks regarding technology and women apply to particular women, and why? Full social approval for many women in many cultures is dependent upon their acting within – and resisting within – interlocking norms of compulsion: compulsory attractiveness, compulsory fertility and social nurturance, and compulsory heterosexuality. These patterns of compulsion determine, for many women, the 'legitimate' limits of attraction, motherhood, and commitment. In these cultural contexts women's attractiveness is defined as attractive-to-men; women's eroticism is defined as non-existent, pathological, deviant, or peripheral when it is not directed to phallic goals; and legitimate motherhood is defined in terms of legally sanctioned and constrained reproductive service to particular men and to particular institutions, such as the nation, the race, the owner, and the class, institutions that are, themselves, more often than not male dominated. Now biotechnology is making beauty, the appearance of youthfulness, fertility, and the appearance of heterosexuality through transsexual surgery accessible to virtually all women who can afford them – and increasingly large numbers of women are making other sacrifices in their lives in order to buy access to the technical expertise.[49]

Why? Why do women's hearts and imaginations resonate with the question posed by Snow White's stepmother – and by the participants and observers in the many Beauty Contests in Life: 'Who is the fairest of all?' What does the public affirmation of beauty, of fertility, bring to women in many cultures? What is frequently the fate of women who are classified among the plain, the ugly, the aged, and the barren in those cultures that prize women's beauty and fertility?

Speaking about their choices in relation to elective cosmetic surgery, the voices and the narratives of the women themselves are seductive. They speak of gaining access to transcendence, achievement, liberation, and power, and we must acknowledge the lived reality of that discourse. Electing to undergo cosmetic surgery not only appears to but often does in reality give a woman a sense of identity that to some extent she has chosen herself. Second, it offers her the possibility of raising her status both socially and economically through increasing her opportunities for heterosexual affiliation (especially with white and/or powerful men). Third, by committing herself to the pursuit of beauty, a woman can give a kind of integrity to her life. This pursuit involves a consistent set of values and choices that she knows will bring her widespread approval and consequently contribute to a more positive sense of herself. Finally, the technologically based pursuit of beauty gives rise to a large range of individuals who will care for that woman and care directly for her body in a way that is often lacking the day-to-day lives of many women in cultures in which direct bodily nurturance and caring between women is devalued or prohibited. In short, the choice to pursue beauty through biotechnological means is directly linked with experience of self-creation, self-fulfilment, self-esteem, and being cared for.

The power of these experiences and accompanying patterns of motivation must not be underestimated.[50] Nevertheless, while I do acknowledge the power and legitimacy of these motivations and see how these choices can confer a kind of integrity on a woman's life, I also believe that they are likely to embroil her in a set of interrelated contradictions that will erode and undermine the very integrity, transcendence, liberation, and self-esteem that she may be seeking. I refer to them as Paradoxes of Choice.

Three Paradoxes of Choice

In introducing these paradoxes I want to integrate the notion of the body as natural artefact with Foucault's concept of the 'docile body.' In *Discipline and Punish*, Foucault introduces the notion of disciplinary power.[51] This is a form of power that is directed at individual bodies and exercises its coercive effect by acting on an apparently active and free body through meticulous control of that body's movements, gestures, attitudes, and speed of motion. Foucault argues that the outcome of the exercise of disciplinary power is the docile body, a body 'that may be subjected, used, transformed, and improved.'[52] While Foucault applies this concept of power to prisons and armies, I believe it is also possible to see how women's cosmetic and fertile bodies are entering 'a machinery of power that explores it, breaks it down, and rearranges it' through recognizable metamorphoses of cosmetic embodiment, conception, gestation, and birthing. I regard these metamorphoses as intrinsically biopolitical in so far as they involve subtle and complicated negotiations of power between women and the relevant technological health care experts in which both sets of individuals are acting in accord with an increasingly coercive set of Technological Imperatives.[53] Coupling Foucault's notion of disciplinary power with docile bodies is also heuristically valuable because it instructs us to search for those experts – theoreticians, ideologues, researchers, health care practitioners, and technicians – whose explicit power mandate is to explore, break down, and rearrange women's bodies in the name of more perfect women and more perfect babies in the larger setting of profit-oriented global capitalism.[54]

Paradox 1. The Choice of Conformity: Aspiring to Be Number '10,' Aspiring to Have 'Perfect' Babies

While the technologies of cosmetic surgery, genetic engineering, and reproduction clearly could be used to create and celebrate idiosyncrasy, eccentricity, and uniqueness, it is clear that they are not at present being used in this way.[55] In the area of cosmetic surgery, surgeons report that legions of women appear in the offices demanding to have 'Bo Derek' breasts[56] (or those of whoever happens to be the most recent mammary goddess of choice in Hollywood). Jewish girls and women appear in their offices demanding reductions of their noses so as to be able to 'pass' as one of their Aryan sisters, who form the dominant ethnic group.[57] Affluent girls and young women in South Korea standardly have their noses lifted, their eyes widened, and their cheekbones shaved in order to 'go Anglo,' despite the conservative naturalism built into the traditions of Confucianism.[58] Asian girls and women in other countries bring in pictures of Elizabeth Taylor and of Japanese movie actresses demanding the 'westernizing' of their faces in hopes of improved employment and marital prospects.[59] What is being created in these instances is often white or light, westernized, Anglo-Saxon bodies in cultures that are racist, anti-Semitic, and increasingly ageist in their norms and practices. Affluence and class privilege are being viscerally inscribed in the visible physiognomy of a woman's skin, facial features, silhouette, and curvature through the needles, the knives, the cannulas, and the implants. 'Designer Labels' of the famous cosmetic surgeons are being stitched, literally, into women's flesh.

Prior to the rise of cosmetic biotechnology, a woman's degree and kind of makeup, her dress, gestures, degree and definition of feminine cleanliness, degree of muscularity, odours, degree of hirsuteness, voice, vocabulary, patterns of silence, hands, feet, skin, hair, vulva, fertility, and gestational life often have been evaluated, regulated, and disciplined in the light of often dominant males and male viewers present in the assessing gaze of other women.[60] Now women can gain the appreciation and approval of other men through demonstrations of achieved femininity by submitting to more invasive procedures of incisions, stitches, staples, anaesthesias, artificial implants, cellular suction and reimplantation, and scar tissue.

Similarly, in the area of fertility, biotechnology has increasing definitional and, by implication, clinical power to identify, monitor, and regulate 'normal conception,' 'normal gestation,' 'normal birthing,' 'responsible motherhood,' and the 'perfect baby.' Fertile women whose babies will be prized in a particular biotechnological culture are encouraged to access biotechnology as a means of liberation, enhanced choice, and greater perfectibility of 'desired fertile outcome.' The result is the production of a sex-selected, genetically monitored or engineered baby whose dangerous gestational development is continuously technologically controlled and whose potentially crisis-laden birth is managed through technological means. Where such technology is 'normalized' and simultaneously restricted to the relatively affluent, the production of the baby/natural artefact will come to be seen as a mark of class and race privilege.

In both these areas the first serious paradox I see is this: that what look like optimal situations of deliberation, maximized choice, and self-determination often simultaneously signal the production of conformity.

Paradox 2. Choosing Dependence in the Name of Autonomy

A woman's desire to create a permanently beautiful and youthful appearance not vulnerable to the threats of externally applied cosmetic artifice or to the ageing processes of the body must be understood as a deeply existential project. So, too, must a woman's desire to choose, to control, and to shape her own fertility and her child be so understood. In both cases these desires deliberately involve a shift from a submission to what is contingent and uncertain in human existence to a posture of rational human control, prediction, and security in some of the most intimately experienced domains of human embodiment – the body as beautiful, the body as fertile. Biotechnology is accessed in the name of transcendence: transcendence of hereditary predestination, of lived time, of one's given 'limitations,' of control over the uncertainties of conception, maternity, and birth. This involves an important metaphysical shift that is important to track: what comes to have primary significance is not the real, given, existing woman but the potentially beautiful, fertile woman. Her present state of embodiment increasingly is viewed as a 'primitive entity' seen only in terms of its (her?) potential, as a kind of raw material or set of fertility functions to be biotechnologically transformed in the name of beauty, fertility, eroticism, and nurturance.[61]

As Foucault and others have noted, practices of coercion and domination often are effectively hidden behind practical rhetoric and supporting theories that claim to be benevolent, therapeutic, and protective of individual choice. I believe that in the areas of cosmetic surgery and reproductive biotechnology precisely this kind of camouflage is practised. In the past, material, psychological, and social colonizing was often done in the name of bringing 'civilization' to 'primitive, barbaric people.' Contemporary colonizers mask their exploitation of 'raw materials and human labour' in the name of 'development.' But who is colonizing here? Often it is a particular man or a variety of men. The woman who wanted to undergo a facelift, a tummy tuck, and liposuction all in one week to win heterosexual approval *from a man she had not seen in twenty-eight years* and whose individual preference she could not possibly know experiences the power involved in heterosexual approval almost in the abstract. Actual men – sons, brothers, fathers, male lovers, male beauty 'experts,' male employers, male colleagues – and hypothetical men, such as 'future husbands,' live in the imaginations and hearts of women.[62] They are present, too, as male engineering students who taunt and harass women and in the form of male cosmetic surgeons who offer 'free advice' in social gatherings to women whose 'deformities' and 'severe problems' could be cured through their healing needles and knives. Their presence is immediate. Some girls and women know, all too well, how their violation of the norms of feminine perfectibility can result in violence, abuse, or abandonment by those men, regardless of class. Or they live more ghostly powerful lives – sometimes as the desired prince who will rescue those girls and women from the violence and the oppressiveness of poverty. But live there they do as a critical locus of coercive power.

In electing to undergo cosmetic surgery, women appear to be protesting against the constraints of the 'given' in their embodied lives and to be seeking liberation from those constraints. Nevertheless, I believe women are, in fact, in danger of becoming more vulnerable, more dependent upon male assessment and the services of those experts who promised to render them liberated, independent, and beautiful. The beauty culture is coming to be dominated by a variety of experts, and consumers of youth and beauty will find themselves increasingly dependent not only on cosmetic surgeons but on anaesthetists, nurses, aestheticians, nail technicians, manicurists, dieticians, hairstylists, cosmetologists, trainers, pedicurists, electrolysists, pharmacologists, and dermatologists.[63] Again, it is a public sign of affluence and privilege to have both the leisure and the income to be able to afford these continuing forms of expert dependence.

In the field of reproductive technologies, similar dynamics can be at work.[64] The official biotechnological rhetoric is often redolent with expressions of care, benevolence, altruism, and enhanced choice, but the reality of women's experiences, when they are accessing the reproductive biotechnologies, is often at sad variance with the official rhetoric. Women report experiencing psychologically oppressive objectifications of themselves through the loss of integrity threatened by repeated procedures such as induced superovulation and the ingestion of powerful medications, surgical interventions requiring anaesthetics, puncturing with needles, invasions of the womb with cannulas, embryo implantations, and bombardment by ultrasound. In addition to feeling physical pain, women report feeling manipulated, personally assaulted, infantilized, and experience anxiety and failure, as the biotechnologists become increasingly fixated on the achievement of fertility. Personal reductionism and reproductive dismemberment and commodification of women's reproductive powers also are reported by women involved with reproductive biotechnologies.[65]

Here again, promised liberation, enhanced choice, and protected autonomy often collapse into lived dependence on a range of biotechnologists who may include fetologists, gynecologists, endocrinologists, bioengineers, biochemists, psychiatrists, anaesthetists, fertility researchers, and pharmacologists. These biotechnologies are controlled primarily by men.

Here then is the second serious paradox: that in choosing to become involved in the biotechnologies in the areas of elective cosmetic surgery and reproduction, women become involved in processes that undermine the integrity-preserving preconditions for full womanly autonomy and lead to greater dependence on experts who are, for the most part, men.

Paradox 3. Coerced Voluntariness and the Technological Imperative[66]

Initially, women who choose to become involved in the biotechnologies of cosmetic surgery and reproduction often seem to represent a kind of paradigm case of a rational chooser. They are coming from an increasingly wide range of economic groups (a rate of participation accelerated by inclusion of these biotechnologies in public health plans) and clearly make a choice, often at significant cost to the rest of their life, to participate in the technologies. They often are highly critical consumers of these services and expect consultation, information with respect to risks and benefits, and professional guarantees of expertise. Unlike most other recipients of health care services, generally they are young and in good health and are not afflicted with any trauma, sickness, or chronic condition that might impair their capacity to make choices. One might even say that they epitomize relatively invulnerable, free, rational agents making a decision under virtually optimal conditions.

In order to illuminate this paradox of choice, I turn first to the reproductive biotechnologies. In this area, the advent of the reproductive technologies has been hailed as enhancing women's self-determination and as increasing the control over and range of women's reproductive choices in an uncontroversial and absolute way. It is certainly clear that owing to the advances with various reproductive biotechnologies, especially *in vitro fertilization*, embryo flushing, freezing, and transfer, and fetal surgery, there are now women with healthy children who previously would not have had children. Nevertheless, there are two important ideological, choice-diminishing forms of pressure at work that affect women's choices in the area of reproductive technology and have analogues in the area of cosmetic surgery.

The first of these is *the pressure to achieve perfection through technology*, signalled by the rise of new forms of eugenicist thinking that stigmatize potential and existing babies, children, and adults with disabilities. More and more frequently, benevolently articulated eugenicist pressures bear down on women to submit to a battery of prenatal diagnostic tests and extensive embryo and fetal monitoring throughout pregnancy in the name of producing 'perfect,' preferably white, middle- and upper-class babies.[67] As the reproductive biotechnologies multiply and are tested on and in the bodies of fertile women, women are pressured by partners, parents, family, obstetricians, and fertility 'experts' to use this technology. The mediating rhetoric emphasizes 'maximized choice' and

'responsible motherhood.'[68] While women who act in accord with this Technological Imperative do not report feeling coerced, women who refuse the reproductive biotechnologies *do* report feeling subjected to increasingly intense
forms of pressure, disapprobation, withdrawal of professional services, and personal self-doubt. Thus, as many feminist theorists have pointed out, the rhetoric
of choice often camouflages the extent to which the Technological Imperative is
leading to an intensifying lack of freedom and the elimination of a full range of
choices.[69]

The second ideological dynamic at work is *the double-pathologizing of
women's bodies*. The history of western science and western medical practice is
not altogether a positive one for women. As voluminous historical and contemporary documentation has shown, scientists, such as cell biologists, endocrinologists, anatomists, and neuroscientists along with their gynecological,
obstetrical, psychiatric, and surgical counterparts, have assumed, hypothesized,
or 'demonstrated' that women's bodies in general are inferior, deformed, imperfect, and/or infantile. Medical practitioners have treated women accordingly.[70]
This is the initial stage of gender pathologizing.

The second stage of pathologizing enters in with the ideology surrounding the
rise of the reproductive biotechnologies. Until the twentieth century, women's
ordinary gestational capacities and processes were regarded as definitional of
normal womanhood and normal human, mammalian reproduction. No more. As
Corea and others have so amply documented, profoundly misogynous beliefs
and attitudes are a central part of the motivation for developing completely
extra-uterine technologies for fetal development.[71] Women's wombs are coming
to be described as 'dark prisons,' as dangerous places, or, with the advent of
ultrasound reductionism, as fetal milieus or uterine environments without reference to women whatsoever. Women-as-pregnant-subjects increasingly are
viewed as threatening, irresponsible milieus that exist in a necessarily antagonistic relationship with the fetus and as bodies that are high-risk sites for the
fetus, since fetal development cannot be continuously monitored and controlled
so as to guarantee the best possible 'fetal outcome.'[72] Now that the entire process of woman-centred pregnancy is coming to be perceived as a less desirable
process of gestation than one that could be technologically controlled in an
extra-uterine site, a double pathologizing of women has taken place.

The normative and political dimensions of coercion are mediated by the concept of 'fully responsible motherhood,' which is made operational, wherever
possible, as acting in accord with whatever technology is available to that
woman. Ideally, this process could include technological management of reproductive cells, zygotes, embryos, fetuses, and newborn babies throughout the
technological management of conception, maternity, and birthing. I believe that

while the new reproductive technologies open up some new alternatives to women, the Technological Imperative is eliminating many of women's previous choices. Moreover, given that many women bear children in an ideological context of obligatory and controlled motherhood, I am reluctant simply to accept the reports of the fertility technologists that their patients 'want access' as a sufficient condition for demonstrating genuinely voluntary choice.[73]

An analogous argument can be made with respect to elective cosmetic surgery. Many women are under enormous pressure to be beautiful and now to achieve perfection through the use of cosmetic biotechnologies. This pressure is on the increase. Cosmetic surgeons report on the wide range of clients who buy their services. They pitch their advertising to a large audience through the use of the media and parade their 'successes' in front of television cameras. They use rhetoric that encourages women to think in terms of seemingly trivial 'nips' and 'tucks' that will transform their lives – or of recycling the 'raw material' of their fat cells from an ugly site to one of beauty such as the lips or breasts. The cosmetic 'success stories' can be seen as more permanent forms of the already normalized 'make overs' that dominate women's media and, like the 'success stories' of the fertility technologies, the cosmetic 'success stories' are displayed on talk shows along with their makers, while surgically transformed women win the Miss America beauty pageants.

Here again, we can see a Technological Imperative take hold through this normalization. Increasingly, women who refuse to submit to the knives and the needles, to the anaesthetics and the bandages are seen as deviant in one way or another. Women who refuse to use these technologies are already becoming stigmatized as 'unliberated,' as 'not caring about their appearance,' as 'refusing to be all that you could be,' or as (the ultimate label of scorn!) 'granola heads.' Not caring about one's appearance as a woman is already taken by patriarchal psychologists, social workers, and psychiatrists as a sign of disturbed gender identity and pathologically low self-esteem. Serious consequences for a woman often can result when she is in the 'care' and control of such professionals.

When greater access to power comes to those women who do 'care about themselves' via cosmetic technologies, more coercive dimensions enter the scene. In the past only those women who were perceived to be *naturally* beautiful (or rendered beautiful through relatively superficial artifice) had access to power, and economic social mobility closed off to women regarded as plain or ugly or old (if there were no overriding factors such as privileged family connections and/or wealth). Now, however, womanly beauty is becoming transformed into a technological commodity for which each and every woman can, in principle, sacrifice and purchase if she wants to succeed in a culture that defines and commodifies womanly beauty and describes these sacrifices as liberation.[74] In such cultures technology is making obligatory the appearance of youth and the reality of 'beauty.' Natural diversity of appearance is being supplanted by biotechnologically produced norms of beauty, which exercise an increasingly coercive effect in the lives and choices of girls and women.

Here too, I argue that we find the dynamic of the double-pathologizing of the normal with respect to women's embodiment. What until recently had been described in both technical and popular literature as normal variations of female bodily shapes or described in the relatively innocuous language of 'problem areas,' are now being described as 'deformities,' 'ugly protrusions,' 'unsightly concentrations of fat cells,' and 'acutely ptotic breasts' – a litany of phrases designed to intensify feelings of disgust and shame and to promise relief at the possibility of technological cures.[75] Cosmetic surgery promises more and more women the creation of beautiful, youthful-appearing bodies. As a consequence, many more women will become labelled 'ugly' and 'old' in relation to this more select population of surgically created beautiful faces and bodies that have been contoured and augmented, lifted and tucked to a state of achieved feminine perfection. We are witnessing a pathological shift here: the naturally 'given' is coming to be seen as the technologically 'primitive' – this is the first stage of pathologizing. The second stage enters in because it will no longer be sufficient to remedy this normal pathology of women's unadorned appearance through artifice; now even the artifice and makeup will be seen as a pathological substitute when women are given the opportunity to achieve status as a beautiful artefact through the surgical technology.

This is the third paradox: that the Technological Beauty and Fertility Imperatives and the pathological double-inversion of the naturally given are coercing increasing numbers of women to 'choose' cosmetic and reproductive technologies; hence the description of Coerced Voluntariness.

Concluding Speculations

In this paper I have tried to show why viewing cosmetic and reproductive biotechnologies through a rights-based bioethical framework – suggested as optimal by the language of 'elective' surgery and the rhetoric of choice, transcendence, and individual self-fulfilment – leaves me puzzled with respect to my central categories of moral questions and fails to illuminate what is deeply problematic about the technology-driven beauty and fertility cultures in the lives of women. I have also tried to show how the autonomy-oriented discourse of rights is inconsistent with the degree of coercion and choice-diminishing pressures that women experience as part of the lived dynamic of these biotechnologies in patriarchal cultures. Finally, I have analysed ways in which women's legitimate aspirations and entitlement to experience self-determination, exercise choice, achieve integrity, and receive dignity and respect can be dangerously compromised and undermined through the ideological commodification of these biotechnologies.

In her influential work *Of Woman Born: Motherhood as Experience and Institution* Adrienne Rich claims that for the first time in history women have the possibility of converting our physicality into both knowledge and power.[76] In order for this to happen in the areas of fertility and beauty I believe we need to

1. challenge the coercive norms of obligatory beauty and fertility that dominate the lives of many women;
2. undermine the power dynamic built into the dependence upon surgical experts who define themselves as the ultimate aestheticians and creators of fertility for women; and
3. responsibly explore, for ourselves as diverse human beings in community, the human potential signalled by our radical creative malleability as human subjects.

I hope the biopolitical reflections in this appear contribute to this collective project.

Notes

Some of the narrative material cited in this essay also has appeared in an earlier companion paper, 'Women and the Knife: Cosmetic Surgery and the Colonization of Women's Bodies,' published in *Hypatia*, Special Issue on the Body, ed. Elizabeth Grosz, Vol. 6, no. 3 (Fall 1991). Particular analytic categories and arguments appearing in the last section concerning various paradoxes of choice play an important heuristic role in my research and have been developed in other contexts as well. In particular, see 'Of Woman Born? How Old-Fashioned! New Reproductive Technologies and Women's Oppression,' in *The Future of Human Reproduction*, ed. Christine Overall (Toronto: Women's Press, 1989).

Earlier versions of this paper were delivered to the Society for Social Philosophy, to the Centre for Applied Ethics and the Department of Philosophy at the University of British Columbia, and to a conference on Feminist Ethics and Social Policy sponsored by the University of Pittsburgh. I am grateful to the members of those audiences for their responses and critical remarks. I wish, too, to acknowledge the support of the members of the Social Science and Humanities Research Council of Canada Research Network in Feminist Health Care Ethics.

1 Nora McCabe, 'Cosmetic Solutions,' *HomeMaker Magazine* (September 1990), 38
2 *Us Air Magazine* (November 1993), 118
3 Margalit Fox, 'A Portrait in Skin and Bone,' *New York Times* (Sunday, November 21, 1993), 8
4 *Mirabella* 'Who is the Face of America?' (September 1994), 14
5 Discussed by Trish Robb, 'The Cutting Edge,' *Washington Post Magazine* (March 24, 1991), 18. Original source *Teen Magazine* (1988)
6 John Williams, MD, and Jim Williams, MD, 'Say It with Liposuction,' Brochure. From a press release reported in *Harper's* (August 1990)
7 Robb, 'Cutting Edge,' 28
8 'Retouching Nature's Way: Is Cosmetic Surgery Worth It?' *Toronto Star* (February 1, 1990)
9 'Falling in Love Again,' *Toronto Star* (July 23, 1990)
10 Quoted from Kathy Davis's empirical research. See Davis, *Reshaping the Female Body: The Dilemma of Cosmetic Surgery* (New York: Routledge, 1995), 127
11 Quoted by Ellen Goodman, 'A Plastic Pageant,' *Boston Globe* (September 19, 1989)
12 Steve, Glain, 'Korean Plastic Surgeons Cash in on 'Go Anglo' Craze,' *Globe and Mail* (December 19, 1993). Reprinted from *Wall Street Journal*
13 'Cosmetic Surgery for the Holidays,' *New York Times* News Service. Reprinted in *The Sheboygan Press* (Wisconsin) (1985)
14 Ibid.
15 Carole Spitzack, 'The Confession Mirror: Plastic Images for Surgery,' in *The Hysterical Male: New Feminist Theory*, eds. A. Kroker and M. Kroker (Montreal: New World Perspectives, 1991), 66
16 Television show, '20–20' (1994)
17 Robb, 'Cutting Edge,' 16
18 Ibid.
19 'The Quest to Be a Perfect 10,' *Toronto Star* (February 1, 1990)
20 'Retouching Nature's Way'
21 Jenny Jones, 'Body of Evidence,' *People Magazine* (March 2, 1992), 62
22 Originally published in Gina Luria and Virginia Tiger, *EveryWoman* (New York: Random House, 1976)
23 For an extended, elegantly nuanced psychological and ethical analysis of elective cosmetic surgery, which acknowledges the sometimes contradictory complexity of personal decision-making and moral assessment, see Davis, *Reshaping the Female Body*. Davis emphasizes identity, agency, and morality as her central themes. Her pathbreaking book is particulary valuable because of her exploration of the dialectic between empirical data derived from three field studies and theoretical feminist analysis. See also Kathy Davis's chapter, 'Cultural Dopes and She-Devils: Cosmetic Surgery as Ideological Dilemma,' in *Negotiating at the Margins: The Gendered*

Discourses of Power and Resistance, ed. Sue Fisher and Kathy Davis (New Brunswick, NJ: Rutgers University Press, 1993), 23–47.

24 'New Bodies for Sale,' *Newsweek* (May 27, 1985)

25 As of 1990 at least twelve deaths have resulted from liposuction complications such as hemorrhages and embolisms. 'All that we know is there was a complication and that complication was death,' was the stark comment about Toni Sullivan, age forty-three. The press described Sullivan as the 'hardworking mother of two teenage children'; 'Woman, 43, Dies after Cosmetic Surgery,' *Toronto Star* (July 7, 1989).

26 There is an astounding silence in the professional mainstream bioethical journals concerning ethical issues raised by elective cosmetic surgery. For example, there is virtually no discussion in the *Hastings Center Report*, the *Lancet*, the *New England Journal of Medicine*, and *Philosophy and Medicine* (which has published one article). Generally, feminist analyses of elective cosmetic surgery appear primarily in aesthetics, cultural studies, social and life science journals, and feminist philosophy journals (see, for example, articles in the *British Journal of Sociology*, *Camera Obscura*, *Feminism and Psychology*, *Hypatia*, *Signs*, *Social Problems*, and *Theory, Culture and Society*). There is, of course, an older body of largely psychiatric literature which pathologizes women's choices of cosmetic surgery procedures. With the advent of the 'normalization' of elective cosmetic surgery, this medical literature is declining. For a more extended discussion of 'normalization', see my 'Women and the Knife.'

27 See, for example, *From Abortion to Reproductive Freedom: Transforming a Movement*, ed. Marlene Gerber Fried (Boston: South End Press, 1990). See in particular the following articles: Angela Davis, 'Racism, Birth Control and Reproductive Rights'; Adrienne Ash and Michelle Fine, 'Shared Dreams: A Left Perspective on Disability Rights and Reproductive Rights'; 'Reproductive Rights Positions Paper' by the National Black Women's Health Project; and Byllye Avery, 'Reproductive Rights and Coalition-Building.' For a more sceptical analysis of the utility of rights, see Patricia J. Williams, *The Alchemy of Race and Rights* (Cambridge, MA: Harvard University Press, 1991).

28 Robert M. Veatch, 'Models for Ethical Medicine in a Revolutionary Age,' *Hastings Center Report* Vol. 2 (June 1972), 5–7

29 For a perceptive analysis of four different political models of doctor-patient relationships: traditional-authoritarian (invariably paternalistic), traditional-egalitarian, traditional-feminist, and radical-feminist, see Sheryl Ruzek, *The Women's Health Movement: Feminist Alternatives to Medical Control* (New York: Praeger, 1978).

30 In an insightful and frightening narrative following a personal ethnographic study in which Professor Carole Spitzack posed as a possible client for elective cosmetic surgery, Spitzack documents the subtle manipulative moves of one such surgeon and their psychological consequence: 'Part of me resists his oppressive view of feminin-

ity, but another part of me is in doubt, ready to acquiesce. He is, after all, the expert'
(66), 'my entire being seems deficient, in spite of myself, apart from my critical sensibilities' (67); 'The Confession Mirror.' See also idem, 'Confession and Significa-
tion: The Systematic Inscription of Body Consciousness,' *Journal of Medicine and
Philosophy* Vol. 12 (1987), 357–69.

31 Cf. R. Iverson, 'National Survey Shows Overwhelming Satisfaction with Breast
Implants,' *Plastic and Reconstructive Surgery* Vol. 88 (1991), 546–7; L. Ohlsen, B.
Ponten, and G. Hanbert, 'Augmentation Mammaplasty: A Surgical and Psychiatric
Evaluation of the Results,' *Annals of Plastic Surgery* Vol. 2 (1978), 42–52. Kathy
Davis's subjects, by and large, also report high levels of satisfaction with their cosmetic surgery procedures; *Reshaping* n9. It is also clear, however, at least with
respect to silicone implants, that the worldwide legal suit being brought against the
makers of silicone implants indicates that definite levels of dissatisfaction exist. For a
poignant and sad narrative, see Jones, 'Body of Evidence.' The important ethical
point here, however, is that the dissatisfaction has resulted from the implants failing,
not from the hoped-for breast augmentation itself. See Lisa Parker's work for a more
extensive critical report of surgeon-patient interactions concerning breast implants;
'Social Justice, Federal Paternalism, and Feminism: Breast Implants in the Cultural
Context of Female Beauty,' *Kennedy Institute of Ethics Journal* Vol. 3, no. 1 (1993),
57–76.

32 See Spitzack, 'The Confession Mirror,' for an excellent description of this blurring.

33 I am not assuming that the term 'medical condition' is unproblematic. It is clear from
a great deal of narrative material that the choice by women to have elective cosmetic
surgery is often preceded by enormous suffering, fragile self-esteem, distorted body
image, and depression – all experienced in a variety of oppressive settings that privilege young, beautiful, fertile, slim, white female bodies. It is only by equating 'medical' with the ideologically narrow constraints of a biomedical model that the above
experiences are not regarded as appropriately 'medical' and worthy of serious therapeutic attention.

34 A new pathologized category of women has now arisen in relation to cosmetic surgery. Referred to as 'scalpel slaves,' these women can be seen either as suffering
from a form of compulsion or, ironically, as kinds of post-modern gender vangardists
appropriating the surgical technology to their own ends. Orlan might be viewed in
this way, as she clearly views herself. So, too, might the imaginative protagonist of
Fay Weldon's powerful and evocative novel *The Life and Loves of a She-Devil* (London: Coronet Books, 1983). For an article on scalpel slaves, see *Newsweek* (January
11, 1988), 58–9.

35 'Retouching Nature's Way'

36 K. Davis, *Reshaping*, presents a persuasive and moving set of personal narratives by
women who have chosen breast augmentation; see Chapter 5. My own reaction of

horror enters in because it is the male *surgeon* who is claiming that performing breast augmentation has high priority for *himself*. That it is important for his female clients appears to have secondary importance relative to his own surgical 'turf wars' over access to scarce surgical territories (i.e., operating rooms) and resources. I also cannot envision any scenario where I would privilege a patient wanting surgery for breast augmentation over a patient needing surgery because of a clearly diagnosed malignancy in the breast.

37　A quintessential expression of this view can be found in the work of Lori B. Andrews; see, for example, 'My Body, My Property,' *Hastings Center Report* Vol. 16, no. 5 (October 1986), 28–38. See also Mary Anne Warren, *Gendercide: The Implications of Sex Selection* (Totowa, NJ: Rowman and Allenheld, 1985).

38　Here I join with Janice Raymond's lucid and, I think, appropriately indignant analysis of current liberal feminist views in the area of reproductive technology; see Raymond, *Women as Wombs* (San Francisco, CA: HarperSanFrancisco, 1993), in particular, Chapter 3, 'A Critique of Reproductive Liberalism,' 76–107. See also Alison Jaggar, *Feminist Politics and Human Nature* (Totowa, NJ: Rowman and Allenheld, 1983), and the papers by Christine Overall and Susan Sherwin in this volume.

39　Hans Jonas, 'Toward a Philosophy of Technology,' *Hastings Center Report* Vol. 9, no. 1 (February 1979), 34–43

40　Ibid., 35

41　See Christine Overall, 'Reflections of a Sceptical Bioethithist,' in this volume for an additional set of arguments supporting the use of politicized bioethical models.

42　For a more extensive analysis of this notion in a larger conceptual framework, see my 'Brave New Baby: Brave New World,' paper presented at the 'Women, Gender, and Science Question' Conference, University of Minnesota, 1995.

43　As Jaggar and others have argued, it is difficult to problematize gender as a central theoretical dimension under classical liberalism partially because of liberalism's explicit commitment to render gender inadmissible (and, hence, invisible) as legitimate impediment to the implementation of formal equality; see Jaggar, *Feminist Politics*.

44　Spitzack, in 'The Confession Mirror,' for example, maintains that gender functions systematically in the area of cosmetic surgery. Often cosmetic surgery for men is designed to enhance their appearance as powerful and young and hence more competitive in the public masculine domain. Where competition does enter in for women, in a heterosexist society, it involves female-female competition for affiliation with privileged males. I think, however, that women's actual motivational accounts call into question Spitzack's gender contrasts, since women are taught and have the experience that their bodily appearance *is* a form of power in competitive settings.

45　For a variety of theoretical discussions of oppressive associations of women and nature in capitalist societies see Brian Easlea, *Science and Sexual Oppression: Patri-*

archy's Confrontation with Women and Nature (London: Weidenfeld and Nicolson, 1981); Donna Haraway, *Primate Visions: Gender, Race, and Nature in the World of Modern Science* (New York: Routledge, 1989); Evelyn Fox Keller, 'The Gender/Science System: Or, Is Sex to Gender as Nature Is to Science?' *Hypatia* Vol. 2, no. 3 (1987), 37–50; and Carolyn Merchant, *The Death of Nature: Women, Ecology, and the Scientific Revolution* (New York: Harper and Row, 1980).

46 The feminist scholarship on this topic is, by now, voluminous. See, for example, Nelly Oudshoorn, *Beyond the Natural Body: an Archaeology of Sex Hormones* (New York: Routledge, 194); Cynthia Eagle Russet, *Sexual Science: The Victorian Construction of Womanhood* (Cambridge, MA: Harvard University Press, 1989); and Londa Schiebinger, *The Mind Has No Sex? Women in the Origins of Modern Science* (Cambridge, MA: Harvard University Press, 1989).

47 'Retouching Nature's Way.' For a recent feminist overview of current developments in genetic engineering, see Pat Spallone, *Generation Games: Genetic Engineering and the Future for Our Lives* (Philadelphia, PA: Temple University Press, 1992).

48 Michelle Stanworth raises this question seriously in 'The Deconstruction of Motherhood,' in *Reproductive Technologies: Gender, Motherhood, and Medicine*, ed. M. Stanworth (Minneapolis: University of Minnesota Press, 1987). Raymond, *Women as Wombs*, rejects Stanworth's optimism.

49 For varying feminist interpretations of transsexual surgery, see Judith Butler, *Bodies That Matter: On the Discursive Limits of 'Sex'* (New York: Routledge, 1993); Margrit Eichler, *The Double Standard: A Feminist Critique of Feminist Social Science* (London: Croom Helm, 1980); and Janice Raymond, *The Transsexual Empire: The Making of the She-Male* (Boston: Beacon Press, 1979).

50 Sandra Bartky makes a very similar point regarding what she calls 'feminine discipline.' She too claims that women will resist the dismantling of the disciplines of femininity because, at a very deep level, it would involve radically altering what Bartky calls our 'informal social ontology.' In her words, 'To have a body felt to be 'feminine' – a body socially constructed through the appropriate practices – is in most cases crucial to a woman's sense of herself as female and, since persons currently can *be* only as male or female, to her sense of herself as an existing individual ... The radical feminist critique of femininity, then, may pose a threat not only to a woman's sense of her own identity and desirability but to the very structure of her social universe.' Bartky, 'Foucault, Femininity, and the Modernization of Patriarchal Power,' in *Femininity and Foucault: Reflections of Resistance*, ed. Irene Diamond and Lee Quinby (Boston: Northeastern University Press, 1989), 78

51 Michel Foucault, *Discipline and Punish: The Birth of the Prison*, trans. Alan Sheridan (New York: Vintage Books, 1979), 136–7

52 Ibid., 136

53 For an examination of how this technological imperative is operating in the context

of genetic counselling, see Abby Lippman's work (Department of Epidemiology and Biostatistics, McGill University). Professor Lippman is also the chair of the Human Genetics Committee of the Council for Responsible Genetics. See, in particular, Lippman, 'Mother Matters: A Fresh Look at Prenatal Genetic Testing,' *Reproductive and Genetic Engineering* Vol. 5, no. 2 (1992) 141–54; 'Prenatal Genetic Testing and Screening: Constructing Needs and Reinforcing Inequities,' *American Journal of Law and Medicine* Vol. 17, nos 1 and 2 (1991), 15–50. In the area of reproductive technologies, a classic article is Barbara Katz Rothman, 'The Meanings of Choice in Reproductive Technology,' in *Test-Tube Women*, ed. R. Arditti, Duelli Klein, and S. Minden (London: Pandora Press, 1984); see also idem, *The Tentative Pregnancy* (New York: Viking, 1986).

54 The theoretical and correlative material breaking down and fragmentation of women's bodies by technology is discussed by many feminist theorists, including Maria Mies, 'From the Individual to the Dividual: In the Supermarket of 'Reproductive Alternatives,''' *Reproductive and Genetic Engineering* Vol. 1, no. 3 (1988), 225–37. Oudshoorn, *Beyond the Natural Body*, n44; and Rosalind Pollack Patchesky, 'Foetal Images: The Power of Visual Culture in the Politics of Reproduction,' in Stanworth, *Reproductive Technologies*, n45. I call this the Fragmentation Model. See my 'Of Woman Born?' for further discussion.

55 Davis's empirical data suggest that women's primary desire in electing to undergo cosmetic surgery is to appear ordinary. This may mark a cultural difference between the Netherlands and North America, where there is a clear emphasis on beauty and prettiness. See Robb, 'Cutting Edge,' for an explicit emphasis on the importance of being among the prettiest girls and ladies. I argue elsewhere that the referents of the terms 'ugly,' 'ordinary,' and 'beautiful' are shifting as a result of the normalization of and increasing pressure to use cosmetic surgery. Remember the McCabe quotation (n1): 'For many women, it's no longer a question of whether to undergo cosmetic surgery – but what, when, by whom and how much.' What today may be accepted as ordinary may well constitute a technologized future's 'ugliness.'

56 'Cosmetic Surgery for the Holidays'

57 Robin Tolmach and Raquel Scherr, *Face Value: The Politics of Beauty* (Boston: Routledge and Kegan Paul, 1984)

58 Glain, 'Korean Plastic Surgeons'

59 'New Bodies for Sale'

60 Frigga Haug et al., *Female Sexualization: A Collective Work of Memory*, trans. Erica Carter (London: Verso, 1987)

61 I don't believe that our biological makeup is somehow more primary than culture. In fact, I am inclined to see our 'biological makeup' as both a theoretical and a cultural construct. I regard our embodiment as both phenomenologically and metaphysically prior to biology and as dialectically and materially connected though not created by

culture. For an extended discussion of this dialectical thesis, see Ruth Bleier, *Science and Gender: a Critique of Biology and Its Theories on Women* (New York: Pergamon Press, 1984); Susan Bordo, *Unbearable Weight: Feminism, Western Culture, and the Body* (Berkeley: University of California Press, 1994); Haraway, *Primate Visions*; idem, *Simians, Cyborgs, and Women; The Reinvention of Nature* (New York: Routledge, 1991); and Marion Lowe, 'The Dialectic of Biology and Culture,' in *Biological Woman: The Convenient Myth*, ed. Ruth Hubbard, Mary Sue Henifen, and Barbara Fried (Cambridge, MA: Schenkman, 1982).

62 Cf. John Berger, *Ways of Seeing* (New York: Penguin Books, 1972); and Bartky, 'Foucault.' Bartky remarks: 'Normative femininity is coming more and more to be centered on woman's body ... The woman who checks her makeup half a dozen times a day to see if her foundation has caked or her mascara has run, who worries that the wind or the rain may spoil her hairdo, who looks frequently to see if her stockings have bagged at the ankle, or who, feeling fat, monitors everything she eats, has become, just as surely as the inmate of the Panopticon, a self-policing subject, a self committed to a relentless self-surveillance. This self-surveillance is a form of obedience to patriarchy' (81).

63 Davis's data indicate that women often choose elective cosmetic surgery with only a single transformation or procedure in mind; K. Davis, *Reshaping*. Again these findings may signal an important cultural difference. In North America total body makeovers or, 'the works,' as one surgeon puts it, are frequently explored as a multi-stage commitment. It may well be that different moral assessments apply to the choice of single procedures in contrast to long-term surgical lifelines with an ongoing commitment to future surgeries.

64 See 'Of Woman Born?' for a fuller development of this claim. There is an extensive body of feminist scholarship in this area.

65 See Laura Shanner, 'Bioethics through the Back Door: Phenomenology, Narratives, and Insights into Infertility,' in this volume.

66 I adopt Rona Archilles' use of this term; see 'What's New about the New Reproductive Technologies?' Discussion Paper, Ontario Advisory Council on the Status of Women, Toronto, Government of Ontario, 1988.

67 See Sandra A. Goundry, for the Canadian Disability Rights Council, 'The New Reproductive Technologies, Public Policy, and the Equality Rights of Women and Men with Disabilities,' in *Misconceptions: The Social Construction of Choice and the New Reproductive and Genetic Technologies*, eds. Gwynne Basen, Margrit Eichler, and Abby Lippman (Toronto: Webcom Ltd, 1993), 154–66. See also two films directed by Basen in the series *On the Eighth Day: Perfecting Mother Nature* (Ottawa: National Film Board of Canada).

68 See Raymond, *Women as Wombs*, for an important critique of identifying commodified multiplicity of choice with self-determining autonomy.

69   See Elisabeth Beck-Gernsheim, 'From the Pill to Test-Tube Babies: New Options, New Pressures in Reproductive Behavior,' in *Healing Technology: Feminist Perspectives*, ed. Kathryn Strother Ratcliff (Ann Arbor: University of Michigan Press, 1989), 23–41. See also Achilles, 'What's New,' Morgan, 'Of Woman Born?' and Rothman, 'Meanings of Choice,' for further discussions of this issue.

70   This is at the core of much of the gender-specific paternalism that is directed at female patients primarily by male physicians. Unfortunately, such paternalism is alive and well and is supported by the dominant messages regarding women's inferior nature which permeate various socializing contexts for physicians, messages that are further distorted by class and race biases. See Joellen Hawkins and Cynthia Aber, 'The Content of Advertisements in Medical Journals: Distorting the Image of Women,' *Women and Health* Vol. 14, no. 2 (1988), 43–59; and Kay Weiss, 'What Medical Students Learn about Women,' in *Seizing Our Bodies*, ed. Claudia Dreifus (New York; Vintage Books, 1978), 212–22. For perceptive discussions regarding paternalism, see Jay Katz, 'Informed Consent – A Fairly Tale?' *University of Pittsburgh Law Review* Vol. 39 (Winter 1977), 137–74; and Carole Pateman, 'Women and Consent,' in *The Disorder of Women: Democracy, Feminism, and Political Theory* (Stanford, CA: Stanford University Press, 1989). In the presence of this misogyny-based medical paternalism, many women share the sentiments of the protagonist in Fay Weldon's novel: 'He was her Pygmalion, but she would not depend upon him, or admire him, or be grateful. He was accustomed to being loved by the women of his own construction. A soft sigh of adoration would follow him down the corridors as he paced them, visiting here, blessing there, promising a future, regretting a past; cushioning his footfall, and his image of himself. But no soft breathings came from Miss Hunter' *Life and Loves*, 215–16. Often many women are not in positions of sufficient privilege and power to withhold those 'soft breathings,' since the 'breathings' are often part of the price of getting access to necessary medical care.

71   Gena Corea, *The Mother Machine* (New York: Harper and Row, 1985)

72   As a limiting case, the pregnant woman drops out of the central description of birthing altogether. See P.A. Treichler, 'Feminism, Medicine, and the Meaning of Childbirth,' in *Body/Politics: Woman and the Discourses of Science*, ed. M. Jacobus, E.F. Keller, S. Shuttleworth (New York: Routledge, 1990).

73   The most sustained and theoretically sophisticated analysis of systemic pronatalism under capitalism is that of Martha Gimenez, 'Feminism, Pronatalism, and Motherhood,' in *Mothering: Essays in Feminist Theory*, ed. Joyce Trebilcot (Totowa, NJ: Rowman and Allenheld, 1984). Gimenez restricts her discussion to working-class women but unfortunately does not develop a more differentiated analysis of pronatalist and antinatalist pressures even within that social and economic group. Clearly, obligatory maternity does not affect all fertile women equally. Women who are regarded as 'deviant' in some respect or other – because they are lesbian or women

living with disabilities or 'too old' or poor or of the 'wrong' race or 'wrong' linguistic/ethnic group – are under enormous pressure from the dominant culture not to bear children; but this antinatalism, too, is an aspect of racialized, heterocentric, patriarchal pronatalism.

74 See Raymond's parallel argument regarding new reproductive technologies. Raymond targets her remarks at reproductive liberals, such as Lori Andrews and John Robertson. See Lori Andrews, *New Conceptions* (New York: St Martin's Press, 1984); and Andrews, David Rankin, Nadine Taub, and Chris Flores, *General Dissent to the New Reproductive Technologies Advisory Committee to State Senator Connie Binsfield* (State of Michigan, March 1987). See also John Robertson, 'Procreative Liberty and the Control of Conception, Pregnancy, and Childbirth,' *Virginia Law Review* Vol. 69, no. 3 (1983), 405–14.

75 As an example of the increasingly pathologizing discourse, complete with pathologizing photographs, see Hilton Becker and J.B. Storm van Leeuwen, 'The Correction of Breast Ptosis with the Expanded Mammary Prosthesis,' *Annals of Plastic Surgery* Vol. 24, no. 6 (June 1990), 489–97. See Laura Shanner for a critical discussion of 'technical medical' material addressing elective breast augmentation in 'Ethical Concerns Regarding Cosmetic Enhancement,' in *Women and Surgery: 1990 Conference Proceedings*, ed. Rosemary Moore (Melbourne, Australia: Healthsharing Women, 1990), 82–4.

76 Adrienne Rich, *Motherhood as Experience and Institution* (New York: W.W. Norton, 1976)

Moral Philosophy and Public Policy: The Case of New Reproductive Technologies

WILL KYMLICKA

1. Introduction

In this paper I will express some reservations about the usefulness of moral philosophy for the analysis of public policy issues. I want to emphasize right away, however, that I am not questioning the importance of morality. On the contrary, I take it as a given that morality is important, that moral considerations should be given their due weight in public policy deliberations, and indeed should have primacy. Policy-makers should do the right thing, morally speaking. Moreover, I believe that constant vigilance is required to ensure that moral considerations are not drowned out by the forces of self-interest, prejudice, or inertia, and that the moral viewpoint is not submerged underneath a more narrowly scientific, economic, or political viewpoint. My question is whether taking *morality* seriously requires taking *moral philosophy* seriously.

This paper focuses on one particular public policy context – namely, government commissions into new reproductive technologies (NRTs),[1] such as Britain's Warnock Committee,[2] Australia's Waller and Michael Committees,[3] Canada's Baird Commission,[4] and many others.[5] These commissions share a number of features: (i) the members of the commission, who usually number from five to sixteen, come from various backgrounds, such as law, social work, medicine, and the church, and they represent a wide range of interests and perspectives; (ii) they are asked to consider the social, legal, economic, and ethical implications of NRTs for the purpose of developing appropriate public policy recommendations; (iii) in the process of developing recommendations, the commissions generally conduct some form of public consultations and often seek out expert advice on various medical, legal, and ethical issues.

Moral philosophers are sometimes asked to participate in these commissions, either as commissioners, staff, or expert advisers. How can moral philosophers contribute to the analysis of public policy recommendations on NRTs? A survey of the literature suggests that there are two main views on this question, one of which is ambitious, the other more modest. The ambitious view says that moral philosophers should attempt to persuade commissioners to adopt the right comprehensive moral theory (e.g., adopt a deontological theory, rather than utilitarianism or contractarianism) and then apply this theory to particular policy questions. The more modest view shies away from promoting a particular moral theory, given that the relative merits of different moral theories are a subject of dispute even among moral philosophers. Instead, it says that moral philosophers should attempt to ensure that the commission's arguments are clear and consistent. On this view, philosophers should focus on identifying conceptual confusions or logical inconsistencies within the commission's arguments, without seeking to influence its choice of the underlying theory.

Now these views seem reasonable enough. Clearly, adequate moral theories are preferable to inadequate ones, and valid arguments are preferable to invalid ones. Moreover, as the authors of these articles point out, government reports are prone to making exactly these sorts of mistakes. An entire issue of the *Journal of Medicine and Philosophy* is devoted to critiques of the 'amateur' way that ethics are dealt with in these reports.[6] So, if government reports are prone to dealing with ethical issues in an amateur way, surely the solution is to have more input from professional moral philosophers, which is just what these articles propose.

However, I am sceptical of these two views. I will discuss the limitations of each and then consider a third way of promoting morally responsible public policy deliberations.

2. The Ambitious View – Selecting a Comprehensive Moral Theory

Proponents of the ambitious view believe that government commissions should adopt a comprehensive moral theory and apply it to the various ethical issues raised by NRTs. A survey of contemporary moral philosophy and bioethics textbooks suggests that the following five theories are the main contenders:

1. utilitarianism
2. deontology
3. contractarianism
4. natural law
5. ethic of care.

There are of course other theories (e.g., virtue-based ethics) that might be included, but this list is enough to begin evaluating the ambitious view.

Would it be useful if government commissions attempted to adopt one of these comprehensive moral theories and then apply it to the various ethical issues raised by NRTs? Let's see what this would involve. In order to select and apply a theory, we would need answers to (at least) the following three questions:

1. What is distinctive to each theory?
2. Which theory is most adequate?
3. What practical conclusions does each theory have for NRTs?

That is, we have to be able to identify, evaluate, and apply each theory. I believe that all three of these questions are so difficult and/or controversial that it is entirely unrealistic to expect government commissions to answer them. Moreover, it is inappropriate for commissions to try to answer them.

a. *Distinguishing Moral Theories*

First, then, what is distinctive to each theory? For example, what distinguishes contractarianism from its four competitors? That is a surprisingly difficult question to answer. Consider John Rawls's theory. It is usually characterized as a contractarian theory (although others deny this, since his 'original position' excludes the possibility of bargaining and differences in opinions or interests). Rawls describes his theory as deontological, however, while others insist that his contractarian method in fact leads to utilitarianism. Yet others argue that the ethic of care is implicit in his account of the original position.[7] Consider another example. Paul Ramsey is a Protestant moral philosopher who is usually characterized as a deontologist (although others insist he is a teleologist). Ramsey himself appeals to natural law, however, while others say that his appeal to Christian love or agape is an example of the ethic of care.[8]

I could give countless other examples of this problem. For any given pair of theories we can find some people who believe that the two theories are identical, or at least consistent. Hence some people would reduce the list of theories by subsuming contractarianism under utilitarianism, or by subsuming natural law under deontology, and so forth. Of course, we can also find other people who insist that the two theories are fundamentally different (although people disagree about what exactly that difference is).

What are we to make of this confusion? As a philosopher, I find it intriguing that there is so much disagreement about the identification and classification of moral theories. I have spent four years trying to determine whether these theories provide genuinely competing approaches to morality, or whether they simply use different vocabularies, and/or operate at different levels (and many years later I'm as uncertain as ever).[9] For public policy makers, however, this kind of confusion is not intriguing. They do not have the time or the inclination to sort it out.

Moreover, these five pure types of moral theory can be combined into various hybrid forms. Given that each of these theories is said to have some counter-intuitive implications, it is not uncommon for moral philosophers to try to combine the more attractive elements of different theories into a new hybrid theory. Hence we find theorists who say that we should combine utilitarianism with deontology, or the ethic of care with the ethic of justice. Mathematically speaking, there are 120 ways of combining these five pure types, and while not all of these combinations are plausible, or even coherent, a thorough search of the literature would reveal that most of them have been endorsed by at least one moral theorist. Moreover, people disagree about which combinations are coherent. For example, is it coherent to combine utilitarianism with deontology, perhaps in some sort of lexical relationship (e.g., guaranteeing some set of minimal rights on a deontological basis but allowing everything else to be decided on a utilitarian basis)? I don't think this sort of mixture is coherent, although others do. If such hybrid forms are coherent, and if we take seriously the project of adopting the best comprehensive moral theory, then clearly commissioners should consider them, since they promise to overcome the counter-intuitive implications of each pure theory.

b. *Evaluating Moral Theories*

Let's assume that we have identified what is distinctive to the various possible theories (whether that be five or 120). How do we go about getting ten commissioners from varying backgrounds to choose one? The relative merits of these theories have been the subject of debate for centuries, and it seems inevitable that reasonable people will continue to disagree. Some people take the persistence of disagreement as evidence that there is no one right answer to moral issues. For example, Mary Warnock, who chaired Britain's government commission into NRTs in the early 1980s, claims that 'It cannot be too strongly emphasized that in questions of morality, though there be better and worse judgements, there is no such thing as a correct judgement.'[10] I disagree with this statement. But even those of us who believe that there are right answers must admit that these answers can be difficult to discover. Moral philosophers have not yet discovered a knockdown argument for or against these different moral theories. Although new theories are developed (e.g., the ethic of care), they do not refute earlier theories in the way that Copernicus is thought to have provided a decisive refutation of Ptolemy.

There have been various attempts to refute moral theories on the basis of logic (e.g., trying to show that a theory is self-contradictory) or sentiment (e.g., trying to show that a theory violates our everyday intuitions about what is right and wrong). The fact that these theories have maintained adherents for centuries, however, suggests that they are not obviously illogical; and while it is not difficult to show that some theories (e.g., utilitarianism) violate some of our everyday moral intuitions, this is not a conclusive argument. For not everyone shares the same intuitions, and in any event, it seems that each of these theories has some counter-intuitive implications. Hence neither logic nor sentiment is capable of providing a conclusive argument for or against a particular comprehensive moral theory.

c. *Applying Moral Theories*

Let's assume that we have agreement on a single moral theory. We now need to know how to apply these theories to the issues raised by NRTs. Proponents of the view that commissions should endorse a single theory often make it sound as if all the hard work is done in choosing the theory. But the hard work is not over, since there is no clear, direct, and uncontroversial line from the very general concepts of 'agreement,' 'utility,' 'care,' and so on found in the moral theory to the nuts and bolts of particular ethical decisions. There is no magical formula for applying any of these theories.

If we decide that morality is a matter of maximizing utility, for example, how do we know what will maximize utility? Should utility be measured in terms of subjective preferences, or are there objective standards by which we can judge some interests to be more important or urgent? Should the principle of utility be applied to acts or to rules or to motivations? Does it apply to personal actions, or only to political actions? All of these questions would have to be answered before we could begin to apply the theory.

Similar questions arise for all the other theories. This is not to deny that there are better and worse interpretations of utility, nature, care, or agreement. Just as reasonable people continue to disagree about which moral theory to adopt, however, so they will continue to disagree about which interpretation of these theories is best.

This disagreement points to an important fact about the way moral and political philosophy have entered public debate. Most people appreciate the level of disagreement *between* the various schools of morality. If anything, people exaggerate these disagreements, and so assume that proponents of different schools will automatically disagree on all issues. Few people seem to recognize how much disagreement there is *within* each of these schools, however, and so they assume that proponents of the same theory will automatically agree on all issues. Hence many people believe that we can draw a one-to-one correlation between moral theories and policy options.

In the case of surrogacy, for example, many people try to situate the five moral theories on a continuum: utilitarians are said to believe in virtually unlimited commercial surrogacy (since the market is the most efficient means of distributing goods); contractarians are said to believe in tightly regulated commercial surrogacy (so as to prevent exploitation); proponents of the ethic of care are said to reject commercial surrogacy but allow for altruistic surrogacy; and proponents of natural law reject all forms of surrogacy.

Similarly, in the case of embryo experimentation, utilitarians are said to believe that non-therapeutic embryo or fetal experimentation is acceptable until birth (since the fetus acquires moral status only at birth); proponents of the ethic of care are said to draw the line at quickening; contractarians draw the line at the acquisition of sentience; proponents of natural law draw the line at conception, and so on.

This is what some people want – that is, a chart that draws a one-to-one correlation between theories and recommendations. But moral philosophy doesn't work that way. Utilitarians disagree among themselves about the acceptability of surrogacy, or the status of the embryo, as do proponents of all the other theories.[11] Adopting a moral theory, therefore, by itself does not provide an answer to any of these difficult issues but simply provides a framework within which to ask them. And utilitarians are as likely to disagree with each other as with the proponents of other theories.

So the idea that a commission could come to a consensus on the selection and application of a particular moral theory is simply unrealistic. Moreover, the idea of seeking a single moral theory is actually quite inappropriate. The fact that commissioners disagree is not simply an unlucky accident. Citizens generally have different views on these issues, and commissioners are chosen to represent different viewpoints.[12] Hence they are expected to come up with recommendations that, so far as possible, are acceptable to a variety of ethical perspectives. Government commissions are instruments within the system of representative democracy. Like elected representatives in parliament, commissions are intended to be representative of the general community, although, unlike elected representatives, they are intended to be insulated somewhat from the day-to-day pressures of interest groups and power politics. This is intended to allow more room for flexibility, for reasonable (as opposed to purely political) compromise, and for long-term (rather than short-term) policy initiatives. This increased room for persuasion and flexibility, however, cannot, and is not intended to, displace the need for recommendations that are acceptable to a wide range of viewpoints. The adoption of a particular ethical theory, therefore, not only is unrealistic, it defeats the purpose of the commission.

3. The Modest View – Philosophers as Technicians

Some philosophers recognize the impossibility of arriving at a consensus on an ethical theory. They focus their attention on the more modest goal of ensuring that a commission's arguments are clear and consistent.

For example, Dan Wikler, who served as the staff philosopher for the President's Commission for the Study of Ethical Problems in Medicine in the United States, argues that philosophers can contribute to health policy through 'conceptual clarification' and 'logic monitoring,' without having to promote a particular moral theory. In his words, 'bioethicists who seek to provide conceptual clarification avoid the need for a theory of their own, for the goal is not ordinarily to present a positive view but rather to "disambiguate" concepts in common currency in health policy circles.' Similarly, in the case of logic-monitoring, 'a bioethicist can effectively argue against a position through criticisms of its internal logic or coherence without having to produce an alternative theory-based point of view.'[13]

Mary Warnock expresses a similar view. After noting that moral philosophers cannot be expected to come up with the right moral theory, she asks: 'What then is the place of philosophy in the proceedings of [government] committee decisions? Philosophers have a role, it seems to me, simply as professional people who by training and habit are accustomed to distinguishing good evidence from bad, sound arguments from fallacies, dogma from experience. They are professionals accustomed to setting out conclusions and preliminary lines of reasoning in an intelligible way.'[14]

Likewise, Peter Singer recommends that moral philosophers have more input on government commissions, on the grounds that 'the distinctive virtue of philosophers is critical thinking – the ability to assess arguments, detect fallacies, and avoid them in their own reasoning.'[15]

If the first view of the role of philosophers is too ambitious, this one is far too modest. These authors make it sound like the role of philosophers is to be technicians, ensuring that the internal plumbing of the report is sound. The problem is that arguments can be clear and consistent and yet be morally bankrupt. An argument can be clear and consistent and yet give no weight to any moral considerations or submerge them beneath economic or prudential considerations. I'm sure that proponents of the modest view believe that morality is important, and that NRTs should be examined from a moral perspective, as well from a scientific, economic, or political perspective. But neither the modest nor the ambitious view actually does much to explain what it means to look at issues from a moral perspective.[16]

What does it mean to look at things morally? One way to answer that question is to return to our five moral theories and ask what makes them theories of *morality*, as opposed to theories of self-interest, or aesthetics, or economics. And in order to answer that question, we need to look, not at what distinguishes the five theories, but at what they share in common – namely, a commitment to what we can call the 'moral point of view.' They all believe that there is such a thing as a moral perspective on issues, which is distinct from a prudential, scientific, or aesthetic perspective and is defined by some notion of respect for persons.

From a prudential point of view, some people's lives may not matter to us, particularly if they are too weak or distant either to harm or to benefit us. From an aesthetic point of view, some people's lives may not matter, particularly if (as with Nietzsche) we think that only a few people are capable of genuine greatness in thought or action. But from a moral point of view, all people matter in and of themselves. It matters how well their lives go, and if our decisions affect their wellbeing, then we must take that fact into account. Adopting the moral point of view, therefore, requires that we sympathetically attend to people's interests and circumstances, try to understand how things look from their point of view, and give due weight to their wellbeing. Adopting the moral point of view requires that we 'put ourselves in other people's shoes' and ensure that our actions are acceptable from their point of view as well as our own.

This, of course, is the basic idea underlying Jesus' 'Golden Rule' (do unto others as you would have them do unto you). This Golden Rule is found not only in Christian ethics, but variants of it are also appealed to by deontologists like Kant, utilitarians like Mill, contractarians like Scanlon, and 'care' theorists like Gilligan. Hence it underlies all five of the theories discussed above.

If this account of the moral point of view is right, then we can see what is wrong with both the ambitious and the modest views of the role of philosophers. Both assume that taking morality seriously requires taking moral philosophy seriously – whether it be a philosophical theory (on the ambitious view), or a philosophical skill (on the modest view). But this assumption is misplaced. Taking morality seriously, in the first instance, requires taking *people* seriously – showing concern for people's lives and interests.[17]

4. A Third Approach

How do we take people seriously? First, by identifying which people are affected by NRTs. Second, by ensuring that NRTs are used in such a way as to promote, or at any rate not to harm, their legitimate interests. This suggestion is only an outline, of course. But I think it helps point out what, in the first instance, is needed to write a morally responsible report. We need a list of affected parties (or 'stakeholders'), and a list of their legitimate interests.

We can call the first list our 'stakeholder list.' The stakeholder list tells us to consider how each recommendation affects the various stakeholders: that is, women; people with disabilities; visible minorities; children; gays and lesbians; as well as doctors and patients. How do we identify these stakeholders? To a large extent, they identify themselves through the public consultations process, either directly or indirectly (e.g., through advocates for children or the disabled). We can identify the stakeholders by listening to the public, and seeing who expresses a concern about the impact of NRTs.

We can call the second list our 'guiding principles.'[18] The guiding principles identify the legitimate interests and goals that must be considered when the impact of NRTs on the various stakeholders is considered. These interests and goals include:

1. autonomy (including informed consent);
2. accountability;
3. respect for human life;
4. equality (both in the general sense of promoting equal respect for all members of the community by combating prejudice and discrimination, and the more specific sense of equal access to health care);
5. the appropriate use of resources (ensuring that funding decisions are made in the light of health care priorities);
6. the non-commercialization of reproduction;
7. protection of the vulnerable (including children).

There is a certain amount of overlap among these seven principles, and some could be combined with others.[19] I think that each identifies a legitimate and distinct goal of public policy, however, and since we are aiming for a useful checklist of interests and goals, they are worth being listed separately.

Where do these principles come from? Evidence from the public consultations held by Canada's Royal Commission suggests that there is in fact a general consensus on these goals, at least in Canada.[20] The principles were endorsed by all sectors of society who appeared before the commission, and I believe the same would be true of most other western democracies.

Of course, the fact that there is a consensus on these principles does not show that they are morally defensible. They could merely reflect arbitrary cultural prejudices. However, there are two reasons for moral confidence in this consensus. First, the fact that these principles were endorsed by such a broad range of groups – professional and lay, men and women, religious and secular, visible minorities, the disabled, doctors and patients – as well as by many international inquiries – suggests that they capture important moral values. The fact that they are endorsed by the marginalized and disadvantaged, as well as the vocal and powerful, suggests that they are not merely the biases of a particular group or tradition.[21]

Second, the principles are consistent with the moral point of view. For example, once we put ourselves in other people's shoes, it is only natural that we will affirm the importance of respecting their points of view (the autonomy principle) and of protecting those who are unable to look after themselves (protecting the vulnerable principle). All of the principles are consistent with, and indeed help spell out, the belief that each person matters in and of herself.[22]

Someone might think that we would have even greater confidence that these principles capture genuine moral values if we could derive them from a comprehensive moral theory. If anything, the direction goes the other way. Our confidence in a particular moral theory will depend largely on whether it makes room for the various mid-level principles we are already strongly committed to. For example, if a moral theory denies that the interests of vulnerable groups (e.g., children) deserve protection, then we are much more inclined to reject the theory than to renounce the principle of protecting the vulnerable. Indeed, this is precisely why most people reject Hobbesian mutual advantage theories as an account of morality. Since mutual advantage theory cannot explain our commitment to principles of protecting the vulnerable and respecting human life, it does not warrant serious consideration as an account of morality.

People do not need to subscribe to a particular moral theory in order to evaluate what counts as a good reason. The fact that a policy will promote the child's interests is clearly a good reason for endorsing that policy. The public and policy-makers accept this as a good reason, even though they may not have adopted or even understand specific moral theories. Anyone who doubts whether promoting the child's interests counts as a moral good is lacking in the most basic ethical sensibilities. He or she has failed to understand what it means to look at things from the moral point of view.

So we don't need to adopt a particular moral theory in order to generate our guiding principles. In any event, it turns out that all five theories endorse roughly the same set of principles. I noted earlier that concepts such as 'agreement,' 'utility,' 'nature,' and 'care' are difficult to interpret and to apply. For this reason theorists who work in the field of applied ethics often need to adopt a set of more concrete principles to guide their deliberations. For example, many utilitarians working in the field of applied ethics argue that it is virtually impossible to measure 'overall utility' in a given situation. The best way to promote overall utility, they believe, is simply to adopt rules that protect specific important interests. It turns out that the kinds of rules endorsed by utilitarians are similar to those endorsed by contractarians and by proponents of the ethics of care or natural law. All endorse principles protecting the child's interests, respecting autonomy, and so on.

This convergence at the level of guiding principles is not complete. But it seems that when practical decisions must be made, each theory relies less on the philosophical nuances that distinguish it from all the others and more on basic principles it shares with all the others. The quest to select a comprehensive moral theory therefore may ultimately be unnecessary. For when we try to apply the theory, we often end up relying on mid-level principles that all theories share.

So we have a list of stakeholders and a list of guiding principles, neither of which requires adopting a comprehensive moral theory. These lists provide the essential basis for a morally responsible government report, because they ensure that the commission will take people's lives and interests seriously. Using these two checklists, a government commission can consider people's interests with empathy. It can consider the fate of the weak and marginalized, as well as the legitimate interests of the more vocal or powerful. A responsible commission will do what it can to put itself in the shoes of all those who are affected by NRTs, to take those effects into account in its recommendations, and to seek creative policies that accommodate them wherever possible.

I believe that a commission that does these things properly cannot go too far wrong, morally speaking, even if it is entirely lacking in philosophical sophistication. Conversely, commissions that do not use these checklists are likely to produce morally flawed reports, no matter how philosophically sophisticated they are. Indeed, this is precisely what is wrong with most previous government reports. Some reports simply ignore relevant interests and stakeholders. For example, the *Warnock Report* does not consider the impact of NRTs on women, the disabled, or children. Instead, it adopts a narrowly medical point of view on various issues. (Warnock has subsequently stated that she views all of the issues in her mandate as 'relatively trivial' compared with the question of embryo experimentation, a view that surely reveals a certain moral blindness.)[23] Other reports identify the relevant interests and stakeholders but fail to consider creative ways in which conflicts between them can be alleviated. For example, many reports that endorse controversial NRTs (e.g., judicial intervention, germ-line gene therapy) fail to consider the possibility that the desired goals can be reached in other ways.

Using this checklist, of course, won't solve all the ethical problems raised by NRTs. Some potential conflicts between principles cannot be eliminated, no matter how creative we are, and then we are faced with a difficult decision regarding the relative weighing of competing principles. In these circumstances the commissioners will have to balance the competing principles as best they can, giving due weight to each. This is similar to the process of balancing values that judges are often confronted with. In both contexts, we have a rough sense of when the process is being carried out impartially and when someone is unduly biased towards particular interests.

Of course, this talk of 'balancing' values, or of giving principles their 'due weight,' is not very helpful from a philosophical standpoint. Without a comprehensive moral theory, the justification for giving priority to some principles over others in a particular context may seem sketchy and unsatisfying. Some philosophers pick up on this fact and insist that because we may face certain kinds of conflicts between principles at the end of the day, and because only a comprehensive moral theory can give a fully satisfactory explanation of why some principles take precedence over others, we therefore should adopt a comprehensive moral theory at the beginning of the day.

There are two reasons for resisting this advice. First, most disagreements over NRTs are not about how to weigh conflicting principles. Rather, the disagreements are about facts. Generally speaking, most of the public's concerns over NRTs are of the 'slippery slope' variety. That is, some people believe that NRTs will (over time) reduce the status of women in society, lead to intolerance of those who are disabled, undermine family stability, lead to eugenics, etc. On this view, the use of NRTs will inevitably lead to the abuse of NRTs. Other people think that NRTs won't have these negative effects, and that society is capable of regulating any possible abuses. This view reflects a deep disagreement in society, but it is not a disagreement over values.[24] Everyone agrees that eugenics is wrong, that prejudice against women or the disabled is wrong, that family instability is undesirable, etc. They simply disagree about whether NRTs will have any of these implications, and this disagreement, in turn, often reflects differences in power – that is, some of those who are most concerned about the implications of NRTs are those who feel that they have no say over the future development.

We can go a long way towards resolving these conflicts by finding more reliable or more conclusive evidence and by establishing regulatory schemes that give all groups in society the feeling that they have some input over the future development of NRTs. Adopting a comprehensive moral theory is neither necessary nor relevant to resolving these conflicts, since the conflicts are not about competing fundamental principles.

Our thinking has been distorted, I believe, by the abortion debate; it is one of fundamental principle, and disagreement would remain even if there was general agreement on the facts. But the debates raised by NRTs are of a different sort. They involve disagreements about the actual impact of NRTs on various groups and about the realistic scope for alternatives. To (mis)interpret these disputes as disagreements of principle lessens the chance for achieving consensus.[25]

Of course, some unresolvable conflicts of principle do exist in the sphere of NRTs, but not all of them need to be resolved by a government commission. If (as I've suggested) a permanent advisory or regulatory body is established, then some conflicts can be left to its deliberations. Since many of the issues raised by NRTs are new, and we are still discovering their implications, this is probably a wise course and one that has worked well in other jurisdictions. Moreover, many of these conflicts have no general solution and so must be left to be resolved more on a case-by-case basis, by either future regulatory bodies, or institutional ethics committees, or individual patients and practitioners.[26]

For all these reasons, I believe that a government commission into NRTs can go a long way in its moral deliberations on the basis of relatively uncontroversial guiding principles. This may not be true of government commissions into other bioethical issues, where conflicts between principles are both more common and more pressing. However, it may be unrealistic to suppose that government commissions would be of much help in these cases, which is why no one (to my knowledge) has proposed a royal commission on abortion in Canada. If the only issue on the table is that of conflicting principles, then we know in advance that any commission that is representative of Canadians will not come to a consensus but rather will divide along familiar lines. A commission on reproductive health care only is useful if there are other kinds of issues, other ways of responding to public concerns that do not entail having to resolve divisive issues of moral philosophy. I think this is precisely the case with public concerns about NRTs.

Appealing to guiding principles may be inadequate as an approach to bioethics in other contexts,[27] but it is, I believe, uniquely appropriate for public policy deliberations on issues such as NRTs. To expect a more sophisticated moral theory in this context is unnecessary and unrealistic.

5. Philosophical Argument in Government Commissions

If this third approach is right, then philosophical sophistication is neither necessary nor sufficient for a morally responsible report on NRTs. In fact, a survey of existing government reports suggests that there is no interesting connection between philosophical sophistication and moral sensitivity. Some of the reports that are most amateurish in their discussion of moral theory have done the best job of identifying and protecting the morally relevant interests. I will consider briefly two examples from recent government reports:

(a) *commercial surrogacy*: The development of NRTs presupposes that it is a legitimate social goal to assist couples in conceiving and bearing children. But few people are willing to accept any and all measures that might be employed to conceive a child. For example, there is relatively little support in most countries for the idea of commercial surrogacy agencies, and most reports have recommended that they be disallowed. Different reports give different justifications for this recommendation. However, one of the most common ones is that children are harmed by being born through a commercial surrogacy arrangement (e.g., the child's sense of self-respect may be harmed if she discovers that she was the product of a commercial transaction). Hence, it is argued, these arrangements should be restricted in the name of protecting the best interests of the resulting child.[28]

This argument is a non-starter. The problem is that the child would not have been born were it not for the surrogacy arrangement. The resulting child may be disadvantaged relative to other children, but being born into disadvantaged circumstances is not against the child's interests where the alternative is not being born at all. So long as the child is glad to be alive, then we cannot say that preventing her conception and birth would have been in her interests. Unless we thought that a child born through a surrogacy arrangement was better off dead, then her conception is not a harm to her.

Here is a fallacious argument, one that most philosophers would pick up on. But it is not a morally unreasonable conclusion – no one has the right to buy or sell children, or their reproductive capacities. Every human society has limited the commodification of reproduction. There are a variety of perfectly good reasons for this restriction: harm to other children, family stability, exploitation, and so on. Anyone who adopts the moral point of view with sensitivity would probably come to the same conclusion. I believe that many government commissions in fact were moved by these genuine moral considerations, even if they were not the ones they ultimately cited in the report. The fact that their ethical argument is amateurish is no evidence, I believe, that the commissioners lacked moral seriousness or sensitivity in their deliberations.

(b) *embryo experimentation*: Consider a second example. Most people believe that human life deserves respect, at all stages of its existence, including its embryonic stage. Few people believe, however, that the degree of moral protection owed to the human embryo is as strong as that owed to human beings after birth. This raises the question of what kind of research, if any, can be conducted on embryos that have been fertilized in vitro. Most government reports have recommended that research is permissible on embryos in vitro, but for only fourteen days after conception.

This recommendation is often defended in terms of the 'potentiality' argument – that is, while embryos are not full members of the moral community, they have the potential to become full members, and this potential is grounds for moral respect.[29] Some such reference to potentiality seems necessary if one wants to argue, as most reports do, that human embryos should receive greater moral protection than sentient animals, since the *actual* capacities of the latter exceed the former.

This potentiality argument has been debated by philosophers for many years. Some people think that the whole argument is implausible, since there is no general moral obligation to bring potentiality to fruition. Moreover, the potentiality argument seems to apply equally to gametes, yet few people think that it is ethically troublesome to do research on sperm.[30] It should be noted that none of the reports makes any attempt to rebut these traditional objections. But let's set them aside; for there is a more obvious problem with this use of the potentiality argument – namely, it cannot explain a fourteen-day limit on experimentation.

Why? Because embryos actually *lose* their potential to become persons after fourteen days. In cases of natural conception, embryos implant in the woman's uterus at around six days. The possibility of successful implantation in utero disappears soon after that date. So the potentiality argument would suggest that there is no moral objection to experimenting on embryos in vitro older than fourteen days. In the words of the Australian Senate Select Committee, if proponents of the potentiality argument wish to leave room for non-therapeutic experimentation on embryos, 'it would appear to make more sense if such experimentation were undertaken *after* the possibility of a future in utero has passed.'[31] If we think that it is permissible to experiment on embryos when they have little or no potential to become persons, then this tells us to experiment on embryos after fourteen days, not before fourteen days.

Here is another fallacious argument, but once again, the conclusion may be quite reasonable. On the one hand, embryos deserve some respect, in virtue of their connection to the human community, but they don't have a right to life; on the other hand, scientific research can provide important benefits, but scientists don't have an unqualified right to experiment on human life.[32] People disagree about the weight of these competing concerns, and the fourteen-day limit may be a good compromise. A charitable interpretation is that the various commissions recognized that the embryo has some kind of status, in virtue of its continuity with the human community, but they simply misdescribed it. As moral philosophers, we know that potentiality is an inaccurate and unsophisticated description of this continuity (for fourteen-day-old embryos). But the basic deliberations could well have been quite reasonable. Hence we cannot conclude that the commissions lacked moral seriousness or sensitivity.

Perhaps my charitable interpretation of this example is incorrect. Many critics believe that the fourteen-day limit reflected the interests of the doctors, since embryos could not be sustained in vitro for more than fourteen days. On this view, the decision was based solely on the interests of one group, or on a narrowly medical view of the issues, and the 'potentiality' argument was just a smokescreen – a way of adding an ethical facade to a basically self-interested decision.

This interpretation is certainly possible. There are many instances where government reports have been accused of being unduly influenced by the medical profession. This shows that when we encounter a fallacious argument, we must consider the possibility that it reflects the undue influence of particular interest groups. But we should do that in any event, even if the argument is consistent. For example, some reports defend the fourteen-day limit on the grounds that this period is when the embryo acquires its 'primitive streak,' which is the precursor of the nervous system and hence the basis for the distinctly human capacity for consciousness and reason. There is no fallacy here. Yet we might well think that the only reason government reports have adopted this limit is that it provided a smokescreen for the interests of doctors. We might think that commissioners didn't really believe that the development of the primitive streak is important in determining the moral status of the embryo but invoked it anyway to provide some ethical window-dressing.

We always need to be wary of the influence of vested interests, and we need to consider the possibility that seemingly ethical arguments are in fact smokescreens for decisions made on other grounds. But this is as likely to be true of valid as invalid arguments. So even if the potentiality argument is a smokescreen, the moral failing is not its lack of philosophical sophistication but its moral hypocrisy.

I have just described two examples of philosophical flaws that are not moral failings and do not reflect any lack of moral seriousness or sensitivity. There are many other examples of this phenomenon (e.g., I believe that many of the arguments for prohibiting cloning are philosophically invalid, yet the conclusion is morally sound).[33] Critics are quite right to say that the commissions have dealt with moral philosophy 'in an amateur fashion.'[34] But they are wrong to assume that these philosophical flaws reflect a failure to take morality seriously. It is one thing to point out an inconsistent argument, but quite another to show that this inconsistency actually leads to a morally flawed recommendation, and critics too often take the former as proof of the latter.

Of course, it is regrettable that government reports make these philosophical errors. For example, it is unfortunate that reports have chosen the misleading notion of potentiality to describe the way that fourteen-day-old embryos are connected to the human community. It would be better if we got the right description of that connection, particularly since government reports often set precedents. In such situations philosophers may well be able to improve the quality of argument through methods such as conceptual clarification and logic-monitoring (see section 3 above).

It is important, however, not to exaggerate the significance of, or scope for, such philosophical fine-tuning. Fine-tuning is less important than the basic structure of stakeholders and principles. If the basic checklists of stakeholders and principles are properly identified and conscientiously applied, then any philosophical confusions are likely to be relatively benign. Conversely, if philo-sophical fine-tuning takes place in the absence of such checklists, it is likely to be entirely without moral benefit, since it may simply extend the impact of an argument that ignored relevant stakeholders or interests.

Moreover, there may be little realistic scope for philosophical fine-tuning. For example, determining the best account of the embryo's continuity with the human community is a very difficult question, and it is probably a fantasy to think that a government commission can come up with a good answer to *that* question. In fact, commissions are constructed in such a way as to reduce the likelihood of philosophical clarity. As we've seen, commissions are designed to represent various ethical viewpoints and to seek some kind of accommodation among them. The need for such accommodation often conflicts with the drive for conceptual precision. For example, the *Warnock Report* has been criticized for the lack of clarity in its discussion of the moral status of the embryo, but as Warnock has explained, 'Every sentence had to be argued over. To reach agree-ment on conclusions was difficult enough. To have arrived at an agreed line of *argument* would have been impossible.'[35] Given that agreement on a specific argument was impossible, but consensus was desired, the solution was to make a vague and confused, but generally acceptable, reference to potentiality. To have expected philosophical clarity to arise from these kinds of compromises is unrealistic.

While it is regrettable that government reports are not likely to achieve philo-sophical clarity, it should not be surprising. It may be that we can't expect philo-sophical acumen from commission reports, no matter how morally committed the commissioners are. Morally serious deliberations in these contexts may often lead to philosophically superficial reports. Conversely, philosophically sophisticated reports may be full of moral hypocrisy and insensitivity. This pos-sibility suggests that a greater understanding of moral philosophy would not necessarily improve government reports on NRTs from a moral point of view. On the contrary, I believe that attempts to immerse policy-makers in academic philosophy may be partly responsible for the lack of moral seriousness and sensitivity found in many government reports. One reason is simply a shortage of time and energy. Time spent mastering the complexity of moral philosophy is time not spent examining the implications of NRTs on people's lives. But there are two other more speculative reasons for thinking that philosophical ambitions may be counter-productive.

First, I worry that getting policy-makers to take moral philosophy seriously may pre-empt the exercise of their everyday moral sensibilities. The problem, as I noted earlier, is that many people believe there is a one-to-one correlation between moral theories and recommendations, such that adopting a particular theory commits one to a set of predetermined recommendations. For example, many people believe that adopting utilitarianism entails a liberalized view of commercial surrogacy and embryo experimentation, whereas adopting natural law or deontology entails opposing all forms of surrogacy and embryo experimentation. In so far as people take these tight connections between theories and recommendations for granted, they are less likely to feel the need actually to put themselves in other people's shoes and see how their lives are affected.

Second, I worry that taking philosophy seriously may undermine people's confidence in their everyday moral sensibilities. The problem, also noted above, is that the five moral theories are very controversial, and the debates between them can be quite confusing. People's confusion at the philosophical level may then erode their confidence at the level of everyday principles. An interesting example of this point is discussed in a 1987 *Ethics* symposium on the President's Commission. Members of the commission had decided that a fund should be set up to compensate people who are injured during medical research. They requested Dan Wikler, the staff philosopher, to explore some ethical implications of this decision. He commissioned a number of papers by other philosophers, representing a variety of viewpoints. One paper, written from a libertarian perspective, argued against the idea of a compensation scheme, on the grounds that people who volunteer for research have consented to the risks and so have waived any rights to compensation for harm. The commissioners were not persuaded by this argument, and the other philosophers disagreed with it. However, the commissioners were unsettled by the existence of this philosophical disagreement. It led them, not to change their moral views, but rather to give less weight to moral considerations. The commissioners began to focus on economic and political considerations, many of which worked against the compensation scheme. In the end, the commission neither endorsed nor rejected the compensation scheme but recommended further study. According to a staff member, the existence of philosophical disagreement meant that commissioners were 'left with the impressions that ethical arguments were conflicting and inconclusive ... Given these impressions, commission members apparently felt themselves "liberated" from any *moral* obligation to support compensation and therefore free to consider other factors.'[36] Given that moral commitment is always threatened by the forces of self-interest, prejudice, and inertia, anything that discourages people from giving morality its due weight should be resisted, including moral philosophy.

For these reasons I would not encourage commissioners to acquire a greater philosophical sophistication regarding controversial moral theories. Rather, I would encourage them to have confidence in the basic values we share but ensure that these values are applied in a more serious and sensitive way – for example, by ensuring that all recommendations are checked against a comprehensive list of stakeholders and principles. This will ensure that the vulnerable are not ignored and that the interests of the weak and marginalized are given the same attention as those of the vocal and powerful. In this way, we can get policymakers to take morality seriously, without getting them to take moral philosophy seriously.[37]

Notes

This is a lightly revised version of a paper that appeared in *Bioethics*, Vol. 7/1, 1993, pp. 1–26. The paper grew out of some work I did for the Royal Commission on New Reproductive Technologies (see note 20). I would like to thank Judith Nolté and Dann Michols at the commission for inviting me to think about these topics. For helpful comments on an earlier draft, I would like to thank Brenda Baker, Elizabeth Boetzkes, Harold Coward, Bernard Dickens, Susan Donaldson, Wayne Norman, Christine Overall, Peter Singer, Wayne Sumner, and Dan Wikler.

1 The term 'new reproductive technologies' often encompasses three different kinds of procedures or technologies: (i) procedures intended to assist individuals or couples to conceive a child (e.g., artificial insemination, in vitro fertilization, and surrogate childbearing); (ii) procedures intended to assess or promote the health of the embryo or fetus after conception (e.g., prenatal diagnosis, sex selection, embryo therapy or fetal surgery, and judicial intervention in pregnancy); (iii) the use of human gametes, embryos, or fetuses in research (e.g., embryo experimentation, or the use of fetal tissue transplants in the treatment of Parkinson's Disease). Some government commissions into NRTs were asked to address all of these procedures; others focused primarily on (i) or (iii). I shall be using the term 'NRTs' to refer to all three of these procedures.

2 Department of Health and Social Security, *Report of the Committee of Inquiry into Human Fertilization and Embryology*, London, 1984.

3 Western Australia Government, *Report of the Committee to Enquire into the Social,*

Legal, and Ethical Issues Relating to In Vitro Fertilization and Its Supervision, Perth, 1986 (the Michael Committee); Victorian Government, Committee to Consider the Social, Ethical and Legal Issues Arising from In Vitro Fertilization, *Report on Donor Gametes in IVF*, Melbourne 1983, and *Report on the Disposition of Embryos Produced by In Vitro Fertilization*, Melbourne 1984 (the Waller Committee).

4 Royal Commission on New Reproductive Technologies, *Proceed with Care: Final Report of the Royal Commission on New Reproductive Technologies*, 2 volumes, Ottawa, 1993 (the Baird Commission).

5 LeRoy Walters identified eighty-five committee statements on NRTs from twenty-five countries in the period from 1979 to 1987, of which he reviewed fifteen in depth; 'Ethics and New Reproductive Technologies: An International Review of Committee Statements,' *Hastings Center Report*, Special Supplement, June 1987, pp. 3–9. The number has at least doubled since then. In researching this paper, I have focused on government commission reports from Australia, Canada, Great Britain, and the United States, of which there are over forty.

6 'Symposium on Bioethics Commissions,' *Journal of Medicine and Philosophy*, Vol. 14, 1989; cf. Birgitta Forsman and Stellan Wellin, *The Treatment of Ethics in a Swedish Government Commission on Gene Technology*, Centre for Research Ethics, Göteborg, 1995 – Studies in Research Ethics #6.

7 Rawls describes himself as both a contractarian and a deontologist in *A Theory of Justice* (London: Oxford University Press, 1971), p. 12 (contractarian) and p. 30 (deontologist). For the claim that Rawls isn't a contractarian, see Jean Hampton, 'Contracts and Choices: Does Rawls Have a Social Contract Theory?' *Journal of Philosophy*, Vol. 77/6, 1980, pp. 315–38. For the claim that his contractarian method leads to utilitarianism, see R.M. Hare, 'Rawls' Theory of Justice,' in *Reading Rawls*, ed. Norman Daniels (New York: Basic Books, 1975). For the claim that his contractarian method presupposes the ethic of care, see Susan Okin, 'Reason and Feeling in Thinking about Justice,' *Ethics*, Vol. 99/2, 1989, pp. 229–49.

8 See the discussion of Ramsey's thought in Lisa Sowle Cahill, 'Within Shouting Distance: Paul Ramsey and Richard McCormick on Method,' *Journal of Medicine and Philosophy*, Vol. 4/4, 1979, pp. 398–417, and the response by Alasdair MacIntyre in the same volume.

9 For preliminary conclusions, see my 'Rawls on Teleology and Deontology,' *Philosophy and Public Affairs*, Vol. 17/3, 1988, pp. 173–90 (on deontology); 'The Social Contract Tradition,' in *A Companion to Ethics*, ed. Peter Singer (Oxford: Blackwell, 1991) (on contractarianism); and *Contemporary Political Philosophy* (Oxford: Oxford University Press, 1990), ch. 7 (on the ethic of care).

10 Mary Warnock, *A Question of Life* (Oxford: Basil Blackwell, 1985), p. 96.

11 It is often said that utilitarians are committed to the view that the fetus acquires full moral status only at birth, whereas proponents of natural law are committed to the

view that the embryo acquires full moral status at its conception. This perception is inaccurate. Many utilitarians argue that the embryo acquires moral status when it is capable of feeling pain and pleasure, and some have even argued that potential embryos prior to conception have moral status, since they would, if conceived and born, contribute to the overall good. Conversely, the natural law tradition gives various answers to the moral status of the embryo. The current position of the Catholic Church is that the embryo acquires personhood upon conception, or at least that we cannot rule out that possibility. Other proponents of natural law, however, including the Catholic Church prior to 1859, have argued that the embryo/fetus is presumed not to acquire personhood until later (see Michael Coughlan, *The Vatican, the Law and the Human Embryo* (London: Macmillan, 1990), pp. 86–8). Some recent Catholic ethicists have considered the possibility that implantation should be taken as the attainment of personhood, since this is when genetic identity is definitively established. A similar range of views about the definition of personhood can be found among proponents of contractarianism or the ethic of care. Since there is no unique connection between moral theories and theories of personhood, adopting a moral theory would not resolve the debate over the status of the embryo.

12 Of course, very few people, other than moral philosophers, identify themselves as 'contractualists' or 'utilitarians.' Most people carry around a mixture of utilitarian, contractarian and other ideas, combined in often unreflective ways. There are important difference in ethical perspective between different groups in society, however, and a government commission must take account of this fact.

13 Daniel Wikler, 'What Has Bioethics to Offer Health Policy?' *Milbank Quarterly*, Vol. 69/2, 1991, pp. 246–7. Wikler also notes that philosophers are adept at 'reasoning from shared premises.' This may be closer to the approach I defend in the next section, depending on how it is described and elaborated (cf. n17).

14 Warnock, 'Embryo Therapy: The Philosopher's Role in Ethical Debate,' paper presented to the International Conference on Philosophical Ethics in Reproductive Medicine, April 1991, pp. 15–16. See also idem, *The Uses of Philosophy* (Oxford: Basil Blackwell, 1992), ch. 4; and idem, 'Philosophy and Public Affairs: A Philosopher's Perspective on Government Committees of Inquiry,' *Irish Philosophical Journal*, Vol. 7/1, 1990, pp. 19–33.

15 Pascal Kasimba and Peter Singer, 'Australian Commissions and Committees on Issues in Bioethics,' *Journal of Medicine and Philosophy*, Vol. 14, 1989, p. 406.

16 In another discussion, Singer does attempt to give an account of the moral point of view that should inform government commissions on NRTs. He says, 'we all agree on enough basic ethical principles to make it unnecessary to prejudice the argument with ... controversial assumptions.' According to Singer, we all can agree on the importance of meeting needs and avoiding suffering: 'To see their validity, all we have to do is to think about the significance our own needs and desires have for us

and then apply the Golden Rule so that we allow to others as much significance for their needs and desires as we would have them allow to ours. The outcomes of this kind of "universalizing" of our own needs and desires is a concern for the welfare of everyone'; Singer and Deane Wells, *Making Babies: The New Science and Ethics of Conception* (New York: Charles Scribner's Sons, 1985), p. 181. This is closer to the approach I defend in the next section. Wikler may have a similar idea in mind when he talks about the value of 'reasoning from shared premises,' rather than from a comprehensive moral theory (see n14). Neither Wikler nor Singer, however, gives this idea of a moral point of view the sort of centrality, or priority, that I think is required. For a related discussion, see Forsman and Wellin, *The Treatment of Ethics*, pp. 34–5.

17 More accurately, morality requires taking sentient life seriously, human or animal. For a discussion of the status of non-human animals within moral theory, see Will Kymlicka and Paola Cavalieri, 'Expanding the Social Contract,' *Etica & Animali* Vol. 8, 1996, pp. 5–33.

18 The term 'principles' is perhaps misleading, since the seven 'principles' state legitimate interests or goals, not decision-making rules. For a helpful discussion of this issue, see Bernard Gert and K. Clouser, 'A Critique of Principlism,' *Journal of Medicine and Philosophy*, Vol. 15, 1990, p. 222.

19 For example, the principle of the non-commercialization of reproduction is largely a conclusion from the other principles, such as protection of the vulnerable, equality, and respect for human life. Similarly, the appropriate use of resources is often connected to the principle of accountability, and the promotion of autonomy is often seen as requiring equal access to NRTs. It may be possible to combine these related principles, although perhaps at the price of losing sight of important issues. Conversely, it may be possible to divide up some of these principles into more fine-grained categories. For example, while most people agree that the requirement of informed consent flows from the principle of autonomy, some people feel that it is sufficiently important to be considered a separate (albeit derivative) principle. It is partly a matter of judgment when it is appropriate either to combine or to disaggregate principles. However, the seven principles listed seem to capture ethical ideas that are both important and relatively distinct. For a more detailed discussion of the content of these principles, and their interrelationships, see my 'Approaches to the Ethical Issues Raised by the Royal Commission's Mandate,' in *New Reproductive Technologies: Ethical Aspects*, Vol. 1 of the Research Studies of the Royal Commission on New Reproductive Technologies Ottawa, 1993, pp. 1–46.

20 For a summary of the views presented in these public hearings, see *What We Heard: Issues and Questions Raised during the Public Hearings*, Royal Commission on New Reproductive Technologies, Ottawa, September 1991. Of the 296 individuals and groups who appeared at the public hearings, seventy-five endorsed a list of specific guiding principles. The seven principles listed in the text constitute clear points of

consensus among these witnesses, representing a wide range of groups in society. For a detailed analysis of the moral arguments made during the public hearings, with particular attention to the principles endorsed by the various sectors of society, see my 'Approaches to the Ethical Issues.'

21 It is important, therefore, to distinguish this sort of genuine consensus from the idea of 'community standards' appealed to in many government reports, which is often nothing more than the arbitrary and unprincipled biases of the majority. For example, many reports recommend that single women and lesbians be denied access to artificial conception procedures. In some cases this recommendation is defended by the claim that children are harmed by being raised in such families. This argument appeals to a widely shared principle concerning the need to protect children from harm, and if the claim of harm could be supported, then it would be a principled (though not necessarily conclusive) argument for restricting access to married couples. There is in fact little or no basis for this claim of harm, however, so other reports simply say that allowing access to single women or lesbians violates 'community standards.' In this case the community's standards are neither shared nor principled but simply reflect the majority's prejudice against a minority. Kasimba and Singer discuss and criticize this sort of appeal to 'community values' in 'Australian Commissions,' pp. 414, 417.

22 What if there is a consensus on principles that violate the moral point of view (e.g., a consensus on racial or sexual discrimination)? In this case a moral philosopher should try to encourage government commissions to question that consensus. Since government commissions are political bodies, however, it would make more sense for someone who sees the consensus as morally illegitimate to work outside the political system entirely. Participating in government commissions presupposes, to some extent, that the political system is legitimate.

23 According to Warnock, the moral questions relating to NRTs fall into two kinds: 'the first kind centers on the concept of the family; the second on the justification, or lack of it, for research using human embryos. My personal belief was, and is, that the second set of questions is both more important and more difficult than the first'; 'Moral Thinking and Government Policy: The Warnock Committee on Human Embryology,' *Milbank Quarterly*, Vol. 63/3, 1985, p. 506. Indeed, she says, 'All the other issues we had to consider seemed relatively trivial compared with this one'; *Question of Life*, p. xvi; cf. 'Philosophy and Public Affairs,' p. 25.

24 For discussions of the deep disagreement between technological optimists and pessimists, see Max Charlesworth, *Life, Death, Genes and Ethics* (Crows Nest, NSW: Australian Broadcasting Corporation Books, 1989), pp. 24–33; Wilbren van der Burg, 'The Slippery Slope Argument,' *Ethics*, Vol. 102/1, 1991, pp. 64–5; and the British Columbia Royal Commission on Family and Children's Law, *Artificial Insemination*, 1975, p. 7. It would be misleading to suggest that this disagreement is

entirely factual. People often search for 'facts' that will support a position that they've adopted on other grounds. For example, people who reject donor insemination (AID) because it is unnatural may, for the purposes of public debate, seek out factual evidence that AID leads down a slippery slope to family instability, partly because the latter argument is more likely to be effective in public debate than the former. Hence moral disagreements can be displaced onto factual ones. Even if slippery slope arguments are sometimes a cover for other concerns, however, it is still true and important that the public debate over NRTs is largely empirical. People appeal to slippery slope arguments not only for strategic reasons, but also because they acknowledge that public policy in a pluralistic society cannot be based on matters of personal belief. Public policy must be based on non-sectarian reasons and arguments that can be understood by all. The prevalence of slippery slope arguments in public debate partly reflects the fact that they pass this test, since they depend on shard values. David Lamb, *Down the Slippery Slope: Arguing in Applied Ethics* (London: Croom Helm, 1988), p. 5. While resolving the slippery slope disputes might not eliminate all moral disagreement over NRTs, it would remove much of that disagreement from the public policy arena to the sphere of personal belief. It is important to note that the slippery slope argument can cut both ways – that is, technological optimists worry that constraints on embryo research or surrogacy may lead down a slippery slope to wholesale restrictions on forms of medicine and scientific research that are perceived by some members of society as 'unnatural.'

25 According to Martin Benjamin, factual disagreements often become perceived as moral disagreements, which 'places gratuitous obstacles in the way of arriving at mutually satisfying accommodation'; *Splitting the Difference: Compromise and Integrity in Ethics and Politics* (Lawrence: University Press of Kansas, 1990), p. 16.

26 Also, some potential conflicts of principle will never arise, because the conflicting principles cannot always be implemented in practice. For example, people may disagree *in principle* about whether a law banning non-medical provision of artificial insemination is legitimate and yet agree *in practice* that any attempt to legislate on this issue would be futile.

27 For discussions of the limits of 'principlism' in bioethics, see Gert and Clouser, 'Critique of Principlism'; Wikler, 'What Has Bioethics to Offer?' pp. 238–40; and Paul Menzel, 'Public Philosophy: Distinction without Authority,' *Journal of Medicine and Philosophy*, Vol. 15, 1990, p. 415. It is worth noting, however, that most of these critics focus on a particular form of principlism, deriving from the work of Beauchamp and Childress, which uses only very vague and indeterminate principles (e.g., 'benevolence'). In so far as the principles endorsed in this paper are more determinate (e.g., 'non-commercialization'), they may be more useful as guides to deliberation and so avoid some of these authors' criticisms. Still, I agree that principlism cannot serve as a complete theory of bioethics. Identifying a checklist of principles

leaves unanswered some of the most philosophically interesting questions about bio-ethics (e.g., how to resolve cases where individual practitioners or institutions face tragic choices between competing principles regarding the treatment of patients). However, the most interesting cases from a philosophical perspective are not always the most interesting or important from a public policy perspective. While principles are not adequate for all bioethical contexts, they are particularly useful in the context of government commissions on NRTs, whose recommendations are aimed at the general structure of public policy, not the specifics of individual cases.

28 This claim is made in a number of Australian government reports. For example, according to the *Waller Report*, 'The Committee has grave doubts whether any such surrogacy arrangements are in the interests of the child whose birth is so planned'; Committee to Consider the Social, Ethical and Legal Issues Arising from In Vitro Fertilization, *Report on the Disposition of Embryos Produced by In Vitro Fertilization*, Melbourne, 1984, pp. 53–4. See also the Family Law Council, *Creating Children: A Uniform Approach to the Law and Practice of Reproductive Technology in Australia*, Canberra, 1986, p. 16; Tasmanian Government, *Report of the Committee to Investigate Artificial Conception and Related Matters*, Hobart, 1985, p. 80; Western Australian Government, *Report of the Committee to Enquire into the Social, Legal, and Ethical Issues Relating to In Vitro Fertilization and its Supervision*, Perth, 1986, p. 78; New South Wales Law Reform Commission, *Surrogate Motherhood* (Report 3), Sydney, 1988, pp. 31–2. But cf. Jonathan Glover, *Ethics of New Reproductive Technologies: The Glover Report to the European Commission* (Dekalb: Northern Illinois University Press, 1989), p. 51 and Australia's National Bioethics Consultative Committee, *Surrogacy: Report 1*, Adelaide, 1990, p. 20.

29 This seems to be the argument of the *Warnock Report*, since it states that 'the objection to using human embryos is that each one is a potential human being'; Department of Health and Social Security, *Report of the Committee of Inquiry into Human Fertilization and Embryology*, London, 1984, Para. 11.22. Warnock now claims, however, that the fourteen-day recommendation reflected a *rejection* of the potentiality argument. She says that the majority of her commission 'were not moved by the argument that these cells could, if certain conditions were satisfied, become human beings. They did not rely, that is to say ... on "potentiality," but on consideration of what the embryo was at a particular time'; *Question of Life*, p. xv. This after-the-fact explanation of the committee's recommendation is disputed by some of her fellow commissioners and by Michael Lockwood in his 'Warnock vs Powell (and Harradine): When Does Potentiality Count?' *Bioethics*, Vol. 2/3, 1988, p. 211, n7.

For clear endorsements of the potentiality argument, see Western Australian Government, *Report of the Committee to Enquire into the Social, Legal, and Ethical Issues Relating to In Vitro Fertilization and its Supervision*, Perth, 1986, pp. 26, 35;

Canadian Bar Association, British Columbia Branch, *Reproductive Technologies*, 1989, p. 34; Senate Select Committee on the Human Embryo Experimentation Bill, *Human Embryo Experimentation in Australia*, Canberra, 1896, p. 25. For obscure justifications of the fourteen-day limit, see Interim Licensing Authority for Human In Vitro Fertilization and Embryology, *Annual Report*, London, 1986, p. 40; Law Reform Commission of Canada, *Biomedical Experimentation Involving Human Subjects*, Working Paper No. 61, Ottawa, 1989, pp. 52–3; Medical Research Council of Canada, *Guidelines on Research Involving Human Subjects*, Ottawa, 1987, p. 33; New South Wales Law Reform Commission, *In Vitro Fertilization*, Report 2, Sydney, 1988, pp. 25–7.

30 For these traditional objections to the potentiality argument, see Lockwood, 'Warnock vs Powell,' pp. 196–7; Warnock, 'Moral Thinking,' p. 518; Singer and Wells, *Making Babies*, p. 74; Charlesworth, *Life, Death*, p. 43.

31 Senate Select Committee, *Human Embryo Experimentation*, p. 27. I should note that at present it is not possible to keep human embryos alive in vitro for over fourteen days.

32 According to Mary Warnock, in the case of infertility treatment to establish a family, 'there was a fairly strong view [among commission members] that the freedom of the individual to take what steps he could had to be respected ... In the case of research, on the other hand, there was general agreement that the issue of individual liberty did not arise ... A scientist who argued that he must be free to carry out whatever research he liked, by whatever methods, would not get much public support, if this involved the use of other human beings'; *Question of Life*, p. xiv. However, see Office of Technology Assessment, *Infertility: Medical and Scientific Choices*, Washington, 1988, p. 211; and the Ethics Committee of the American Fertility Society, *Ethical Considerations of the New Reproductive Technologies*, Supplement 2 to *Fertility and Sterility*, Vol. 53, 1990, p. 22S.

33 Many reports view cloning as so obviously immoral that no justification is required. One committee that does seek to justify that recommendation is the National Health and Medical Research Council of Australia. It argues that cloning is immoral because higher forms of life almost always reproduce sexually (by fusion of haploid nuclei), and only rarely reproduce asexually (by fission of a diploid cell). Hence, it says, 'cloning may therefore be seen to contravene a biological principle that has strong fundamental claim to ethical sanctity'; *Ethics in Medical Research*, Canberra, 1983, p. 38. Unlike the first two examples, this argument is not so much fallacious as simply absurd.

34 John Williams, 'Commissions and Biomedical Ethics: The Canadian Experience,' *Journal of Medicine and Philosophy*, vol. 14, 1989, p. 441. Cf. Wikler, 'What Has Bioethics to Offer?' p. 246.

35 Warnock, quoted in Lockwood, 'Warnock versus Powell,' p. 188.

36 Alan Weisbard, 'The Role of Philosophers in the Public Policy Process: A View from the President's Commission,' *Ethics*, Vol. 97/4, 1987, p. 781.
37 Or rather, without getting them to take seriously the sort of moral philosophy that currently dominates Anglo-American philosophy departments. In so far as the articulation and application of guiding principles can be seen as in part a philosophical task, then of course policy-makers should take that sort of 'moral philosophy' seriously.

Public Moral Discourse

DAN W. BROCK

What is the nature of public moral discourse as it is done by ethics commissions charged with addressing ethical or moral issues in medicine and biomedical science and technology?[1] In what ways does it differ from the methods of moral philosophy and moral philosophers when they address such issues? Can public ethics commissions provide reasoned solutions to these ethical issues, and if so how? I shall first discuss some features of the nature of ethics commissions – the different goals they pursue, their typical charge and composition, and the role in public policy that they typically play. These features distinguish the processes they employ in some respects from moral reasoning as it is done by either moral philosophers or ordinary citizens. I shall argue that these differences are relatively superficial and that how ethics commissions address and reason about moral issues is not fundamentally different from the method, when it is properly understood, of moral philosophy used in addressing substantive moral issues of practice and policy. I shall show as well the respects in which this method can provide solutions to moral issues in public policy, or more specifically the respects in which an ethics commission's process of public moral reasoning warrants the claim that the substantive conclusions reached by that process are justified.

Some Features of Public Moral Discourse as Done by Ethics Commissions

Goals of Ethics Commissions

What are some of the different goals or aims that public ethics commissions typically have? First, they often are charged with developing relatively discrete legislation to deal with a particular ethical issue. For example, the President's Commission for the Study of Ethical Problems in Medicine and Biomedical and

Behavioral Research (hereafter President's Commission) addressed in its first study the definition of death and developed a proposal for a uniform statutory definition, which has subsequently been adopted by nearly all states. Even with this relatively narrowly focused outcome, the President's Commission evaluated alternative definitions of death, for example the 'whole brain' account, which it supported, and the 'higher brain' account, which it rejected, and offered philosophical and policy arguments in support of its choice of the whole brain formulation.

Second, ethics commissions are sometimes charged with addressing specific unethical practices and recommending governmental responses to correct those practices. For example, the National Commission for the Protection of Human Subjects of Biomedical and Behavioral Research (hereafter National Commission) was established in large part as a response to a number of well-publicized examples of abuses of human subjects in research and to an influential article detailing such abuses.[2] A central component of the National Commission's recommendations was the establishment of Institutional Review Boards, whose task is to assure that human subjects are properly protected. The National Commission also developed detailed guidelines and recommendations governing the use of specific populations in research. Here, too, the National Commission offered arguments in defense of its recommendations and indeed in its *Belmont Report* developed the general moral principles on which its recommendations rested.

Third, an ethics commission may seek to have a broad and diverse influence on policy and practice with regard to a particular moral issue. For example, the President's Commission in its report, *Deciding to Forego Life-Sustaining Treatment*,[3] sought a multifaceted impact on such practices and policies as institutional, especially hospital, policies that guide practice within particular health care institutions; court decisions that set the legal framework of permissible practice; and the beliefs and practices of physicians and other health care professionals. A part of the influence of the Presidents Commission's work on this issue derived from its prestigious nature as a nationally constituted body, as has no doubt been true of other ethics commissions. But the influence of its recommendations also derived importantly from the force and persuasiveness of the moral reasoning the commission offered for its conclusions and recommendations.

Finally, an ethics commission may sometimes have aims rather less focused on public policy. It may see its role more as influencing ongoing public debates on specific moral issues. In doing so, it may seek to have quite different kinds of influence on different occasions, for example, on the one hand sharpening the issues in dispute or on the other hand seeking to forge a consensus on those issues. These roles too, of course – whether sharpening the issues or forging consensus – require provision of the ethical analysis and arguments that either sharpen the issues or on which a new consensus might rest.

Consensus building, broadly understood, is an important part of each of these four different aims of ethics commissions. In part, this is simply because in a democratic society public policy is forged in political processes requiring majority, or at least broad, support of a proposed policy. However, there are deeper reasons why consensus is seen as especially important in the work of an ethics commission. For many public policy issues, the fact that a majority of policymakers, reflecting a majority of citizens, support a particular policy position is reason enough to warrant its adoption (for example, decisions to expend public resources on particular projects, such as public parks or medical research). It is not that supporters and opponents will have no reasons for their respective positions on such issues (of course they will have reasons), but that we consider it appropriate to settle the disagreement by some form of majority rule decision process; within limits, the position that should be adopted is what the majority supports. On a moral question, however, it would be at the least odd or problematic for a commission to declare that it found by a vote of six to five that, for example, patients have a moral right to forego life-sustaining treatment. Many political questions and legal disputes may be reasonably decided by majority decision procedures, whether on legislatures or courts, but whether a public policy is moral cannot be settled by counting votes. A political or legal solution to a moral dispute might be settled by majority vote in a legislature or court. But a majority vote cannot determine what is the morally correct or justified solution to that conflict, that is, what is right. In some sense, the moral question can be settled only by the quality of the arguments that can be offered for different positions on it. There are no authoritative bodies to settle moral questions and disputes such as exist in politics and the law for settling political and legal disputes. It is in part for this reason that the development of moral arguments and positions is common to all the diverse goals of ethics commissions noted above. The nature of the argumentation that commissions should employ is therefore at the heart of understanding their work.

Typical Scope of Ethics Commissions' Concern

Ethics commissions are typically charged with addressing the social, ethical, and legal issues concerning a particular topic like genetic screening or informed consent. To the extent that moral philosophy addresses only the moral or the ethical issues, the scope, and perhaps in turn the methods, of ethics commissions' work will have apparently to be different from moral philosophy. However, I believe it is a mistake to see this typical charge to ethics commissions as instructing them to go beyond the moral or ethical issues and to take up independent social and legal issues as well. Instead, this charge is usually best understood as instructing the commission to address the moral issues of public policy in their broader social and legal context rather than to engage in social and legal analysis independent of the moral issues. This typical charge reflects as well a widespread confusion as to exactly what the domain of the moral or ethical is in the context of public policy, a confusion that has contributed in turn to two views – both of them, I believe, mistaken – that assign a more restricted scope to ethics commissions' proper concerns. The first view understands ethical analysis to be addressed to individual actions, whereas policy analysis applies to many cases and institutional practices and so must in some way extend beyond ethical analysis. The second view understands moral considerations, as well as the method of moral reasoning employing those considerations, to be only a part of the overall considerations relevant to evaluation of public policy. In the latter view, moral philosophers and the methods of moral philosophy may analyze the morality of some policy, but overall policy analysis and evaluation must take into account additional nonmoral considerations such as economic costs, political feasibility, legal constraints, and so forth. Consequently, the distinctly moral or ethical analysis of an ethics commission would not yield 'all things considered' judgments or recommendations about public policy. To do that the ethics commission would have to consider these additional nonmoral economic, political, and legal considerations as well, which it has no special expertise to do. On the other hand, if these nonmoral economic, political, and legal considerations are part of the proper province of ethics commissions and ethical analysis, then it seems all policy analysis has been collapsed into ethical analysis, an unwarranted ethical aggrandizement of the policy field. I shall address each of these related, but, I believe, mistaken, views in turn.

In the first view, ethical analyses and judgments apply only to particular cases, not to the general practices that are the province of public policy. This view is sometimes expressed by a distinction between when one is 'doing ethics' and when one is 'doing policy.' This putative ethics-policy distinction rests on what can be called the one-many assumption about the relation of ethics to policy. Policy evaluation, in this view, is not ethics, because it must address policies that apply to many cases. In the evaluation of what action is ethically justified or permissible in a particular case, it is natural to believe that only the particulars of that case are relevant, though those particulars will include the social context in which the case takes place, the social and professional roles of the various involved parties, the causal impact of what is done in that case on what will be done in future cases, and so forth. For example, if the case concerns a dying patient suffering from pain that has proved impossible to relieve adequately who requests euthanasia from her physician, it would appear that it is only the particulars of this case that are morally relevant to its moral evaluation. Different people will disagree about which features of the case are morally significant or important, and about what moral principles or reasons bear on it. For example, some people might hold that euthanasia would be morally wrong in this case because it would be the deliberate killing of an innocent person, which they believe is always morally impermissible; others might see it as morally permissible because it is an exercise of an individual's moral right to self-determination. Still others, of more consequentialist or utilitarian leanings, may evaluate the act by its impact on the well-being of all affected by the action. If doing it would make the physician more likely to perform euthanasia in other similar cases as well, then that too is a consequence of this particular action. But all these are differences about how the act in question should be morally evaluated.

The moral evaluation of a social or legal policy, for example, permitting euthanasia, is, of course, not unrelated to the moral evaluation of particular instances of euthanasia.[4] But a person's moral position about such a policy need not follow directly from his or her moral position about a particular case. Many people who grant that there are individual cases in which euthanasia would be morally justified nevertheless oppose a public or legal policy permitting it because of worries about how that policy might or would be abused, leading to other wrongful performances of euthanasia. Because the policy must apply over time, in many circumstances and to many persons, the policy's effect in these other cases is relevant to its moral evaluation as well. Many of the differences in the substantive moral principles and reasons different people applied to the individual case will resurface in the moral evaluation of policy as well. But both evaluations – of the particular case and of the general policy – can be equally and fully moral evaluations to which one's moral principles and reasons apply. The typical object of moral evaluation by ethics commissions, namely, one or another public policy, does not entail a fundamental difference in the moral principles or reasons used in making the evaluation, or in the methodology of moral reasoning and argument employed.

There is reason then to remind ethics commissions to attend to the broader social and legal context of the ethical issues they address. The general practices that are the proper province of concern of ethics commissions exist in a social context, often in diverse social contexts involving individuals with diverse motivations and knowledge. These actions and practices also are often regulated by law. Although the law is only one form of influence on and regulation of practice, public policy, as opposed to forms of private regulation of behavior and practice, is often distinguished by the presence of legal or quasi-legal over-

sight. Because ethics commissions typically address policy and general practices, not individual actions, various empirical questions regarding practice are
relevant to their deliberations: What is the nature of current practice in the area
under consideration? What are the possible means of policy and institutional
change? What are the means of enforcement of specific policies? What would
be the economic and other costs of different policy alternatives? The answers
are relevant and integral to an ethical analysis of the policy issue.

This ethical analysis must also address questions like the following. What
ethical principles and values bear on the ethical evaluation of current practice in
the areas of behavior in question? What would be ethically more desirable practice in the areas of behavior in question? What means are available to shift practice in those desirable ways? Thus, the consideration of economic costs,
political feasibility, legal constraints, potentials for abuse, and so forth, all bear
on and must be considered as part of the ethical case for a particular policy. But
this brings us directly up against the second mistaken view noted above about
the proper scope of ethics commissions' concern. That view rejects a conception of ethical analysis that encompasses these economic, political, and legal
considerations and restricts the ethical analysis to only the distinctly ethical consideration. It follows that the ethical recommendation on policy in a particular
area cannot be an 'all things considered' recommendation regarding the policy,
what John Rawls claimed for justice in characterizing it as the 'final court of
appeal' in practical reasoning.[5] Instead, in this second view of the restricted
scope of ethics commissions' concern, the ethical analysis takes account of only
some considerations relevant to what policy should be. This implies that when
the ethical analysis is completed, additional relevant considerations will remain
that have not yet been taken into account, but that must be, before drawing a
conclusion about what, all things considered, practice and policy ought to be.

Why is this view mistaken? It is certainly correct that moral philosophers are
not experts on the economic, political, and legal considerations about which
economists, politicians, lawyers, and social scientists typically are consulted.
Consequently, an ethics commission will still have to consult with these experts
when economic, political, and legal considerations form a significant part of its
policy analysis and recommendations. But why should an ethics commission be
burdened with these additional concerns which apparently go beyond its ethical
expertise? In part, because ethics commissions are asked to make public policy
recommendations, 'all things considered' recommendations about what policy
should be, not just restricted recommendations about what would be ethical in
some restricted sense. To fulfill this role, they cannot restrict themselves to only
the considerations that most people would intuitively identify as ethical. But
this common intuitive distinction between ethical and nonethical considerations

itself is misleading. Perhaps a very simple example will most clearly make the point. If you promise to meet a friend tomorrow at 3:00 p.m., that promise gives you a moral reason to do so. But then tomorrow, quite unpredictably, it turns out that you must finish some project or take some action to avoid a very substantial financial loss. Doing so will prevent you from meeting your friend whom you cannot now reach. Ought you morally to keep your promise at very substantial and unexpected financial cost to yourself? If we apply the intuitive distinction assumed above between ethical and economic considerations, then the promise is ethical and the financial cost is economic. Could the ethical analysis concern only the ethical consideration – the promise? It should be clear that this would make no sense. The moral question is simply the 'all things considered' question of whether you must keep the promise in the face of the very substantial unexpected financial cost to you of doing so. The moral analysis must weigh these two considerations against each other; it cannot consider only the ethical consideration of keeping promises.

The same is true of policy analysis. It is not that the common intuitive distinction between moral considerations, such as promise-keeping, and nonmoral considerations, such as financial costs, is mistaken. The mistake in thinking that moral judgments can avoid weighing the two when they come into conflict; when that conflict occurs, the financial cost becomes a morally relevant consideration in the moral judgment about whether the promise ought to be kept. The same will be true of moral judgments about the public policies that ethics commissions address; for example, apparently nonmoral considerations (financial costs) are morally relevant to the moral question of how much equality of opportunity (the moral consideration) requires society to do to improve opportunities for the handicapped. Does this account make 'all things considered' policy evaluations and recommendations ethical, and so result in unwarranted aggrandizement of the policy realm by ethics or morality? And why are only some policy questions then seen as ethical and given to an ethics commission?

My view here does not lead to ethics swallowing up policy. Many policy choices remain essentially nonethical because ethical considerations are not significantly affected by them and so are not relevant to them. For example, on the policy questions of what rate of growth of the money supply and what economic stimulus packages are compatible with holding inflation to a three percent level, the economic analysis is appropriately sought from bodies such as the Federal Reserve and the Council of Economic Advisors, not an ethics commission. (This is not to deny, of course, that there are ethical implications of policies to control inflation, but that is a different policy question.) If there is no neat and clear division of labor for ethical and nonethical considerations, which policy questions should go to an ethics commission for analysis and which should go elsewhere? Very roughly, policy questions are appropriately referred to an ethics commission when the considerations commonly and intuitively considered ethical have a significant role or impact in the policy question. But the ethics commission cannot then do its job of analysis and recommendation without weighing those considerations that are quite appropriately considered ethical against other considerations with which they come into conflict that are intuitively seen as nonethical.

Membership of Ethics Commissions

The principal ethics commissions in the United States in recent decades were deliberately established with widely diverse members. Typically, only a small minority of members are professional ethicists or moral philosophers with extensive professional training in ethics and moral philosophy. But this does not mean that what an ethics commission does when it addresses moral issues, or how it does so, is different in kind or method from how professional ethicists would or do address the same issues. Professional ethicists and other commissioners together will be engaged in ethical reasoning on the issue at hand. Ethical reasoning and argument is done in the ordinary circumstances of everyday life by ordinary persons without academic or scholarly training in moral philosophy. It is not an esoteric subject like cell biology or quantum mechanics, accessible only to experts. Ordinary people make ethical judgments when they morally evaluate different states of affairs, different individuals' actions and character, and different social and political institutions. We employ such judgments in morally justifying our own actions to ourselves and to others, as well as in moral evaluations of the actions of other people.

Professional ethicists and moral philosophers, who are typically at least represented among commissioners and staff members on ethics commissions, do bring a certain expertise to the work of ethics commissions – typically, at least the results of having studied ethical reasoning and alternative ethical theories in a full-time, formal, and rigorous manner. They should be trained in the careful, critical evaluation of the soundness of arguments. They should have systematically studied and evaluated arguments for and against different moral theories, principles, reasons, and positions. Nevertheless, the methods by which professional ethicists or moral philosophers address substantive moral issues do not differ in kind from the methods used to address those issues by ordinary persons unschooled in the formal study of moral philosophy. Ethics commissions typically have diverse membership in order to ensure diverse experience, training, and viewpoints required by the diversity of considerations noted above that bear on their overall recommendations, not to represent diverse approaches or methods of doing ethics. I shall have more to say about the role of this diversity below.

Methods of Moral Reasoning – in Moral Philosophy and in Ethics Commissions

One reasons some believe that moral reasoning as done in moral philosophy is different from public moral reasoning as done by ethics commissions is what I consider a mistaken view about the nature of moral reasoning in moral philosophy or in public ethics commissions, or in both. Understanding the respects in which these accounts are mistaken or confused will help to clarify the appropriate common method that both moral philosophy and public moral reasoning can and do employ.

Deductivism

Some believe the method of reasoning by which public ethics commissions address ethical issues in public policy is different from the method of moral reasoning employed in moral philosophy from a mistaken view about the later. In this view, which I shall call deductivism, the philosophical approach to moral reasoning in applied and policy contexts ideally consists in employing the true or correct moral theory and principles, together with the empirical facts relevant to their application, to deduce logically the correct moral conclusion for the case or policy in question. When the issue is not what it is morally correct to do in a particular case, but instead is what public policy should be on an ethical question, such as whether voluntary euthanasia should be permitted, the moral calculus will be more complex. Assume for the sake of illustration that the correct moral theory is some form of consequentialism or utilitarianism, according to which an action is morally right just in case it has at least as good consequences for human well-being as any alternative action open to an agent. When the moral issue is about the evaluation of a public policy, the calculation is much more complex, since it is then necessary to estimate the effects over time of alternative policies on the well-being of all who would be affected by the alternative policies. In the case of voluntary euthanasia, the possible effects to take account of would include positive effects, such as the relief of suffering and giving people control over the circumstances of their dying, together with negative effects, such as possible abuse of the policy for purposes of controlling costs or possible erosion of trust in the medical profession. The empirical determination of the consequences would be difficult, complex, and controversial, and there would be much ineliminable uncertainty. But deductivism provides a method of moral reasoning that at least in principle yields right answers to the moral problems of policy that ethics commissions face.

Once the likely effects on the well-being of the various affected parties are determined, the consequentialist moral principle can be used straightforwardly and deductively to determine which alternative policy is morally right or justified. The truth or correctness of the consequentialist theory would solve the problem of justifying the commission's policy recommendations by transferring its truth to the conclusion that whichever alternative policy will best promote well-being is morally right or correct. Nothing about the general method of deductivism depends, of course, on the correct theory's being consequentialism. If instead the correct moral principle is that the intentional killing of an innocent person is always wrong, that principle, together with the premise that euthanasia is the intentional killing of an innocent person, deductively yields the conclusion that euthanasia is morally wrong.

Is deductivism a feasible and defensible account of how moral reasoning is and should be done either in policy contexts or in moral philosophy? One obvious problem is that it does not seem an accurate account of how ethics commissions in fact function. Most people, including most members of such commissions, have no relatively comprehensive, or even more limited, moral theory that they know, or even believe, to be true or correct, and so it is hardly a surprise that we do not find them using and applying one in practical contexts. Most people are largely ignorant of philosophical work in developing general moral theories and principles; yet they nevertheless do reason and have moral views about concrete moral issues like euthanasia. So deductivism is certainly not an accurate description of the moral reasoning that real people typically do in applied or policy contexts. Defenders of deductivism, nevertheless, might respond that it is the method used in moral philosophy and is how people ought to do moral reasoning. Is deductivism a defensible account of moral reasoning?

The central difficulty with deductivism is that there is no single comprehensive moral theory, or even theories or principles of more limited scope, which is agreed to be true or correct and so could be deductively applied to policy issues. For example, even if there were agreement that the overall effects on human well-being of permitting voluntary euthanasia would be positive, some people nevertheless would still believe that because euthanasia is the deliberate killing of an innocent person, it is morally wrong and should not be permitted. What began as a specific disagreement about what public policy should be about euthanasia has shifted to a more fundamental disagreement about whether consequentialism is the correct or true moral theory, or whether instead duties to protect innocent human life are paramount. Those who disagree on the policy will frequently do so because they do not agree about which moral principles or theories are correct. Consequently, so long as the different moral principles and theories are being correctly applied, moral disagreement about a particular policy will be reproduced in disagreement about the correct broader principles or theory. So if moral reasoning should begin with the correct general moral theory and its principles, which are then deductively applied to the particular policy in question, we face the embarrassment of having no agreement about what are the correct theory and principles to employ. To make matters worse, if a moral theory or moral principles can be true or false, correct or mistaken, as deductivism requires, then even were there agreement about which principles and theory are true or correct, it would be compatible with all parties to that agreement being mistaken.

The existence of disagreement about which general moral principles and theory are true or correct would not be an insuperable barrier to deductivism if there were agreement about the criteria for determining which principles and theory are true or correct. Disagreement about which principles and theory are correct then might reflect only a mistaken application of those criteria by one party to the disagreement. I shall not canvass here the different views on this issue but will note only that there is no agreement in philosophical ethics, or in ordinary morality, about the criteria that would establish general moral principles or a general moral theory to be true or correct. A final important barrier to deductivism is that, even if there are basic moral truths, there is no agreement or assurance that they are to be found or established at the level of general moral principles or theories, which through application could then transfer their truth to conclusions about particular policies ethics commissions address.

Deductivism as a method of moral reasoning takes a position on how the justification of moral judgments is secured that is commonly called foundationalist. A foundationalist account of justification in moral reasoning requires that some moral beliefs, which might be at any level of generality – the most general moral principles (like the consequentialist principle), very specific judgments about concrete cases, or moral beliefs at any level of generality in between – can be established to be true or correct.[6] These foundational moral truths, as we might call them, have foundational status in moral reasoning in the sense that all other moral judgments gain their justification by being derived through sound reasoning from them. Foundationalism assigns privileged epistemic status regarding truth or correctness to some moral beliefs – foundational status – with the justification of all other moral beliefs coming from their being deductively derived from the foundational beliefs.

Deductivism is the particular version of foundationalism that assigns this foundational status to general moral principles or to a general moral theory. Deductivism fails as an account of moral reasoning and justification not only because we lack any agreement either on the true moral principles or theory or any method for determining the true general moral principles or theory, but also because foundationalism more generally is a mistaken account of the nature of justification in ethics. No version of foundationalism is a correct account of justification in ethics, as I shall argue shortly, and that includes deductivism, which accords foundational status to general principles or theories.

One further problem with deductivism should be mentioned. Consequentialism, in the very simple form specified above, appears to be a comprehensive and fully determinate theory for the moral evaluation of both actions and social policies – all are justified to the extent they promote human well-being. But in fact there are many possible versions of consequentialism depending on how some key terms are interpreted. If we assume a single determinate interpretation there should always be, at least in principle, a correct answer to the moral evaluation of any action or policy. This simplicity and comprehensiveness is bought, however, at the unacceptably high cost of sharp conflict with many important components and complexities of most people's considered moral judgments. Moral principles and theories that incorporate these other components and complexities do have their own costs. They typically have significant indeterminacies in their content, which tend to occur at just the points of significant moral conflict and intrapersonal and interpersonal controversy – for example, where different moral rights, duties, or important values within the theory come into conflict.

In the absence of strict priority rules or other determinate methods for resolving these conflicts and the moral issues in which these different moral considerations come into conflict (essentially all the interesting or hard moral cases), deductivism will be impossible to apply in exactly the cases in which we most need it.

Particularism

The polar extreme position about moral reasoning and moral knowledge or justification I shall call particularism. It holds that moral reasoning in practical and policy contexts begins and remains with the specific concrete case under consideration. If some moral judgments are true or correct, and so others false or mistaken, moral knowledge is achieved only at the level or particular cases. Some particularists hold that there is no standard for evaluating our moral judgments external to the particular judgments themselves. Others hold that moral knowledge resides at the level of particular paradigm cases, with moral reasoning in new cases then consisting of fitting the new cases to the paradigms closest to them.[7] Thus, in the example of the commissioners' policy dispute about euthanasia, reasoning remains at the level of a particular case, or a particular paradigm case, of euthanasia, with no external appeal to moral principles or theory from which, in foundationalist fashion, a conclusion could be derived and justified about euthanasia.

One problem for the particularist is moral disagreement, illustrated in the example about euthanasia. If moral reasoning remains only with the particular case, with no external appeal to moral theory or principles, then we shall have no external appeal by which the disagreement might be resolved. Moreover, if two conflicting judgments about a paradigm case of euthanasia both cannot be true, then particularism seems to provide no standard by which we might determine which position is true or correct. Because particularism locates moral knowledge only at the level of particular judgments and confines moral reasoning only to the particular case, it seems to provide no standard for determining which particular judgments are true when they all cannot be true. But the most serious difficulty for particularism is that it is incompatible with the very process of giving reasons for moral judgments at all. It is important to see why this is so.

Moral judgments are unlike some judgments of taste, and moral disagreements are unlike some disagreements over matters of taste, because moral judgments must be backed by reasons. If you like vanilla ice cream and I like chocolate, we can just accept this as a difference in taste – there is no correct preference about flavors of ice cream, and if asked why I prefer chocolate, I may be able to repeat only that it tastes better to me. Unlike matters of taste, moral judgments, for example, about whether voluntary euthanasia is wrong, must be backed by reasons. A moral discussion between a proponent and an opponent of euthanasia might only begin, not end, with claims that it is right or wrong. An opponent of euthanasia might challenge its proponent by arguing that the deliberate killing of an innocent person is wrong. A proponent might respond that voluntary euthanasia is different from most killing because the victim wants to die and consents to being killed.

So their discussion might continue. Their initial disagreement quickly turns into a process of giving and clarifying reasons for their respective moral views about why euthanasia is or is not morally justified. Their discussion rapidly moves to more general issues about when killing is wrong, and for what reasons. This is inevitable. Their discussion could not remain at the level of a particular instance of euthanasia. *Whenever* we offer reasons in support of a particular moral judgment, we do so by picking out properties of the object of the judgment that support or are the basis for the moral judgment. Any feature of an object of moral evaluation that is offered as a reason supporting a positive or negative moral evaluation of it will be a property which, on another occasion, could be a property of other objects of evaluation. Both being an innocent human being and having consented to be killed are properties that can apply in other possible cases – to other innocent human beings and to other persons who consent to be killed.

Now clearly neither the proponent nor the opponent of euthanasia need appeal to a comprehensive moral theory in supporting his or her position about euthanasia, but both appeal to moral principles or reasons with some degree of generality – they can be applied to other particular actions, that is, other possible killings, as well. Indeed, if one of the two was a consequentialist and was then pressed about why killing human beings was wrong, she would respond that it is wrong when, and only when, it has worse overall effects for human well-being than not killing the person in question. Then she would have been driven to appeal to her most basic moral beliefs, her comprehensive moral theory, in providing her reasons for supporting or opposing the particular case of euthanasia. Of course, most people are not consequentialists and would stop the process of offering reasons for their moral position about euthanasia well short of any comprehensive theory, if for no other reason than that most people do not have any explicit, comprehensive theory that they accept; they might stop instead with an appeal to a basic moral duty not to kill, or a basic moral right not to be killed. But while not a comprehensive theory, a principle specifying a general moral duty or right of this sort can be thought of as a potential part of a broader theory, or a theory fragment.

The central and fatal problem for particularism, then, is that it is incompatible with the very process of having and offering reasons for our moral judgments, which is the principal feature distinguishing morality from mere expressions of simple taste or preference. Some at least partial or fragmentary moral theorizing is an unavoidable part of moral reasoning, of making and offering reasons for moral judgments in practical and policy contexts. What level of generality the reason-giving process in fact reaches on a particular occasion of moral reasoning or disagreement will depend both on theoretical factors, such as how deep and general the parties' reasons for their positions are, and on practical factors, such as the depth of one's own uncertainty or another's challenge on the issue in question. Even if a person's reasons for a particular moral judgment are so many and complex that as a matter of fact they fully fit few if any other real cases, the reasons must be such that they at least in principle can apply to other cases. Particularism, which locates moral reasoning and knowledge only at the level of the particular judgment regarding an individual case, is not a feasible alternative.

Justification with Considered Moral Judgments

A Critical Screening Process

Neither deductivism, which gives a foundational role to general moral principles or theories in moral reasoning, nor particularism, which purports to give no role to general moral principles or theories in moral reasoning, is a plausible account of the nature of moral reasoning and justification. We need an account of moral reasoning that is neither too ambitious in the role it gives to moral principles and theories, as deductivism is, nor too dismissive of their role, as particularism is. One grain of truth in particularism is that people's moral thinking does typically begin with particular practical moral choices and cases. A discussion of euthanasia, for example, usually would begin with a particular instance of it but proceed with the participants' providing reasons in support of their positions. But how might their different moral judgments and positions be evaluated in order to determine which are true or false, correct or mistaken, or justified or unjustified? I now want to address more directly the problem of justification. If not deductivist or particularist, what method or process of moral reasoning could ethics commissions use that would warrant a claim that their conclusions are morally justified?

John Rawls introduced the notion of 'considered moral judgments,' which can be of use here, though I shall add features to it beyond those Rawls specified.[8] The idea is to characterize an idealized process at which both individuals and an ethics commission could aim in their moral deliberations. How do considered moral judgments differ from simply moral judgments? What does *considered* add? In answering this question, I shall develop what I shall characterize as a critical screening process through which individuals can put their moral views and judgments. Considered judgments generally, not only considered moral judgments, are, first, judgments that are not made in conditions that we know from experience often lead to mistakes. Here are some examples of such conditions: when we have insufficient time to consider the matter carefully; when we lack significant, relevant information bearing on the question at hand; when we have a relatively fixed commitment to a particular position on the question at hand that makes us inadequately open to a fair consideration of other positions; when the question at hand requires technical knowledge or training that we lack; when we must make a decision while distracted or emotionally overwrought; when we lack sufficient relevant experience to appreciate fully some considerations and to integrate them adequately into our decision making; and so forth. Notice that none of these features are in any way special to *moral* judgments – they are features that, if present, should equally weaken our confidence in judgments about empirical matters of fact. There is in addition at least one important feature that should likewise weaken our confidence specifically in our moral judgments, a condition that experience tells us often leads to moral judgments we later come to believe were mistaken. It is that what we decide morally to believe or do will importantly affect our own interests – this often leads us to rationalize in the pejorative sense, that is, to find some purported rationale for why *we* are not morally required to do a burdensome or unwanted action that we would have no trouble concluding others morally must do. Of course, when our important interests are at stake, we are often led to give more careful attention to the issue at hand. This condition does not rule out considered moral judgments, but warns us to look carefully for such a form of rationalization. With this qualification, considered moral judgments then are, first, judgments made in the absence of conditions like those just noted that we know from experience often lead to mistakes.

There is a second aspect of considered moral judgments that needs to be brought out. With empirical judgments about matters of fact, our confidence in a judgment is increased, other things being equal, the more fully we have been able to consider all relevant evidence that bears on the issue. While disputes about empirical matters of fact often bear on moral questions as well, moral judgments have specifically moral reasons that support them. Considered moral judgments, then, are also judgments made as a result of having fully considered the reasons that support them. In the ideal or limiting case, this would involve fully considering to the deepest level possible the nature of the reasons to which one would appeal in attempting to justify one's judgment. In the example above of voluntary euthanasia, this would involve fully probing one's moral views about killing and any factors that bear on one's views about killing in the context of euthanasia. Any example like this in which different people disagree brings out another important feature of evaluating the reasons in support of our moral judgments – this evaluation involves not only exploring as fully as possible the reasons in support of one's own judgment or position, but also considering all possible reasons and arguments *against* one's own position and in support of alternative positions. Until one has examined what can be said both for and against all plausible alternative positions on a particular issue, one will not fully have considered all alternatives, and all that can be said for and against all alternatives, to one's own position.

A third aspect of considered moral judgments and the critical screening process that produces them is that the process of considering alternative positions and evaluating the reasons that support them on any issue typically has both an intrapersonal and an interpersonal component. It will often begin as an intrapersonal process as one initially thinks about the issue oneself; but then it should expand to an interpersonal process as well, because we know from experience that our moral vision if often enlarged by discussion and reasoning with others and by confronting the positions and arguments of others, either in discussion or in print. Thus at the limits, arriving at one's considered moral judgments about a particular action or policy will involve considering all the reasons that can be offered by anyone for and against any alternative position, choice, or decision on the matter at hand. A practical implication for ethics commissions is that having diverse membership helps ensure a process in which diverse moral perspectives, experience, and views are brought to bear in the commission's deliberations.

Reflective Equilibrium

In criticizing particularism, I argued that it is impossible to give reasons for moral judgments while at the same time restricting the implications of judgments solely to the particular case at hand. By their very nature, moral reasons can apply to other cases beyond the specific case in which they are being employed. Sometimes these reasons have substantial scope or generality and so potentially apply to many other moral choices and evaluations that people face. We might therefore say that people's moral beliefs, and in turn their considered moral judgments that have survived the critical screening process I have just sketched, come at all levels of generality. Now a substantive or normative moral theory can be briefly characterized for my purposes here as a small body of relatively general principles applying to the objects of moral evaluation in a given domain. While the domain of a maximally comprehensive moral theory would be all possible objects of moral evaluation, most people at best hold less comprehensive theories, or what are partial theories or theory fragments from the more comprehensive perspective. This means that, although deductivism may be mistaken in holding that moral reasoning and justification begin from a moral theory already and independently established as true, which then could be somewhat mechanically applied to particular cases, it is correct that at least parts or fragments of moral theories are either implicitly or explicitly appealed to in reasoning about particular cases. It is this scope of moral reasons – that they always can apply to cases beyond the one at hand – that gives considerable force to the requirement of consistency in moral reasoning: consistency requires accepting the implications of the reasons or principles to which one appeals in a particular case for the other cases to which they also apply. A few important additional aspects of the appeal to general moral principles need to be emphasized.

Since our considered moral judgments and beliefs include general moral principles, these principles often can be appealed to in reasoning about particular cases or policies. For example, some principle of equality of opportunity is an important component of American moral and political culture and can be used to help decide what kind of inequalities are morally acceptable in access to health care. This much is true about deductivism – sometimes we may have greater moral conviction or confidence about a general moral reason or principle than we do about a particular judgment concerning a concrete case or policy, and so we largely form or revise our moral judgment about the case or policy to fit the more general reason or principle that applies to it. Our moral conviction about the case or policy then is derived principally from our conviction about the more general reason or principle. Different moral judgments about particular cases or policies, as well as different general moral principles, are held with different degrees of conviction by any individual, even at the end of the critical screening process. This is important for understanding how internal conflicts within an individual's moral views should be resolved.

When there is conflict between our moral judgments about particular cases or policies and our moral principles, as often occurs, no systematic priority can be assigned either to the judgments about the particular cases and policies or to the general principles regarding which should be retained and which revised or abandoned in the attempt to eliminate the inconsistency in our moral views. In removing the inconsistency in order to reach what Rawls has called 'reflective equilibrium' between an individual's particular judgments and general principles, the revision should be made so as to leave the individual with a consistent view that retains as much overall conviction as possible. Sometimes the initial judgment about the particular case or policy will be revised or abandoned, sometimes the more general principle. When an ethics commission is seeking interpersonal consensus among its members or in the broader society, the resolution of conflicts will be more complex than, but in some respects similar to, this intrapersonal process. Compromises between individuals should be sought that require different individuals to make concessions at points of least conviction, scope, and importance in their views, and with a presumption for some rough equality in the concessions that individual members make to the others.

Foundationalist accounts of justification, of which deductivism is one instance, hold that some moral beliefs have privileged status regarding truth and/or justification, and so are not subject to revision in the case conflict with other judgments lacking this privileged status. In the different account of justification sketched here, usually called coherentist, no judgments are assigned such privileged status that they never should or could be abandoned or revised. In any instance of conflict between particular judgments and general principles, it is an empirical matter, to be determined on a case-by-case basis, which carries least conviction and could be revised with least cost to a particular individual's other moral convictions. To seek reflective equilibrium is to seek the consistent, comprehensive set of considered moral judgments at all levels of generality, including both judgments about particular cases and general moral principles, that carries for the individual the greatest overall conviction.

Besides this role in reflective equilibrium, general moral principles and theories also play a more direct role in justifying moral judgments about particular cases or policies which is analogous to how scientific theories provide explanatory force to a domain of phenomena. A central function of theories in natural and social science is to provide order and structure to a body of observations or data about the world that would otherwise be merely a large set of unconnected data. Scientific theories thereby produce gains in understanding: by displaying a structure and order in the data, they show us the variables an causal relations that explain what would otherwise be a disordered and unrelated mass of observations or phenomena. In this respect, it is the same with moral theories. In morality, the analog to the observation statements and data that a scientific theory explains is the particular moral judgments about some range of cases that the more general principles of a moral theory, or of a partial moral theory, explain.

Because the principal role of moral judgments is to guide action – unlike both data and theories in science, whose principal roles are to guide belief – moral judgments are subject to a special worry. The worry is that they may be no more than a hodgepodge of thinly veiled rationalizations and biases reflecting our own self-interest, prejudices, and arbitrary preferences. General moral principles or theories can help allay this worry by explaining these judgments: they are shown to fit, and to be derivable and made from, a coherent, unified moral conception. We come to see that our particular moral judgments have a coherent identifiably moral source, heretofore likely only implicit, and are not merely a cover for our prejudices and self-interest. The principles and theory display those judgments as recognizably moral and make their moral basis subject to explicit critical evaluation. This can in turn increase our conviction in particular judgments because we come to see that they fit within or have the same basis as, other judgments about which we may have additional and/or more confidence. In this coherentist account of justification no particular part of a person's overall moral beliefs or conception has any privileged status with regard to truth, correctness or justification. Instead, each component of the comprehensive moral conception gains part of its justification from all the rest of the moral conception of which it forms a part.

Fully coherent and comprehensive general principles or theories covering all of one's moral judgments are more than most people can in fact achieve. For most of us, there is no single, unified moral framework from which all our particular moral judgments are made or can be shown to follow. In fact, I believe that for most people there are multiple different independent sources of moral value, or parts of their overall moral view, with no single deeper unified account of those parts. One of the central problems for applied ethics and practical moral thinking and deliberation is giving an intelligible account of how the unity of moral deliberation and action is possible, even for a single individual, in the face of this lack of unity or full coherence in the individual's moral beliefs or overall moral conception created by these different, independent components of the person's morality.[9] Of course, if we look across a culture or society, this diversity of sources of moral value is greater still – and is one of the greatest challenges public ethics commissions face.

This process of reaching one's considered moral judgments in reflective equilibrium is an ideal that in practice can only be more or less approached. Besides the obvious limitation of time and effort, there are always limitations at any time on the alternative positions on any issue that we and others can imagine, as well as on the arguments that we and others can think of for and against any alternative. So even if this ideal were fully realized at any time, we could never be sure that in the future we or others would not think of new alternatives and/or arguments, perhaps on the basis of new experience, that would change our minds. This critical screening process, even in its ideal form, never warrants absolute certainty about any particular moral judgment that could put it beyond further question. While this ideal of considered moral judgments in reflective equilibrium is never fully achievable in practice, it is useful nevertheless because it specifies an ideal process by which all possibly relevant reasons and arguments available to anyone and bearing on a moral issue can be given due consideration; the shortcomings and more restricted focus of moral reasoning in the real world can be measured against this ideal.

There is one important respect in which the ideal process of moral reasoning at which a public ethics commission should aim differs from what I have just sketched for individuals. It will rarely, if ever, be appropriate for an ethics commission to seek, much less present in its reports, a single fully comprehensive and determinate moral conception in support of its analyses and recommendations, even if it thought that possible. It will usually be enough to present the principal reasons and arguments that bear on and support the specific policy recommendations it makes. Often this process will require criticizing alternative positions and/or responding to natural objections to its own positions and recommendations. In the example of euthanasia discussed above, the commission might at most offer a general analysis and argument on the wrongness of killing and on the kinds of cases, if any, in which killing can be morally justified that bear on euthanasia. Exploring the implications of the commission's argument and position for other cases of killing, for example, killing in war or capital punishment, would be unnecessary, indeed undesirable, because it would be a source of unnecessary controversy and a diversion of attention from the commission's policy focus on euthanasia. For the same reasons, presenting an entire moral theory or a complete set of moral principles would be all the more unnecessary and uncalled-for given the policy focus. Nevertheless, the process of moral deliberation in which the commission engages, together with the results of that process it presents to the public in its reports, is properly understood within this broader account of moral deliberation, reasoning, and justification.

I noted above that one respect in which general principles and theories help justify particular moral judgments is by showing them to be made from a coherent and unified moral conception. There are two further respects in which moral judgments that have survived the critical screening process and reflective equilibrium are justified. First, they are justified because they are made in relatively ideal conditions for judging, that is, in the absence, to the extent possible, of conditions that we know from experience often lead to mistakes; as noted above, these will include conditions leading to mistakes in judgments generally, as well as conditions leading to mistakes in moral judgments in particular. Second, they will have survived a process of critical examination in which all arguments both for and against them, as well as in support of and against alternative conflicting positions, have received due consideration. In both of these respects, considered moral judgments in reflective equilibrium are justified because they have survived a maximally broad critical screening process. To repeat, this is not to say that we may not later come to change our view, and/or come to believe that our earlier conclusions were mistaken. Even when our moral judgments have been maximally subjected to arguments for and against both them and other alternative positions, there are limitations in our and others' moral thinking at any point in time. Thus, just as in the case of justified empirical beliefs, justification does not provide any guarantee of the truth or correctness of our moral beliefs.

Some readers may object that this account of moral reasoning and justification, which begins from the moral beliefs we happen to have at any time, is unduly conservative. Our moral beliefs are a result of our experience and the socialization process to which we have been subject. Consequently, those beliefs will likely reflect the values and moral beliefs predominant in our culture and society and be biased in favor of the status quo. But this objection is misplaced. The critical screening process for reaching considered moral judgments, which describes an ideal of considering all arguments for and against both the particular moral judgment or position with which one began as well as all judgments or positions that are alternatives to it, asks us to consider all criticism of and alternative perspectives on the status quo, no matter how radical. Failures to consider sufficiently radical criticisms or alternatives will be failures of our critical and moral vision or will, to some degree unavoidable, but not failures fostered by the method of moral reasoning that I have described.

Relativism and the Subjectivity of Moral Judgments

Is the method of moral reasoning that I have sketched for use both by individuals and by public ethics commissions objectionably relativist? Moral relativism is usually understood as the view that different incompatible moral beliefs can be true for different individuals, groups, or societies. In this view, whether a moral judgment is true or correct will depend on who is making it. One of the central problems of moral methodology is how the justification, rather than the truth or correctness, of the moral judgments of either an individual or a group, such as an ethics commission, can be established. From the standpoint of justification, the problem of relativism is whether incompatible moral judgments each can be justified for different individuals or groups. It is a familiar point that even in the case of judgments that most people believe are noncontroversially capable of being either true or false, or correct or mistaken, such as empirical judgments about matters of fact, one individual may be justified in accepting a judgment as true that another individual can be justified in rejecting as false. This is because different people may have different evidence available to them bearing on the judgment in question, and an individual's justification for accepting a belief depends on the relevant evidence he or she has, or should have. If evidence tending to confirm or disconfirm a particular belief is available to one individual but unavailable to another, each can be justified in holding beliefs both of which cannot be true.

So the question about the relativism of moral judgments is whether different individuals possessing the same empirical or factual information and beliefs relevant to a moral issue can be justified in holding incompatible moral judgments on that issue. Another way of putting this question is whether some moral disagreement can be in principle, not just in practice, rationally irresolvable. Much moral disagreement is in practice irresolvable when people cling irrationally to beliefs in the face of evidence of their falsity, make mistakes in their reasoning that cannot be corrected, and so forth. Moral disagreement that is irresolvable in principle is clearly a more serious problem for any account of public moral discourse because it means that even when different people fully conform to the standards for that moral discourse, there may in the end be no way of resolving their moral disagreement.

It should be clear that the account of moral reasoning and justification sketched above, which employs a critical screening process together with reflective equilibrium, does allow for the possibility of moral disagreement that is in principle rationally irresolvable, and for the possibility that different individuals each may be justified in holding incompatible moral judgments; we can call this justificatory relativism. Of course, we shall not know that any particular moral disagreement, such as that among members of an ethics commission, is in fact irresolvable, either in principle or in practice, until their different views have gone through the critical screening process and achieved reflective equilibrium. Any conclusions that a particular moral disagreement is in principle irresolvable should come only at the end of a full, but failed, attempt to resolve the disagreement. The possibility that moral disagreement can be even in principle irresolvable is compatible with moral disagreements rarely, or even never, in fact turning out to be such. Some moral disagreement does, I believe, turn out to be irresolvable even in principle, but not as often as many people today suppose. Very often disagreement that initially appears to be moral turns out on closer analysis to be empirical disagreement about matters of fact.

Justificatory relativism implies that moral judgments are correctly understood to be in one sense subjective. Claims about the subjectivity and objectivity of morality and moral judgments are commonly so poorly defined and used in so many different senses that they often bring more confusion than clarity. What I have in mind here by the claim of subjectivity is as follows. At the end of the day, so to speak, after the process of moral reasoning and justification that I have sketched here has been completed, a particular individual's moral judgments, principles, or theory will depend on what that person is prepared on reflection to accept, to try to live by, and to judge him- or herself and others by. The same is true for groups of people living together in a society, and for bodies like ethics commissions they establish to help them address moral issues of public policy. Choice of and commitment to a way of life in this broad sense cannot in the end be avoided, and different individuals can choose and pursue different ways of life. But this hardly implies, as R.M. Hare pointed out long ago, that such choice is ungrounded or arbitrary; the choice I am describing here is choice after everything of relevance to the choice has been given due consideration, which is exactly the opposite of arbitrary choice understood as choice for which we have no basis.[10]

The Appeal to an Overlapping Consensus

One important qualification must be put on the account of moral reasoning I have sketched above for its use in public moral discourse in contexts in which identifying or forging a consensus about public policy, or making recommendations about public policy, is the goal. In more recent development of his theory of justice, John Rawls used an 'overlapping consensus' to capture the idea that people who hold quite different comprehensive moral, religious, philosophical, and cultural views might share an overlapping consensus about principles of justice and about the political reasons that support those principles.[11] If people appeal to their comprehensive moral conceptions, including the full moral, religious, philosophical, and cultural underpinnings of those views, they will often give different and conflicting reasons or support for particular substantive positions on which they agree. The 'fact of pluralism' – that different citizens hold different comprehensive moral, religious, and philosophical conceptions – is a permanent feature of free liberal democracies. It implies that the ethical and political bases that all citizens can reasonably accept for public policies in a liberal democracy cannot rest on these full comprehensive conceptions. The task of ethics commissions is often to try to find a common public moral discourse that can yield a consensus on which public policy can be formed among individuals and groups otherwise in disagreement on many important matters.

The role of an overlapping consensus for policy raises complex and controversial issues that cannot be explored here, but one point needs at least to be mentioned. In a liberal democracy, public policy that requires everyone to act in specific ways should not be based on sectarian views reasonably rejected by substantial segments of the population. This is a goal that cannot always be realized for all policy, certainly in practice, but I believe in theory as well; still, it is an important goal nonetheless. It implies, for example, that public policy should not be based on specific religious beliefs that many do not share. Not only public policies themselves, but the reasons that are offered in their support in policy debate, whether in ethics commissions or other settings, should not be reasons that others can reasonably reject as a basis for public policy in a pluralistic society. The common agreement to search for an overlapping consensus in public policy, a search in which an ethics commission can sometimes play a significant role, should be understood to mean not only that we seek to find or forge a consensus on particular policy issues, but also that we seek consensus on the kinds of reasons that we shall offer in support of policy positions. One crucial aspect of the latter is the consensus on what reasons are appropriate for policy debate.

This is a qualification on the account of public moral reasoning on policy questions sketched above for ethics commissions, since the full exploration of one's reasons for one's moral positions and judgments will take one deeply into the details of one's comprehensive religious, philosophical, and moral views. To appeal to those comprehensive views is to go beyond what should be the basis of public policy. This restriction on reasons that are appropriate in the policy debates of an ethics commission is an implication of wanting public policy in a liberal democracy to be justified as far as possible by shared reasons that all could accept as reasonable.

Conclusion

I shall emphasize only two general points in conclusion. The first is that the process of public moral discourse in which an ethics commission engages is not fundamentally different in its nature from the moral reasoning in which individual members of the society engage in public and private contexts. The second points is that while the process of public moral discourse, even properly carried out, does not guarantee the truth or correctness of the conclusions it yields, it can provide us with a warrant for accepting them as a justified basis for public policy.

Notes

1 While some people make a distinction, although usually not a clear one, between 'ethics' and 'morality,' I shall use them interchangeably in this paper.

2 D. Rothman, *Strangers at the Bedside: A History of How Law and Bioethics Transformed Medical Decision Making* (New York: Basic Books 1991); Henry Beecher, 'Ethics and Clinical Research,' *New England Journal of Medicine* 74 (1966) 1354–60.

3 President's Commission for the Study of Ethical Problems in Medicine and Biomedical and Behavioral Research, *Deciding to Forego Life-Sustaining Treatment*, (Washington, DC: U.S.Government Printing Office 1983).

4 D.W. Brock, 'Voluntary Active Euthanasia,' *Hastings Center Report* 22 (March–April 1992) 10–22, and reprinted in Dan W. Brock, *Life and Death: Philosophical Essay in Biomedical Ethics* (Cambridge: Cambridge University Press 1993).

5 J. Rawls, *A Theory of Justice* (Cambridge, MA: Harvard University Press 1971).

6 Foundationalists differ on how this privileged truth status can be secured for some moral judgments, as well as on what the privileged status is, for examples contingent or necessary truth. Intuitionists like H.A. Prichard and W.D. Ross held that some moral statements are necessary truths, although they disagreed about whether the moral statements that had this privileged truth status were concrete, all things considered, moral judgments about particular actions, or general principles specifying moral duties, such as to keep promises and not to deceive, which could be overridden in some particular circumstances.

7 A.R. Jonsen and S. Toulmin, *The Abuse of Casuistry: A History of Moral Reasoning* (Berkeley: University of California Press 1988). To what extent Jonsen and Toulmin are examples of what I call particularists is unclear. They do endorse a 'stronger claim – namely that *moral knowledge is essentially particular* so that sound resolutions of moral problems must always be rooted in a concrete understanding of specific cases and circumstances ... The stronger account sees the primary locus of moral understanding as lying in the recognition of *paradigmatic examples* of good and evil, right and wrong' p. 330 (italics in original). This suggests that they do accept the epistemic aspect of what I call particularism that moral truth or knowledge is to be found at the level of particular cases, their '*paradigmatic examples.*' It may be that their account of the actual *process* of moral reasoning, which is centrally a matter of fitting specific actual cases to the paradigmatic examples, does make room for gen-

eral principles in the manner of reflective equilibrium discussed below, although I am unsure of this. But it is unlike Rawlsian reflective equilibrium in giving judgments about particular cases privileged epistemic status, and that is the only respect in which I am interpreting them to be particularists here.

8 Rawls, *Theory of Justice*.
9 Thomas Nagel has stressed this point in 'The Fragmentation of Value,' in *Mortal Questions* (Cambridge: Cambridge University Press 1979).
10 R.M. Hare, *Freedom and Reason* (Oxford: Oxford University Press 1963).
11 J. Rawls, *Political Liberalism* (New York: Columbia University Press 1993).

Contributors

Tom L. Beauchamp is Professor in the Philosophy Department at Georgetown University, with a joint appointment at the Kennedy Institute of Ethics. He wrote, with James Childress, *Principles of Biomedical Ethics* (4th edition, 1994) and is one of three international editors of the critical edition of the philosophical works of David Hume.

Joseph Boyle is Professor of Philosophy at St Michael's College and a Member of the Joint Centre for Bioethics, University of Toronto. He works on moral theory, natural law ethics, the history of ethics, and applied ethics. He has written numerous articles on bioethics.

Dan W. Brock is University Professor of Philosophy and Biomedical Ethics and Director of the Center for Biomedical Ethics at Brown University. He served as Staff Philosopher on the Present's Commission for the Study of Ethical Problems in Medicine in 1981 and 1982, and on the White House Task Force on National Health Care Reform in 1993. He is the author of *Deciding for Others: The Ethics of Surrogate Decisionmaking* (with Alan Buchanan, 1986) and *Life and Death: Philosophical Essay in Biomedical Ethics* (1993) as well as many articles in biomedical ethics, ethics, and political philosophy.

Daniel Callahan is President of the Hastings Center, Briarcliff Manor, New York. He is the author or editor of thirty-one books, most recently *The Troubled Dream of Life: In Search of a Peaceful Death* (1993).

Norman Daniels is Goldthwaite Professor in the Department of Philosophy at Tufts University. He is the author of *Thomas Reid's Inquiry* (1974), *Just Health Care* (1985), *Am I My Parents' Keeper?* (1988), and *Seeking Fair Treatment*

(1981) and has written widely in ethics and political and social philosophy. His newest book is *Justice and Justification: Reflective Equilibrium in Theory and Practice*, forthcoming from Cambridge University Press.

R.M. Hare was until his retirement in 1995 Graduate Research Professor at the University of Florida and before that White's Professor of Moral Philosophy at Oxford. His books include *The Language of Morals* (1952), *Freedom and Reason* (1963), *Moral Thinking* (1981), and *Essays in Ethical Theory* (1989), and he is the author of many articles on ethical theory and applied moral philosophy.

Albert R. Jonsen is Professor of Ethics in Medicine and Chair of the Department of Medical History and Ethics, School of Medicine, University of Washington. He is the author of *The New Medicine and the Old Ethics* (1991) and, with Stephen Toulmin, *The Abuse of Casuistry: A History of Moral Reasoning* (1988).

Will Kymlicka is the Research Director of the Canadian Centre for Philosophy and Public Policy, Department of Philosophy, University of Ottawa. He is the author of *Liberalism, Community and Culture* (1989), *Contemporary Political Philosophy: An Introduction* (1990), and *Multicultural Citizenship* (1995). In 1991–2 he worked on the staff of the Canadian Royal Commission on New Reproductive Technologies.

Kathryn Pauly Morgan is Professor of Philosophy and Women's Studies and a Member of the Joint Centre for Bioethics at the University of Toronto. She is a co-author of *The Gender Question in Education: Theory, Pedagogy, and Politics* (forthcoming from Westview Press) and has written various articles in feminist ethics, feminist social philosophy, philosophy of sexuality, and feminist bioethics. She is currently a member of the Social Sciences and Humanities Research Council of Canada Strategic Research Network in Feminist Health Care Ethics.

Christine Overall is Professor of Philosophy at Queen's University, Kingston. She is the author of *Ethics and Human Reproduction: A Feminist Analysis* (1987) and *Human Reproduction: Principles, Practices, Policies* (1993). She is also the editor of *The Future of Human Reproduction* (1989) and co-editor of *Feminist Perspectives: Philosophical Essays on Method and Morals* (1988) and *Perspectives on AIDS: Ethical and Social Issues* (1991).

Laura M. Purdy is Professor of Philosophy at Wells College. She is the author of *In Their Best Interest? The Case against Equal Rights for Children* (1992) and co-editor of *Feminist Perspectives in Medical Ethics* (1992). A collection of her essays in reproductive ethics, *Reproducing Persons*, will be published by Cornell University Press in 1996.

Laura Shanner is I'Anson Assistant Professor in the Department of Philosophy and a Member of the Joint Centre for Bioethics at the University of Toronto. Her training includes a year of research in Australia funded through the Fulbright competition. Her main areas of interest include issues in reproduction and genetics, feminist approaches to bioethics, bioethics education, and international perspectives on bioethics. Articles on these topics have been published in journals and books in philosophy, law, and medicine.

Susan Sherwin is Professor of Philosophy and Women's Studies at Dalhousie University. She is the author of *No Longer Patient: Feminist Ethics and Health Care* (1992) and a co-editor of *Moral Problems in Medicine* (2nd edition, 1983) and *Health Care Ethics in Canada* (1995). She is currently engaged in an interdisciplinary research project on feminist health care ethics.

L.W. Sumner is Professor of Philosophy and Law and a Member of the Joint Centre for Bioethics at the University of Toronto. He is the author of *Abortion and Moral Theory* (1981) and *The Moral Foundation of Rights* (1987), as well as numerous articles in ethics, applied ethics, and political philosophy. His latest book is *Welfare, Happiness, and Ethics* (1996).

Earl Winkler is Professor and Head of the Philosophy Department and Senior Research Fellow at the Centre for Applied Ethics, University of British Columbia. He is co-editor of *Ethics and Aging* (1989) and *Applied Ethics: A Reader* (1993), as well as the author of numerous articles in philosophical journals, particularly in ethical theory and applied ethics. He is a member of the Advisory Council on Ethical Issues in Health Care for the British Columbia provincial government.